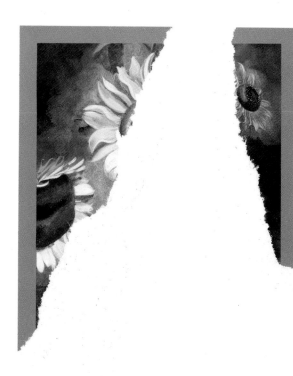

Awareness of Deficit
After Brain Injury

Awareness of Deficit After Brain Injury

Clinical and Theoretical Issues

Edited by

GEORGE P. PRIGATANO

Barrow Neurological Institute
St. Joseph's Hospital and Medical Center
Phoenix, Arizona

DANIEL L. SCHACTER

Department of Psychology
University of Arizona
Tucson, Arizona

New York   Oxford
OXFORD UNIVERSITY PRESS
1991

Oxford University Press

Oxford New York Toronto
Delhi Bombay Calcutta Madras Karachi
Petaling Jaya Singapore Hong Kong Tokyo
Nairobi Dar es Salaam Cape Town
Melbourne Auckland

and associated companies in
Berlin Ibadan

Library of Congress Cataloging-in-Publication Data
Awareness of deficit after brain injury : clinical and theoretical issues
edited by George P. Prigatano and Daniel L. Schacter.
p. cm. Includes bibliographical references.
ISBN 0-19-505941-7
1. Brain damage. 2. Anosognosia.
I. Prigatano, George P. II. Schacter, Daniel L.
[DNLM: 1. Brain Injuries—complications. 2. Cognition.
3. Cognition Disorders—etiology. WL 341 A964]
RC387.5.A93 1991
617.4′81—dc20
DNLM/DLC for Library of Congress 90-6782

9 8 7 6 5 4 3 2

Printed in the United States of America
on acid-free paper

This book is dedicated to different sources of inspiration.

G.P.P. recognizes the insight of
D. O. Hebb concerning "what psychology is
about" and the creative genius of C. G. Jung regarding
the complexity of the consciousness/unconsciousness continuum.

D.L.S. recognizes Théodule Ribot and
Pierre Janet for the insight that disorders of cognition
and awareness provide a unique window on normal functioning.

Preface

This book has two different but related sources of inspiration. Rehabilitative efforts to return young adult brain-injured patients to work, or at least to a productive lifestyle, amply documented the clinical importance of altered awareness associated with cerebral dysfunction. Clinical experience indicated that brain-injured patients are often unaware of the very deficits that impair their performance in everyday life. Despite the clinical importance of the phenomenon, a theoretical understanding of it was entirely lacking. At the same time, scientific research concerning normal and abnormal cognitive processes, including memory and memory disorders, began to focus on the role of awareness. For example, memory researchers addressed implicit memory processes, where effects of recent experiences are expressed without awareness of those experiences. Issues concerning forms of awareness and unawareness, therefore, began to develop in this field as well.

The editors of this volume, although coming from quite different backgrounds, shared a common interest in exploring what they felt was an important clinical and theoretical phenomenon: altered awareness after brain injury. A relocation of primary work sites led both of us to Arizona and, with the combined support of the Barrow Neurological Institute and the University of Arizona, we began to organize this volume. In October 1988, the contributing authors met in Scottsdale, Arizona for a three-day conference to discuss the issues and ideas presented in this volume. Funding for that conference and related costs involved in developing the book was initially provided by the Barrow Neurological Institute, St. Joseph's Hospital and Medical Center. Additional funding was obtained from the Faculty of the Social and Behavioral Science, University of Arizona. Major support was obtained from the Stephen Patrick Hagan Fund for Neurological Rehabilitation at the Barrow Neurological Institute. Dr. Joseph C. White, Jr., then Chairman of the Department of Neurology, was instrumental in arranging for the use of these funds. The editors wish to express special thanks to Dr. White for his efforts in this regard as well as to the Hagan family for providing monies to make this book a reality.

Administrative support from Dr. Robert Spetzler, Director of the Barrow Neurological Institute and Sister Nancy Perlick, Vice President of Neurosciences is also appreciated. Finally, we wish to thank Dean Lee Sigelman of the University of Arizona for his support.

It is hoped that the information obtained from studying disorders of self-awareness will ultimately lead not only to greater scientific insights into the nature of disturbed awareness following brain injury, but also to improved rehabilitation of patients with brain dysfunctions.

Phoenix, Arizona   George P. Prigatano
March, 1990   Daniel L. Schacter

Contents

Contributors

WILLIAM B. BARR, PH.D.
Hillside Hospital
Long Island Jewish Medical Center
Glenn Oaks, New York 11004

EDOARDO BISIACH, M.D.
Istituto di Clinica Neurologica
Università di Milano
Milan, Italy

MERRILL F. GARRETT, PH.D.
University of Arizona
Cognitive Science Program
 and Department of Psychology
Tucson, Arizona 85721

GIULIANO GEMINIANI, M.D.
Istituto di Clinica Neurologica
Università di Milano
Milan, Italy

ELKHONON GOLDBERG, PH.D.
Division of Neuropsychology
The Medical College of Pennsylvania
Philadelphia, Pennsylvania 19129

KENNETH M. HEILMAN, M.D.
Department of Neurology
University of Florida
College of Medicine
Gainesville, Florida 32610

MARCIA K. JOHNSON, PH.D.
Department of Psychology
Princeton University
Princeton, New Jersey 08544

ALFRED W. KASZNIAK, PH.D.
Department of Psychology
University of Arizona
Tucson, Arizona 85721

JOHN F. KIHLSTROM, PH.D.
Department of Psychology
University of Arizona
Tucson, Arizona 85721

LISA LEWIS, PH.D.
The Menninger Clinic
Topeka, Kansas 66601

SUSAN M. MCGLYNN, M.A.
Department of Psychology
University of Arizona
Tucson, Arizona 85721

GEORGE P. PRIGATANO, PH.D.
Barrow Neurological Institute
St. Joseph's Hospital and Medical Center
Phoenix, Arizona 85013

ALAN B. RUBENS, M.D.
University of Arizona
Health Sciences Center
Tucson, Arizona 85721

DANIEL L. SCHACTER, PH.D.
Department of Psychology
University of Arizona
Tucson, Arizona 85721

DONALD T. STUSS, PH.D.
Departments of Psychology
 and Medicine (Neurology)
Rohman Research Institute of Baycrest Centre
North York, Ontario, Canada

BETSY A. TOBIAS, J.D.
Department of Psychology
University of Arizona
Tucson, Arizona 85721

EDWIN A. WEINSTEIN, M.D.
7603 Holiday Terrace
Bethesda, Maryland 20817

Awareness of Deficit
After Brain Injury

1
Introduction

GEORGE P. PRIGATANO
AND DANIEL L. SCHACTER

At the turn of the century Herman Munk (1881), Sigmund Freud (1891), Jean-Martin Charcot (1894), Constantine von Monakow (1885), Gabriel Anton (1899), Arnold Pick (1908), and Joseph François Flex Babinski (1914) made experimental and clinical observations that greatly influenced thinking on the nature of impaired human awareness. Coupled with more recent observations, their work has led to novel hypotheses concerning brain disorders that alter patients' ability to perceive important changes in their behavioral and mental capacities. This book, extending the ideas and observations of these historical figures, presents a variety of contemporary approaches to the problem of altered awareness following brain injury.

In 1881 Munk (cited by Blakemore, 1977) reported that experimental lesions in the association cortex lying between primary visual and auditory cortex produced temporary "mind-blindness" in dogs (Figs. 1–1 and 1–2). The animals' behavior after the operation indicated that they could "see" objects (i.e., they did not bump into them) but failed to recognize their significance. That is, they failed to exhibit typical reactions to objects that once frightened or attracted them (Bauer and Rubens, 1985). Soon the term "mind-blindness" was replaced by the term *agnosia*. Bauer and Rubens (1985) credited Sigmund Freud with introducing this term in 1891. Freud's contribution, however, was soon to be considered more for the description of psychiatric patients than neurological ones.

After the term "agnosia" came into use to denote an impairment in recognition secondary to brain damage that could not be explained on the basis of primary sensory or motor impairment, the term *anosognosia* was coined. Although this term refers literally to a lack of knowledge about a recognition deficit, it was first used to describe a somewhat different clinical syndrome.

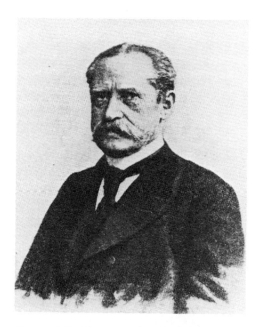

Figure 1–1. Hermann Munk (1839–1912). From Blakemore, C. ed.: *Mechanics to the Mind.* London: Cambridge University Press, 1977, p. 62. Reprinted with permission of Wellcome Institute Library, London.

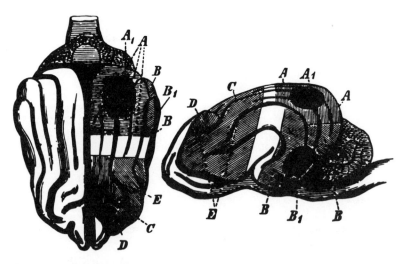

Figure 1–2. Hermann Munk's (1881) diagram of the dog's brain showing areas of the cerebral hemispheres where damage (on both sides) produced temporary "mind-blindness" (A_1) and "mind-deafness" (B_1). These regions lie within the visual and auditory receiving areas of the cortex. From Blakemore, C. (ed.): *Mechanics of the Mind.* London: Cambridge University Press, 1977, p. 63. Reprinted with permission of Wellcome Institute Library, London.

Joseph François Félix Babinski (Fig. 1–3) introduced the term anosognosia in 1914 to describe an apparent loss of recognition or awareness of left hemiplegia following an abrupt brain insult. Yet the clinical phenomenon of unawareness of startling neurological deficits was described before that time. Constantine von Monakow described a patient's failure to recognize cortical blindness in 1885. Gabriel Anton (Fig. 1–4) described a similar case in 1889 and "emphasized the relationship of unawareness of disease and focal cerebral lesions" (Friedland and Weinstein, 1977). Anton was making the point that a lack of awareness could result from a focal lesion as opposed to diffuse brain injury, producing a general decline in higher cerebral functioning (Friedland and Weinstein, 1977). Arnold Pick (Fig. 1–5) has been given credit as the first to actually report unawareness of hemiplegia (Gerstmann, 1942); but as noted above, it was Babinski who introduced the term anosognosia.

Since these pioneering studies, several papers have been published on the nature of anosognosia. Weinstein and Kahn (1955) provided a brief historical

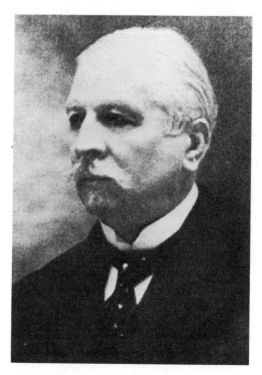

Figure 1–3. Joseph François Félix Babinski. (From Haymaker W., ed: *The Founders of Neurology: One Hundred and Thirty-Three Biographical Sketches.* Springfield, IL: Charles C Thomas, 1953, p. 235. Courtesy of Dr. Maurice Genty, Académie de Médecine, Paris, France. Reprinted with permission of Charles C Thomas.)

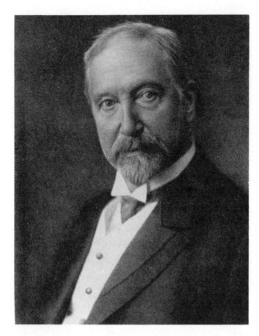

Figure 1–4. Gabriel Anton. (From *Archiv Für Psychiatrie Und Nervenkrankheiten.* Berlin: Verlag von Julius Springer, 1982. Reprinted with permission.)

overview of many of them. At the turn of the century, one common view was that anosognosia was a part of a disturbance of "body schema." Weinstein and Kahn suggested that this view was directly attributed to the work of Head and Holmes (1911) and Pick (1908). Also around that time, Redlich and Bonvicini (1908) suggested that Anton's syndrome or denial of cortical blindness was not in fact an agnostic defect. They suggested, as Weinstein and Kahn (1955) reported, that this problem was a form of Korsakoff syndrome in which confabulation of denial was occurring in a blind person. There were also psychoanalytically based interpretations. For example, Schilder (1932) suggested the concept of "organic repression" to explain the anosognostic phenomenon. Goldstein (1939) considered anosognostic reactions as possible attempts to avoid the catastrophic reaction and related to problems of abstract reasoning. This point was also underscored by Sandifer (1946). During the 1920s, 1930s, and 1940s, therefore, there were no new major theories to explain anosognosia.

As Weinstein and Kahn (1955) also reported, autopsy studies at this time revealed that there was frequently extensive neuropathology involving subcortical structures (particularly the thalamus) as well as the parietal lobe when anosognosia for hemiplegia existed.

Over the years, however, most of the debate on anosognosia seems to have centered around three topics: Is this disturbance a result of some type of focal cognitive/perceptual impairment or a result of disruption of overall intellectual abilities (Sandifer, 1946)? Is this phenomenon determined by motivational or nonmotivational factors (Weinstein and Kahn, 1955)? Does anosognosia reflect a specific disturbance in higher cerebral information processing (Bisiach et al., 1986)?

Bisiach and Geminiani (see Chapter 2) provide a historical review of literature dealing with these problems. However, the specific question of whether unawareness of deficit is determined by motivational or nonmotivational factors seemed especially relevant to research in this area. Even before Babinski described anosognosia for hemiplegia in 1914, Jean-Martin Charcot (Fig. 1–6) demonstrated disturbances in awareness in patients who were apparently free from brain lesions. Charcot, an eminent French neurologist, was interested in the differences between "organic" and "hysterical" paralysis. While investigating these differences, Charcot observed a number of striking instances of disturbed

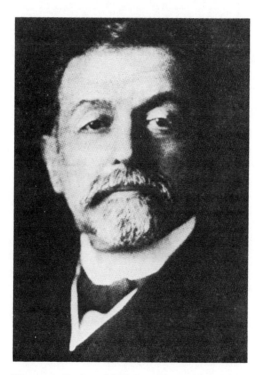

Figure 1–5. Arnold Pick. (From Haymaker W., ed: *The Founders of Neurology: One Hundred and Thirty-Three Biographical Sketches.* Springfield IL: Charles C Thomas, 1953, p. 203. Courtesy of Prof. F. Jahnel and Lt. Col. H. Sprinz, M.C., Munich, Germany. Reprinted with permission of Charles C Thomas.)

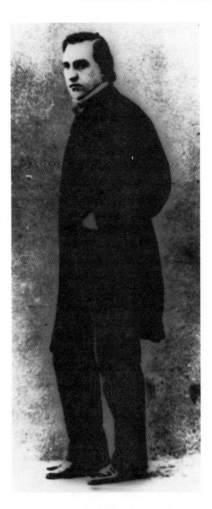

Figure 1–6. Jean-Martin Charcot (1825–1893). (Courtesy Professor Paul Castaigne, Paris. From Ellenberger HF: *The Discovery of the Unconscious.* New York: Basic Books, 1970. Reprinted with permission.)

awareness in his patients. Ellenberger (1970) provided a lucid account of these observations.

> In 1884 three men afflicted with a monoplegia of one arm following trauma were admitted to the Salpêtrière. Charcot first demonstrated that the symptoms of that paralysis, while differing from those of organic paralyses, coincided exactly with the symptoms of hysterical paralyses. The second step was the experimental reproduction of similar paralyses under hypnosis. Charcot suggested to some hypnotized subjects that their arms would be paralyzed. The resulting hypnotic paralyses proved to

have exactly the same symptoms as the spontaneous hysterical paralyses and the posttraumatic paralyses of the three male patients. Charcot was able to reproduce these paralyses step by step, and he also suggested their disappearance in the reverse order. The next step was a demonstration of the effect of the trauma. Charcot chose easily hypnotizable subjects and suggested to them that in their waking state, as soon as they were slapped on the back, their arm would become paralyzed. When awakened, the subjects showed the usual posthypnotic amnesia, and as soon as they were slapped on the back, they were instantly struck with a monoplegia of the arm of exactly the same type as the posttraumatic monoplegia. Finally, Charcot pointed out that in certain subjects living in a state of permanent somnambulism, hypnotic suggestion was not even necessary. They received the paralysis of the arm after being slapped on the back without special verbal suggestion. The mechanism of posttraumatic paralysis thus seemed to be demonstrated. Charcot assumed that the nervous shock following the trauma was a kind of hypnoid state analogous to hypnotism and therefore enabling the development of an autosuggestion of the individual. [Ellenberger, 1970, p. 91]

This clinical demonstration made clear to the scientific and medical communities that one could manipulate psychologically a patient's conscious perceptions and thereby produce what appeared to be neurological symptoms. Also, patients who were characterized as existing in a state of "permanent somnambulance" (in contemporary terms, a reduced arousal level) seemed especially prone to the development of symptoms similar to neurological ones.

If this situation were the case, it followed naturally that psychological disturbances could have a direct impact on conscious perception and could influence how individuals view themselves after suffering neurological impairment. Certainly Freud's *The Interpretation of Dreams,* published in 1900, made a cogent argument for the role of psychological defense mechanisms in blocking unpleasant thoughts from awareness. Freud, who reportedly spent 4 months at the Salpêtrière during 1885 and 1886 (Ellenberger, 1970), believed that many "neurotic" symptoms arose from factors outside the patient's awareness. He argued that human consciousness made use of a "filtering system" that kept unpleasant thoughts about the self out of awareness. Freud made a number of penetrating observations about the problem of self-awareness in neurotic states.

I have noticed in the course of my psychoanalytical work that the psychological state of a man in an attitude of reflection is entirely different from that of a man who is observing his psychic processes. In reflection there is a greater play of psychic activity than in the most attentive self-observation; this is shown even by the tense attitude and the wrinkled brow of the man in a state of reflection, as opposed to the mimic tranquility of the man observing himself. In both cases there must be concentrated attention, but the reflective man makes use of his critical faculties, with the result that he rejects some of the thoughts which rise into consciousness after he has become aware of them, and abruptly interrupts others, so that he does not follow the lines of thought which they would otherwise open up for him; while in respect of yet other thoughts he is able to behave in such a manner that they do not become conscious at all—that is to say, they are suppressed before they are perceived. In self-observation, on the other hand, he has but one task—that of suppressing criticism; if he succeeds in doing this, an unlimited number of thoughts enter his consciousness which would otherwise have eluded his grasp. With the aid of the material thus

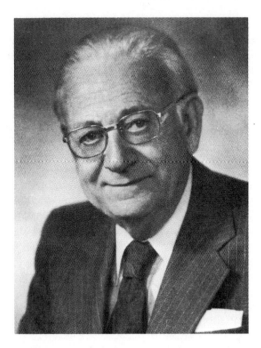

Figure 1-7. Edwin A. Weinstein, M.D.
(Courtesy of Dr. Edwin Weinstein.)

obtained—material which is new to the self-observer—it is possible to achieve the
interpretation of pathological ideas, and also that of dream-formations. [*The Interpretation of Dreams,* 1900. Translated by Brill, 1938, p. 192]

These reflections highlight the point that self-observation or self-awareness
is not an easy task even for the human adult without brain damage; they also
underscore the notion that thoughts/perceptions may not reach conscious
awareness for psychological (not neuropsychological) reasons. This line of reasoning led Edwin Weinstein (Fig. 1-7) and Robert Kahn (1955) to postulate that
motivational factors indeed have a great influence on the symptom picture
patients demonstrate in various anosognosic states.

Our findings indicate that the various forms of anosognosia are not discrete entities
that can be localized in different areas of the brain. Whether a lesion involves the
frontal or parietal lobe determines the disability that may be denied, not the mechanism of denial. Thus the patterns of anosognosia for hemiplegia and blindness do
not differ from those in which the fact of an operation or the state of being ill is
denied. Under the requisite conditions of brain function the patient may deny the
paralysis of an arm whether it results from a fracture, an injury to the brachial
plexus, a brain stem or cortical lesion. The effect of the brain damage is to provide
the milieu of altered function in which the patient may deny *anything* that he feels
is wrong with him. Some motivation to deny illness and incapacity exists in everyone
and the level of brain function determines the particular perceptual-symbolic organization, or language, in which it is expressed. [Weinstein and Kahn, 1955, p. 123]

Weinstein and Kahn's (1955) redescription of phenomena that had been previously referred to as "anosognosic" with the term "denial of illness" produced a major conceptual shift in explaining these complex symptoms. The use of the term denial implied that a patient with anosognosia was motivated to block distressing symptoms from awareness with a defense mechanism of the kind hypothesized by the psychoanalysts. This description of the phenomenon of anosognosia implies the need for a psychological or psychodynamic level of explanation that is absent from theorizing about traditional neurobehavioral problems such as aphasia and amnesia. As pointed out by McGlynn and Schacter (1989), research concerning anosognosia declined over the years following the publication of the monograph by Weinstein and Kahn (1955).

Although all of the reasons for this decline are not entirely clear, we speculate that two factors may have been particularly important. First, the appeal of Weinstein and Kahn (1955) to psychodynamic variables as explanatory constructs and their use of the term *denial* instead of *anosognosia* may have led to the perception that anosognosia is a psychiatric problem rather than a purely neurological or neuropsychological one, even though they acknowledged that brain damage plays a role in the genesis of denial. Second, in view of the dominance of psychology by behaviorism at that time, experimental psychology and neuropsychology had little to say about such "mentalistic" issues as awareness or awareness disturbances. Thus as the neurological literature on anosognosia declined, neither experimental psychology nor neuropsychology could provide an alternative conceptual/empirical framework within which the issue could be approached.

REEMERGENCE OF INTEREST IN DISTURBANCES OF AWARENESS

Several factors have led to a reemergence of interest in anosognosia. First, with the decline of behaviorism, the phenomena of consciousness have once again become a respectable target of investigation in academic psychology (Mandler, 1975; Hilgard, 1977; Kihlstrom, 1987). Thus, for example, the construct of consciousness has played an important role in models of attention (Posner, 1978), perception (Marcel, 1983), and memory (Tulving, 1985; Schacter, 1989). These developments have provided new empirical and conceptual tools that can be usefully applied to the analysis of anosognosia.

Second, the study of brain–behavior relations has highlighted the importance of consciousness in neuropsychological theory. Luria (1966) defined the higher cerebral functions as being complex reflex processes that were "mediate" (i.e., symbolic) in structure, social in origin, and *conscious* and voluntary in their mode of interaction. He emphasized the important role of consciousness in higher cerebral functioning. Stuss and Benson (1986) subsequently identified the anterior regions of the brain as playing an important role in "executive" functions such as planning, monitoring, and anticipation. They also described the emergence of self-awareness as the highest of all integrated activities of the brain. Thus the term self-awareness is now actively utilized by "respectable" neurologists and neuropsychologists.

In addition, research on split-brain or commissurotomy patients revealed a variety of striking disorders of consciousness that may occur when the corpus callosum is surgically sectioned (Sperry, 1974). For example, patients who could verbally identify objects placed in the right hand could not do so with the left hand. However, by pointing to objects they were able to show that they could successfully perceive information processed by the right cerebral hemisphere that apparently lacked access to the speech centers of the left cerebral hemisphere. These observations indicated that verbal reports alone are not the sole measure of conscious information processing.

In a related development, research on a variety of neuropsychological syndromes began to demonstrate that patients may have intact implicit knowledge within a specific domain even when they exhibit impaired conscious or explicit knowledge in that domain (Schacter, McAndrews, and Moscovitch, 1988). Thus, for example, amnestic patients who lack explicit, conscious memory for recent experiences nevertheless possess intact implicit memory for various aspects of those experiences (for review, see Shimamura, 1986; Schacter, 1987). Similarly, prosopagnosic patients do not exhibit conscious recognition of familiar faces yet show preserved covert or implicit recognition of facial familiarity in a variety of task situations (e.g., Bauer, 1984; DeHann, Young, and Newcombe, 1987; Tranel and Damasio, 1985); patients with lesions in the striate cortex who do not experience conscious perceptions of their environment demonstrate unconscious perception or "blindsight" (Weiskrantz, 1986) on appropriate tasks; and similar dissociations have been observed in aphasic, alexic, and other patients (Schacter et al., 1988; see also Chapters 8 and 11). These findings suggest that specific disturbances in consciousness may be associated with specific disturbances in brain function and have already stimulated a great deal of interest that is reflected in several chapters of this volume.

A third possible reason for the reemergence of interest in anosognosia is that clinicians attempting rehabilitation of brain-injured patients have found that although the patients may be motivated to return to work they often lack insight into (or awareness of) the nature and severity of their neuropsychological impairments (Prigatano et al., 1986; Ben-Yishay and Prigatano, 1990). Success at returning these patients to a productive life style appears to be contingent on improved awareness of their residual strengths and deficits. The need to treat and rehabilitate growing numbers of brain-damaged patients thus helped to reintroduce altered awareness phenomena to clinical neuropsychology. Fourth, and finally, theoretically oriented investigations have introduced and developed the notion that anosognosia has important implications for major issues in behavioral neurology, particularly as they relate to the organization of the higher cerebral functions (see Chapter 2).

TOWARD A DEFINITION OF CONSCIOUSNESS AND AWARENESS

In his thoughtful review of the term consciousness, Frederiks (1969) reminded us that:

Etymologically, the word consciousness derives from *cum* (with) and *scire* (to know). In other words, it is not simply a "knowledge of," but also a certain "knowledge with," a particular state. The state of consciousness and the consciousness of something indeed emerge as two essential aspects of consciousness suitable for consideration from the psychological and physiological-anatomical standpoints. [pp. 48–49]

The above quote suggests that consciousness has both an objective and a subjective quality to it. The *knowledge of* something can be considered the objective side of consciousness, whereas the *knowledge with* something can be considered the subjective quality. For example, a traumatically brain-injured patient may know that he has a "memory problem." When asked to describe how significant the problem is in his daily life, however, he may state that it is a relatively "small" problem—one that does not significantly affect his day-to-day functioning. In contrast, family members who live with him assert that the memory problem has substantial negative impact on his day-to-day activities.

The patient has, in a sense, "knowledge of" his memory disability but seems to lack "knowledge with" its true extent and personal and interpersonal impact. This failure to subjectively appreciate the significance of his "memory problem" reflects a true impairment of one aspect of consciousness: the subjective, phenomenological, or experiential component. This "knowledge with" can be separated from "knowledge of" his existing memory problem. Clearly, both aspects of consciousness are important for clinical and theoretical reasons (Marcel and Bisiach, 1988).

Agreeing with Frederiks (1969), we find it exceedingly difficult—if not impossible—to provide a clear, concise, universally acceptable definition of consciousness or awareness. However, in the effort to move toward a definition that could be of use in advancing the field, we make the following suggestions.

Self-awareness is the capacity to perceive the "self" in relatively "objective" terms while maintaining a sense of subjectivity. It is a natural paradox of human consciousness. On the one hand, it strives for "objectivity," that is, perceiving a situation, object, or interaction in a manner similar to others' perceptions, while at the same time maintaining the sense of a private, subjective, or unique interpretation of an experience. The latter aspect of consciousness implies a feeling state as well as a thought process. Self-awareness or awareness of higher cerebral functions thus involves an interaction of "thoughts" and "feelings." We agree with Stuss and Benson (1986) that it is the highest of all integrated functions. Moreover, we see it not as a unitary phenomenon but one that may reflect the highest level of organization in specific cerebral subsystems, as Bisiach et al. (1986) have suggested.

As a highly integrated function, however, it may well depend on the integrity of multiple brain regions and involve areas considered by Mesulam (1985) as "heteromodal" cortex. These cortical association areas are thought to integrate inputs from primary sensorimotor systems with limbic or paralimbic systems. This theoretical point of view is expanded by Prigatano in Chapter 7.

Clearly, there are no simple definitions of the terms awareness or consciousness, which are used interchangeably in this text. However, this volume does reflect an effort to examine this important topic from various clinical and experimental vantage points. A volume by Marcel and Bisiach (1988) provided a stimulating review of the concept of consciousness in contemporary science. It provided an in-depth theoretical analysis of the uses of the term consciousness, its subjective component, and the manner in which it may be approached scientif-ically. The reader is referred to that text for a thorough discussion of the term "consciousness."

BRIEF OVERVIEW OF THE TEXT

Given that no book since 1955 has been devoted to altered self-awareness after brain injury, the primary purpose of this volume is to bring together contem-porary reviews of this subject. We sought an interdisciplinary perspective encompassing neuropsychology, cognitive psychology, clinical psychology, neu-rology, and psychiatry. The emphasis has been on integrating data and present-ing theoretical perspectives. The clinical and theoretical implications of aware-ness deficits are presented throughout the text.

The early chapters deal with anosognosia from a behavioral neurologist's perceptive. Bisiach and Geminiani provide a historical overview of the phenom-enon. Focusing on anosognosia for hemiplegia and hemianopsia, they raise a number of important questions for cognitive scientists to address. Rubens and Garrett discuss altered awareness in aphasic patients and its implications for the study of aphasia. Heilman presents a model for explaining anosognosia and relates it to hemiplegia, Anton's syndrome, and Wernicke's aphasia.

Following these chapters, a clinical neuropsychological view is presented. Stuss discusses the relation of the frontal lobe system activity to the perception of the self. He describes various types of disturbed awareness observed in "fron-tal lobe patients" and explains their implications for rehabilitation. McGlynn and Kaszniak describe empirical observations of impaired awareness in patients with various forms of dementia. They connect their observations to the field of schizophrenia as well, reflecting once again the historical struggle to evaluate such phenomena in so-called organic versus psychiatric patients. Various psy-chological research methodologies are considered in this chapter.

Prigatano approaches the problem of impaired self (and social) awareness in patients with severe chronic brain damage of traumatic origin. These patients are commonly seen in neurological and neuropsychological rehabilitation cen-ters. They have suffered varied neuropathological insults, which often affect the "heteromodal" cortex (Mesulam, 1985). A model for conceptualizing impaired awareness using Mesulam's theoretical framework is presented.

Schacter considers the problem of altered self-awareness in amnestic patients and relates his ideas to recent concepts of explicit and implicit memory. Goldberg and Barr consider three possible neuropsychological mechanisms underlying awareness of deficit.

Following these discussions, the chapters by Johnson and by Kihlstrom and Tobias relate contemporary theories in cognitive psychology to different forms of self-awareness deficits. Johnson uses a multientry modular memory system to explain confabulatory deficits. Her chapter shows how the phenomenon of real-ity monitoring can be studied from a modern cognitive psychology perspective. Kihlstrom and Tobias also emphasize how cognitive psychological research may shed light on certain awareness phenomena.

The chapter by Lewis integrates clinical psychological insights with the traditional psychoanalytical view of repression and denial. Weinstein, whose seminal work in 1955 described altered awareness after brain injury in terms of denial of illness, reflects on the use of the term anosognosia versus denial of illness. The chapter summarizes his current thinking on relevant observations associated with altered awareness after brain injury. Finally, the last chapter considers the theoretical and clinical reasons forms of unawareness of deficits after brain injury warrant further investigation.

REFERENCES

Bauer, R. M. (1984). Autonomic recognition of names and faces in prosopagnosia: a neuropsychological study. *Neuropsychologia* 22:457–469.

Bauer, R. M., and Rubens, A. (1985). Agnosia. In K. M. Heilman and E. Valenstein (eds.), *Clinical Neuropsychology.* New York: Oxford University Press, pp. 187–241.

Ben-Yishay, Y., and Prigatano, G. P. (1990). Cognitive remediation. In E. Griffith and M. Rosenthal (eds.), *Rehabilitation of the Adult and Child with Traumatic Brain Injury.* Philadelphia: Davis, pp. 393–409.

Bisiach, E., Vallar, G., Perani, D., Papagno, C., and Berrti, A. (1986). Unawareness of disease following lesions of the right hemisphere: anosognosia for hemiplegia and anosognosia for hemianopia. *Neuropsychologia* 24:759–767.

Blakemore, C. (1977). *Mechanics of the Mind.* Cambridge: Cambridge University Press.

DeHann, E. H. F., Young, A., and Newcombe, F. (1987). Face recognition without awareness. *Cogn. Neuropsychol.* 4:385–415.

Ellenberger, H. (1970). *The Discovery of the Unconscious. The History and Evolution of Dynamic Psychiatry.* New York: Basic Books.

Frederiks, J. A. M. (1969). Consciousness. In P. J. Vinken and G. W. Bruyn (eds.), *Handbook of Clinical Neurology. Vol. 3: Disorders of Higher Nervous Activity.* Amsterdam: Elsevier/North-Holland, pp. 48–61.

Freud, S. (1938). *The Interpretation of Dreams.* In A. A. Brill (ed., trans.), *The Basic Writings of Sigmund Freud,* New York: Random House, pp. 181–549 (original work published 1900).

Friedland, R. P., and Weinstein, E. A. (1977). Hemi-inattention and hemisphere specialization: Introduction and historical review. In E. A. Weinstein and Friedland R. P. (eds.), *Advances in Neurology (Vol. 18): Hemi-inattention and Hemisphere Specialization.* New York: Raven, pp. 1–13.

Gerstmann, J. (1942). Problem of imperception of disease and of impaired body territories with organic lesions; relation to body scheme and its disorders. *Arch. Neurol & Psychiat* 48:890–913.

Goldstein, K. (1939). *The Organism: A Holistic Approach to Biology Derived from Pathological Data on Man.* New York: American Book Co.

Head, H., and Holmes, G. (1911). Sensory disturbances from cerebral lesions. *Brain* 34:102–254.

Hilgard, E. R. (1977). *Divided Consciousness.* New York: Wiley.

Kihlstrom, J. F. (1987). The cognitive unconscious. *Science* 237:1445–1452.

Lebrun, Y. (1987). Anosognosia in aphasics. *Cortex* 23:251–263.

Luria, A. R. (1966). *Higher Cortical Functions in Man.* New York: Basic Books.

Mandler, G. (1975). Consciousness: respectable, useful, and probably necessary. In R. L. Solso (ed.), *Information Processing and Cognition: The Loyola Symposium.* Hillsdale, NJ: Lawrence Erlbaum Associates, pp. 229–254.

Marcel, A. J. (1983). Conscious and unconscious perception: experiments on visual masking and word recognition. *Cogn. Psychol.* 15:197–237.

Marcel, A. J., and Bisiach, E. (1988). A cautious welcome: an introduction and guide to the book. In A. J. Marcel and E. Bisiach (eds.), *Consciousness in Contemporary Science.* Oxford: Clarendon Press, pp. 1–15.

McGlynn, S. M., and Schacter, D. L. (1989). Unawareness of deficits in neuropsychological syndromes. *J. Clin. Exp. Neuropsychol.* 11:143–205.

Mesulam, M-M (1985). *Principles of Behavioral Neurology.* Philadelphia: F. A. Davis.

Pick, A. (1908). Ueber storungen der orientierung am eigenen Korper, in Arbeten aus der Psychiatrischen. *Klin Prag.* 1.

Posner, M. (1978). *Chronometric Explorations of the Mind.* Hillsdale, NJ: Lawrence Erlbaum Associates.

Prigatano, G. P., and Others (1986). *Neuropsychological Rehabilitation After Brain Injury.* Baltimore: Johns Hopkins University Press.

Prigatano, G. P., et al. (1988). Anosognosia, delusions, and altered self-awareness after brain injury: a historical perspective. *BNI Q.* 4(3):40–48.

Redlich, E., and Bonvicini, G. (1908) Ueber das Fehlen der Wahrnehmung der eigenen Blindheit bei Hirnkrankheiten. *Jahrb. Psychiatr.* 29:1–134.

Sandifer, P. H. (1946). Anosognosia and disorders of body scheme. *Brain* 69:122–137.

Schacter, D. L. (1987). Implicit memory: history and current status. *J. Exp. Psychol.* [*Learn. Mem. Cogn.*] 13:501–518.

Schacter, D. L. (1989). On the relation between memory and consciousness: dissociable interactions and conscious experience. In H. L. Roediger and F. I. M. Craid (eds.), *Varieties of Memory and Consciousness: Essays in Honor of Endel Tulving.* Hillsdale, NJ: Lawrence Erlbaum Associates, pp. 355–389.

Schacter, D. L., McAndrews, M. P., and Moscovitch, M. (1988). Access to consciousness: dissociations between implicit and explicit knowledge in neuropsychological syndromes. In L. Weiskrantz (ed.), *Thought Without Language.* Oxford: Oxford University Press, pp. 242–278.

Schilder, P. (1932). Localization of the body image (postural model of the body). *Assoc. Res. Nerv. Ment. Dis.* 13:466–484.

Shimamura, A. P. (1986). Priming effects in amnesia: evidence for a dissociable memory function. *Q. J. Exp. Psychol.* 38A:619–644.

Sperry, R. W. (1974). Lateral specialization in the surgically separated hemispheres. In F. O. Schmitt and F. G. Worden (eds.), *The Neurosciences.* Cambridge: Massachusetts Institute of Technology, pp. 5–19.

Stuss, D. T., and Benson, D. F. (1986). *The Frontal Lobes.* New York: Raven Press.

Tranel, E., and Damasio, A. R. (1985). Knowledge without awareness: An autonomic index of facial recognition by prosopagnosics. *Science* 228:1453–1454.

Tulving, E. (1985). Memory and consciousness. *Can. Psychol.* 25:1–12.

Weinstein, E. A., and Kahn, R. L. (1955). *Denial of Illness: Symbolic and Physiological Aspects.* Springfield, IL: Charles C Thomas.

Weiskrantz, L. (1986). *Blindsight.* New York: Oxford University Press.

Welman, A. J. (1969). Right-sided unilateral visual spatial agnosia, asomatognosia and anosognosia with left hemisphere lesions. *Brain* 92:571–580.

2
Anosognosia Related to Hemiplegia and Hemianopia

EDOARDO BISIACH
AND GIULIANO GEMINIANI

In one of the letters addressed to his friend Lucilius (*Liber* V, *Epistula* IX), L. A. Seneca dealt with beliefs related to the self. Although primarily interested in moral implications of such beliefs, he related the following anecdote.

> You know that Harpastes, my wife's fatuous companion, has remained in my home as an inherited burden. . . . This foolish woman has suddenly lost her sight. Incredible as it might appear, what I am going to tell you is true: She does not know she is blind. Therefore, again and again she asks her guardian to take her elsewhere. She claims that my home is dark.[1]

Further on, Seneca remarked that there are instances in which "it is difficult to recover from illness just because we are unaware of it."[2]

Almost 2000 years were to elapse before von Monakow (1885) reported a similar observation in a 70-year-old patient with bilateral extensive damage to the posterior regions of the brain. Although in retrospect this patient's symptoms were somewhat unclear, they seemed to include loss of sight, of which the patient was not aware and which, like Harpastes, he attributed to ambiental darkness. Von Monakow's paper is a landmark in the history of clinical neurology. It is not merely the first clinical report of lack of awareness of severe loss of sight. By underscoring the difference between his case and cases in which imperception of disease might have been explained on the basis of a global mental deterioration due to diffuse brain damage, von Monakow implicitly raised the issue of the pathological dissociation of beliefs related to the self. Although still in bare out-

---

[1] *Harpasten, uxoris meae fatuam, scis hereditarium onus in domo mea remansisse. . . . Haec fatua subito desiit videre. Incredibilem rem tibi narro, sed veram: nescit esse se caecam; subinde paedagogum suum rogat ut migret, ait domum tenebricosam esse.*
[2] *. . . et ideo difficulter ad sanitatem pervenimus quia nos aegrotare nescimus.*

line, the stage was set for subsequent neurological investigation of the highest cognitive functions.

The selectivity of anosognosia was definitively proved in Anton's famous paper of 1899. Knowledge of this paper is universal, so it is superfluous to give any in-depth account of it in these pages, although specific points are mentioned where appropriate in subsequent sections of the chapter. It is worth remembering, however, that in the case of Ursula Mercz (Anton's only case of anosognosia related to cortical blindness, the two other cases he described in that paper being instances of unawareness of cortical deafness) the disorder of sight affected the whole visual field.

It is less known that in a previous paper (1893) Anton had referred to a disordered awareness of the left side of the body in a patient suffering from a vascular lesion of the posterior regions of the right hemisphere. According to Anton, the patient (Johann K.) had left hemianopia and hemianesthesia and did not move his left limbs spontaneously. In addition to showing obvious symptoms of left hemineglect, the patient manifested what is probably the first recorded instance of productive (in contrast to merely defective) phenomena of unilateral misrepresentation: He claimed that his daughter was lying to his left, making sexual advances.

An unequivocal case of lack of awareness of left-sided motor and visual disorders was later described by Pick (1898). His patient, Adolph W., a 31-year-old alcoholic, had a cerebrovascular accident that resulted in left hemiparesis and hemianopia associated with neglect dyslexia. The patient explicitly denied the disorder.

The first serious attempt at giving a psychological explanation of the syndrome of which anosognosia is one of the main symptoms was made by Zingerle in 1913 (see Bisiach and Berti, 1987, for a revaluation of this important contribution). Hemineglect, lack of concern for hemiplegia, and delusions circumscribed to the contralesional side of egocentric space were considered by Zingerle to be a local disorder of mental representation and consciousness, for which he used—borrowing from Jones (1910)—the comprehensive term "dyschiria" (impairment of one side). The importance of Zingerle's early breakthrough for such issues as representation, beliefs, consciousness—which constitute the highest problems of cognitive science—is self-evident: Selective disorders of thought processes caused by focal brain lesions can indeed offer important clues as to the structure of such processes. In particular, the study of these disorders may, as argued later, shed light on thought processes that appear to be instantiated in the functional architecture of the human brain as analogues of outer reality.

Babinski's discussions of anosognosia related to hemiplegia at the meetings held by the French Société de Neurologie in June 1914 and December 1918 are a further outstanding landmark. The term "anosognosia" was coined there, and the clarity and elegance of Babinski's exposition was such as to obscure previous contributions, with the sole exception of Anton's paper of 1899.

The subsequent development of studies on anosognosia has now been reviewed by McGlynn and Schacter (1989), and there is no need to duplicate it here.

CONCEPTUAL PROBLEMS: NEGLECT VERSUS MISREPRESENTATION AND IRRATIONAL BELIEFS

A satisfactory definition of anosognosia per se is perhaps impossible, attributable to the fact that the term anosognosia, rather than referring to a truly distinct symptom, may be (and has indeed been) used to denote aspects of patients' behavior in relation to their illness that are heterogeneous in appearance and unlikely to depend on a specific set of causes exclusively related to them.

Recall Seneca's observation that Harpastes *"nescit esse se caecam"* (she *does not know* she is blind). Even assuming that she had never denied blindness verbally, the truth of Seneca's statement seems to be irrefutable given the behavior she displayed after the onset of her illness. However, patients who verbally deny their hemiplegia usually do not object to being confined to bed. In contrast, patients who verbally admit of paralysis on one side may attempt to stand and walk or ask for tools they are patently unable to handle as they did prior to their illness. Anton (1899) used the term *"dunkle Kenntnis"* (dim knowledge) with reference to such instances; it seems, however, more appropriate to talk of *dissociation* of knowledge (see Chapters 11 and 14).

In other cases—indeed, in most cases—unawareness of hemiplegia or hemianopia, whatever the basis on which it is inferred, is clearly secondary to the fact that patients ignore one side of their body and environment. Other cases exist in which deficient knowledge of illness is inferred from the apparent lack of adequate emotional reactions, the condition Babinski (1914) named "anosodiaphoria."

These definitional issues cease to be a problem if anosognosia related to hemiplegia and hemianopia—rather than being treated as a separate subject—is viewed as one of the peculiar symptoms of a circumscribed brain lesion disrupting a single substrate of cognitive activities. Such concepts as attention, representation, beliefs, and consciousness are related, within a circumscribed domain of spatial reference, to this area. This view is defended in a later section of this chapter.

CLINICAL PRESENTATION AND ASSESSMENT OF ANOSOGNOSIA RELATED TO HEMIPLEGIA AND HEMIANOPIA

As foreshadowed in the preceding section, the symptomatology of unawareness of hemiplegia and hemianopia is not uniform; and it is inextricably interwoven with the manifestations of neglect and misrepresentation of objects on one side of egocentric space. As regards hemiplegia, the patients' imperfect knowledge of all it entails is suggested in minimal cases by an emotional indifference and unthinking resignation. Sometimes the motor defect is acknowledged but explained away, even when it is massive, as being due to some less threatening disease such as rheumatism. Other patients deny outright any motor impairment. Requested to make a given movement with a paralyzed limb, they may suddenly appear absent-minded, their attention is distracted elsewhere, or they move the unaffected limb on the other side. Often they make such statements as

"Here you are," implying the purported execution of the required movement. In such instances, it is seldom possible to force the patient to acknowledge that no movement had actually been made by the paralyzed limb. In the exceptional instance in which the patient admits the lack or insufficiency of movement, he may sometimes explain it in various ways as being due to the fact that the involved limb is the left and therefore weaker one (Bisiach et al., 1986). Trying to rationalize the immobility of the paralyzed limb may entangle the patient in a web of bizarre arguments, the fallacy of which can hardly be demonstrated to him (Bisiach, 1988a). It is worth emphasizing that, in general, whether the patient looks at his paralyzed limbs during examination makes no difference. As mentioned above, despite the denial of illness, the patient as a rule does not ask why he is bedridden and appears satisfied with his unusual condition.

Unawareness of hemiplegia is sometimes complicated by the coexistence of somatoparaphrenic phenomena (Gerstmann, 1942). A minimal form of these disorders may be seen in the feeling of alienness of the limbs contralateral to the brain lesion, explicitly referred to by the patients or inferred by the peculiar nicknames they apply to them or from statements they make (Critchley, 1955; Weinstein and Kahn, 1955). With the severe form of somatoparaphrenia the patient maintains that the contralesional limb belongs to someone else, e.g., to the examiner. The content of delusional beliefs may be utterly bizarre: The patient may claim that the contralesional arm belongs to a fellow patient previously transported by ambulance, or that it had been forgotten in the bed by a previous patient. Sometimes the patients have a tolerant attitude to the repudiated limbs, whereas in other instances they are irritated by their presence and insist on having them taken away. In some cases, albeit infrequently, there is furious hatred toward the alien limbs, and even physical violence may be observed. Critchley (1974) termed this condition "misoplegia." Delusional beliefs do not always clearly refer to the patients' limbs (e.g., Anton, 1893; Zingerle, 1913): The patient may claim that some other person lies at his side (the side contralateral to the lesion); and sometimes this "person" is an uncanny presence, engaged in objectionable activities. In such instances, there seems to be a transition from somatoparaphrenia toward a misrepresentation encompassing the whole contralesional side of the environment.

The semiology of the unawareness of hemianopia is much poorer. This is likely to depend on the fact that overt symptoms of the latter are much less salient compared with those that characterize the unawareness of hemiplegia, and much less attention has been devoted to them by investigators. Unawareness of hemianopia may also range from imperception of the defect until it is revealed by the examiner to incorrigible denial.

From what has been said about the clinical presentation of anosognosia, it follows that no satisfactory standard assessment of this condition can be suggested. Anosognosia deserves assessment tailored to each individual case, comprising faithful records of all relevant spontaneous behavior as well as of that instigated by the examiner's queries, the limits to which are set only by the examiner's inventiveness and the patient's mood and intelligence. Usually, even when the patients are not dull, the clinical interview is quickly foiled by their unwillingness to oppose the examiner's counterarguments.

For specific purposes, i.e., for purposes of crude classification during studies on a large population of subjects, unawareness of hemiplegia and hemianopia may be evaluated following a simple standard procedure such as that used by Bisiach et al. (1986). This procedure scores anosognosia according to a 4-point scale ranging from 0 to 3.

0 = The disorder is spontaneously reported or mentioned by the patient in reply to a general question about his complaints.

1 = The disorder is reported only following a specific question about the affected function.

2 = The disorder is acknowledged only after its demonstration through routine techniques of neurological examination.

3 = No acknowledgment of the disorder can be obtained.

ANATOMY

Even today little can be said about clinicoanatomical correlations regarding anosognosia related to hemiplegia and hemianopia. To a large extent, the issue merges with the problem of the anatomy of unilateral neglect (Vallar and Perani, 1987; Bisiach and Vallar, 1988). Most authors agree that the region most frequently involved is the inferoparietal cortex (Gerstmann, 1942; Critchley, 1953). However, lesions apparently confined to the frontal lobes may also involve anosognosic behavior, as suggested by Zingerle's (1913) case 3.

In a study on a fairly large population of right-brain-damaged patients who had undergone CT scan examination (Bisiach et al., 1986), anosognosia related to left hemiplegia and left hemianopia was found in association with both corticosubcortical lesions and lesions confined to deep structures. Superficial lesions mainly involved the inferoposterior parietal cortex. Lesions of the thalamus or the lenticular nucleus were diagnosed in anosognosic patients, in whom the lesion was confined to deep structures. This finding is in agreement with previous reports (Gerstmann, 1942; Watson and Heilman, 1979; Healton, Navarro, Bressman, and Brust, 1982). Although unawareness of hemiplegia and hemianopia may be found in dissociation from one another (see next section), no clear clinicoanatomical basis for such a dissociation has been found. Hemianopic patients who have been unaware of their visual-field defect have tended, however, to have lesions involving the occipitotemporal region. Nonetheless, exceptional instances can be found in which hemiplegic and hemianopic patients with large lesions involving the inferoparietal cortex are not anosognosic (e.g., patients Z.M. and B.D. of Figure 3 in Bisiach et al., 1986).

INCIDENCE, ASSOCIATIONS, AND DISSOCIATIONS

The issue of left/right differences in the incidence of unawareness of hemiplegia and hemianopia is a thorny one, even more than for unilateral neglect. The reason is fairly obvious: In left-brain-damaged patients, language disorders may conceal unawareness of disease much more effectively than symptoms of neglect. Although an overview of the available literature suggests a higher frequency of unawareness of hemiplegia after right brain damage, thus confirming the conviction shared by most clinicians, some studies challenge this view. As for unawareness of hemianopia, left/right differences might even be less pronounced. Because the aim of this chapter is to discuss implications of anosognosia not strictly related to hemispheric functional asymmetries the latter subjects are not further investigated; the reader who wishes to pursue the subject is referred to the available literature (Gross and Kaltenbäck, 1955; Battersby, Bender, Pollack, and Kahn, 1956; Cutting, 1978). It is worth noting, however, that phenomena that are most likely to be intimately connected with anosognosia, such as overt manifestations of somatoparaphrenia, are undeniably expressions of right hemisphere disease. Nonverbal behavior congruent with denial of ownership of one limb, such as excited indication of that limb or gestures requiring its removal, are seldom (if ever) observed in left-brain-damaged patients. Moreover, if there is any reason to believe that the etiology of unawareness of hemiplegia and of unilateral spatial neglect are essentially the same, the largely uncontroversial left/right asymmetry of the latter [see Bisiach and Vallar (1988) for an appraisal of the issue] points to a similar asymmetry of unawareness of hemiplegia.

Within the population of right-brain-damaged patients, associations and dissociations between anosognosia and other disorders may be assessed without the impediments set by dysphasia. Following is a compendium of the findings published in the previously mentioned paper (Bisiach et al., 1986), in which awareness of motor and visual disorders was investigated in a sample of patients selected for the presence of severe paralysis of the left upper limb, severe left hemianopia, or both. This selection was necessary because the scale adopted to quantify anosognosia would have had a different meaning if applied to disorders having different degrees of severity.

Medium or severe anosognosia related to motor impairment (scores 2 and 3, as defined in the preceding section) was found in 12 of 36 patients with paralysis of the left upper limb. Medium and severe anosognosia related to severe left hemianopia was found to be much more frequent: It was present in 28 of 32 patients. This difference cannot be completely explained by the fact that hemianopia is much less obtrusive than hemiplegia in the patient's self-perception. In fact, 5 of 36 patients denied a motor defect and 24 of 32 a visual defect, despite clear demonstration of the impairment (grade 3 anosognosia). The most plausible explanation is that brain lesions resulting in hemianopia are more likely to encroach on structures that, when affected by a lesion, cause impairment of awareness of visual (or visual and motor) disorders.

Although anosognosia related to motor deficit was found to be positively correlated with both (tactile) somatosensory impairment and homonymous visual-field defects, there were clear instances of double dissociations. This point is particularly interesting as regards somatosensory disorders, whose usual association with unawareness of motor impairment, rather than suggesting a necessary causal link, might thus depend in part on the anatomical contiguity of structures having different functional roles. Indeed, although loss of sensory information about a paralyzed limb is likely to contribute to the causation of anosognosic phenomena, our data—taken together with the case of Pick's patient Adolph W., who was severely anosognosic despite retained somatosensory function—seems to be a clear demonstration that somatosensory impairment is by itself neither sufficient nor necessary to generate anosognosic states.

The pattern of association between anosognosia for motor impairment and somatosensory impairment or homonymous visual-field defects did not change if these disorders were considered, respectively, at the level of the lower limb and the lower quadrant of the visual field.

The positive correlation between anosognosia related to motor impairment and unilateral neglect, both personal and extrapersonal, was evident. Instances of double dissociation were found, however. As expected, they were more frequent with extrapersonal than with personal neglect. Denial of paralysis in the absence of neglect of the paralyzed limb is theoretically important (see next section).

No significant correlation was found between unawareness of hemianopia and sensorimotor disorders. This finding is far from surprising and does not seem to have any theoretical implications.

More interesting is the fact that unawareness of left hemianopia was double-dissociated from personal and extrapersonal neglect. The correlation between unawareness of hemianopia and unilateral neglect (both personal and extrapersonal) came closer to zero more than in any other correlation. However, the greater incidence of extrapersonal, in contrast to personal, neglect that characterized the group of patients with unawareness of paralysis was also found in patients with unawareness of hemianopia; indeed in these patients it was even more evident.

Our population comprised only 12 patients who had both paralysis of the left upper limb and severe hemianopia. Two patients were not anosognosic, six were unaware of both disorders, and four denied hemianopia even after the examiner had tried to demonstrate its presence; the latter were minimally, if at all, anosognosic as regards their motor impairment. This fractionation of awareness of illness has strong theoretical implications, as discussed in the last section.

Of the 36 patients with complete paralysis of the upper limb, 27 had their lower limb affected to the same degree. Only five of these patients showed a different degree of awareness of the upper and lower limb deficit, their scores being 0-1, 0-2, 1-3, 2-3, and 2-1 (the first and second number in the score of each patient referring to the upper limb and lower limb, respectively). This finding suggests that unawareness of motor impairment might more easily be induced as regards the lower limb.

Another thorny issue that afflicts the study of anosognosia much more than the issue of left/right asymmetries is the association of lack of awareness, or denial of illness, with general confusion and general mental deterioration. This point is of crucial theoretical relevance and is worth serious consideration. Many authors have stressed the intimacy of such associations. However, although it is often difficult to ascertain on the basis of clinical descriptions whether and to what extent a patient is anosognosic, it is much more difficult (except in extreme instances) to infer from those descriptions the presence or absence of *general* confusion and *general* intellectual impairment. Sometimes, for example, the label "confusion" is applied to highly selective and insulated cognitive disorders such as reduplicative paramnesia, i.e., phenomena that may co-occur with anosognosia and might even be caused by the same basic, selective disorder of thought. [See Black and Kertesz (1984) for a case of reduplicative paramnesia due to a focal lesion of the right hemisphere and associated with unilateral neglect.]

Implicit in the idea of an intimate association of anosognosia with general confusion or intellectual deterioration is the temptation to explain away anosognosia as one aspect of a global, undifferentiated disorder of cognitive function. This point leads us to the next section.

INTERPRETATION OF ANOSOGNOSIC PHENOMENA RELATED TO ONE SIDE OF THE BODY

The fact that anosognosia might be accompanied, in some instances, by manifestations of "mental confusion" or intellectual impairment is hardly surprising, given that the patient suffers from more or less widespread brain damage. It is even possible that some general factors such as depressed vigilance might favor the appearance of anosognosic phenomena. However, there are instances in which no confusion or intellectual impairment can be detected in patients with severe and irreducible manifestations of anosognosia. This point was already suggested by von Monakow's observation and has been well known since Babinski's (1914, 1918) reports. More recent and striking examples are provided later in the chapter (patients L.A.-O. and P.R.), and a detailed overview of the literature concerning this important point may be found in the report of McGlynn and Schacter (1989). On the other hand, as remarked by Angelergues and coworkers (1960), global impairment of brain functions does not necessarily imply unawareness of deficit resulting from superadded, circumscribed damage to one cerebral hemisphere.

Two further pieces of evidence against an interpretation of anosognosia in terms of general confusion or intellectual impairment can be found among the arguments listed below against an interpretation of the disorder in terms of a goal-directed reaction. One is the selectivity of anosognosia: the fact that a patient may be anosognosic with respect to one defect but not to another. The second argument is based on the observed disappearance of the anosognosic state after vestibular stimulation.

The explanation of anosognosia in terms of a nonconscious, goal-directed reaction has had several proponents [see McGlynn and Schacter (1989) for a description]. It has been couched in slightly different terms, sometimes with a biological orientation (e.g., Schilder, 1935) and sometimes with a psychological slant (e.g., Goldstein, 1939; Sandifer, 1946; Weinstein and Kahn, 1955). Essentially, it views anosognosia as a defensive adaptation against the stress caused by the illness. Of course, it is possible, even likely, that repressive mechanisms contribute to producing and shaping anosognosic behavior, especially as regards diseases that are not due to brain damage. In their classic study, Weinstein and

Kahn (1955) argued convincingly for the existence of mechanisms of this kind. However, several considerations show that this explanation per se fails to account for eight important facts concerning anosognosia related to neurological disorders that affect one side of the body.

1. Unawareness of such disorders is usually present only during the acute stage of the illness, when the patient's vigilance may be clouded and his evaluation of the pathological event is still incomplete, whereas it often disappears after a few hours or a few days, when the patient comes to fully realize all the consequences of his condition. A goal-directed denial of illness should be characterized by an evolution opposite to that commonly observed by the clinician.

2. As a rule, patients are fully aware of their neurological disorders if the latter are the consequence of a lesion that does not involve neural structures responsible for higher cognitive functions (e.g., of lesions confined to the pyramidal pathways or to primary visual cortex).

3. It was argued in the preceding section that there are grounds for believing that unawareness of hemiplegia is more frequent and severe after damage to the right than to the left hemisphere. As noted by Friedland and Weinstein (1977), a motivational explanation totally fails to account for this asymmetry. It is worth adding that the hypothesis that qualitative and quantitative left/right differences in anosognosia depend on interhemispheric differences in the organization of intellectual and emotional function (Gainotti, 1972) is contradicted by the fact that patients who deny their left hemiplegia or seem to be totally unaware of it may be intolerant of minor disorders affecting the right side of the body. There are even patients who vividly complain about ailments which, though actually affecting the left side, are referred by such patients to the right; this extreme form of allochiria may, for example, be observed in the presence of phlebitis of the left lower limb, whereas in the case of patient L.A.-O. (see next section) it concerned the motor defect itself.

4. Anosognosia may be selective. Anton's (1899) patient Ursula Mercz. denied blindness but was fully cognizant of her mild dysphasia. In most instances, all pathology related to one side of the body may be disavowed or ignored (maybe even retrospectively: see the case of patient P.R. in the next section). However, anosognosia related to one side of the body may itself be dissociated. It was noted in the preceding section that denial of severe left hemianopia (irreducible despite the examiner's demonstration of the disorder) may not be associated with denial of left hemiplegia. It was also remarked that in our sample different degrees of awareness could be observed in the *same* patient as regards paralysis of the upper and lower limb, the latter being more liable to be denied. A similar dissociation was reported by von Hagen and Ives (1937) in a patient who denied paralysis of the left lower limb while being aware of her memory disorders and paralysis of her left upper limb.

5. As already mentioned, unawareness of disease may be apparent in the patient's verbal, but not in their nonverbal, behavior or vice versa. This double dissociation too cannot be accounted for by a motivational interpretation.

6. Theories envisaging self-defensive mechanisms (as well as hypotheses based on cognitive and affective dissimilarities of the two cerebral hemispheres) cannot give a satisfactory explanation as to why, apart from cases in which the patients seem to have banished their paralyzed limbs from their mind, there are instances in which utter dislike and even aggression is displayed to the offending limbs.

7. Anosognosia, sometimes, far from affording the patients a factitious peace of mind, creates serious impediments and even danger. Unawareness of hemianopia makes the patients unable to foresee and avoid obstacles in one side of the environment;

unawareness of hemiplegia exposes them to disastrous falls. Unawareness of language disorders suppresses any possibility of communication between the jargon aphasic, who sometimes retains an intact language comprehension (Kinsbourne and Warrington, 1963), and the interlocutor. In Kinsbourne's words (1987), ignoring or denying disability is "implicitly failing to modify one's actions and reorganize one's surroundings in view of the disability." This attitude, as already pointed out by Seneca, undermines recovery from illness at its very roots.

8. Finally, the observed remission of severe, intractable unawareness of left hemiplegia (Cappa, Sterzi, Vallar, and Bisiach, 1987), if confirmed, definitively rules out the applicability of motivational explanations.

A theoretical model of anosognosia for hemiplegia and hemianopia, and indeed the simplest way of conceiving of unilateral neglect of space in all its clinical manifestations, is postulation of a disorder at the topmost neural level ["analyzer" being the term adopted by Kinsbourne (1980) to refer to this level] at which a part of the organism or one of its functions is represented and its activity monitored to other components of the nervous system.

An oversimplified, idealized neuronal model of a function-specific representational device has been outlined (Bisiach and Berti, 1987) that, if lesioned in slightly different ways, can account for unilateral defective phenomena such as neglect and unawareness of hemiplegia and hemianopia, as well as for the unilateral, productive disorders of representation that can be observed in association with them. Although the model was originally addressed to visuospatial processing, it can be generalized for use in other domains, such as somatosensory or auditory areas. It can also be adapted to incorporate intersensory processes (e.g., visuo-somatosensory) that, especially in the case of unawareness of hemiplegia, may complicate the clinical picture. The model largely ignores the problem of its actual implementation in the two cerebral hemispheres, including the problem of left/right asymmetries, although a suggestion was made by Bisiach and Vallar (1988).

The afferent component of the model (Fig. 2–1, layer I) is a sensory transducer transmitting information relative to that portion of the stimulus array that at any given instant falls within the field of a sensory receptor. The transducer projects information into a representational network that reconstructs and keeps in active memory an internal image of the stimulus array explored by the receptor during a given time interval. The process of reconstruction is needed to unfold and reassemble overwritten sensory messages that result when a receptor (e.g., the retina) is successively oriented toward different sectors of the stimulus array or when the content of the latter changes relative to a stationary receptor. An example of the second occurrence is the reconstruction of the shape of an object seen in motion behind a fissure (Bisiach, Luzzatti, and Perani, 1979). The inner image is generated according to analogue principles. With respect to spatial properties, it means that a topological correspondence is maintained between the external object and the neural activity that constitutes its inner representation in approximately the same way in which such correspondence is evident at the receptor surface or in the primary sensory areas of the cerebral cortex. Anatomical data about the topological maps of the brain support the plausibility of this

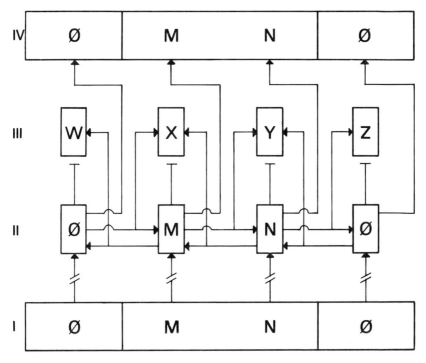

Figure 2-1. Model of two-dimensional visuospatial processing. (From Bisiach, E., and Berti, A. Dyschiria: an attempt at its systemic explanation.   In M. Jeannerod, ed: *Neurophysiological and Neuropsychological Aspects of Spatial Neglect.* Amsterdam: Elsevier, 1987, pp. 183–201. With permission.)

assumption (e.g., Merzenich and Kaas, 1980). Cellular groupings within the *same* representational network of the model may be activated through a top-down mechanism. This activation corresponds to the generation of modality-specific "mental" representations such as waking and hypnagogic images, hallucinations, and dreams. The existence of a common substrate for sensory and mental representation has not been expressly postulated for the purposes of the present model but has been inferred by different authors on different grounds (e.g., Finke, 1985).

Under normal waking conditions, the sensory-driven neuronal groupings (layer II) are assumed to inhibit the *topologically corresponding,* internally activated groupings (layer III), so that the activity of the latter is either prevented or recognized by the system as being fantastic in nature. In this case, the output of the representational network (layer IV) faithfully mirrors outside reality.

Two kinds of lesions of the model may be envisaged with reference to anosognosia and, more generally, unilateral misrepresentation including hemineglect.

In one case (Fig. 2–2), one side of the topologically organized representational network is completely destroyed or at least inactivated. In this case, only

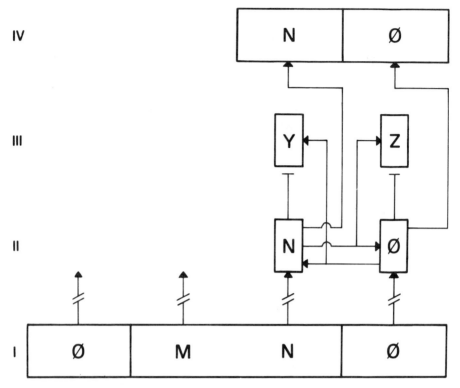

Figure 2–2. Dysfunction underlying hemineglect. (From Bisiach, E., and Berti, A. Dyschiria: an attempt at its systemic explanation.   In M. Jeannerod, ed: *Neurophysiological and Neuropsychological Aspects of Spatial Neglect.* Amsterdam: Elsevier, 1987, pp. 183–201. With permission.)

one side of the stimulus array is normally perceived. The missing side cannot even be *conceived,* and therefore the organism cannot compensate for the defect through exploratory behavior; that is, it has no access to the remedial tactics that can be observed, for example in a case of pure hemianopia (e.g., eye and head turning toward the blind field). This condition corresponds to unilateral neglect proper. As regards anosognosia, the behavior from which it may be inferred reflects, in this case, a global lack of representation of one side of the body and its surroundings. Apparent unawareness or explicit denial of illness related to one side of the body is therefore, in this case, only one aspect of hemineglect.

    In the other case (Fig. 2–3), the dysfunction is confined to sensory-driven activities. In these circumstances, processes occurring in top-down activated cellular groupings are no longer under bottom-up control in a sector next to that in which representational processes develop in a regular manner. The result of this type of dysfunction is a condition in which the output of the representational network is characterized by the presence of phenomena of pathological representation that are confined to one side of egocentric space. The simplest and most frequent instance of this condition is pathological completion such as is observed in perceptual tasks using incomplete drawings (Warrington, 1962) or in neglect dyslexia (Kinsbourne and Warrington, 1962). The normal representation of one side of the body and environment is in particularly striking contrast with the representation of the opposite side when the colorful manifestations of somatoparaphrenia, or analogous phenomena referring to the extrapersonal environment, are released. In these circumstances, unawareness or denial of illness is the consequence of parasitic representations and beliefs related to one side of the patient's body and may occur in the absence of neglect phenomena.

The model enjoys at least two kinds of empirical support. The first relates to the findings from research on sensory deprivation, which show that hallucinated representations can arise when brain activity ceases to be modulated by information sent by sensory receptors. A review of such findings was undertaken by Zubec (1969). The second, deriving from the neurophysiological studies by Sprague and colleagues (1961), is even more cogent. After lesioning the lemniscal system in the cat, these authors noted an association of symptoms of spatial neglect and stereotyped hyperexploratory activity, which they interpreted as having a hallucinatory origin.

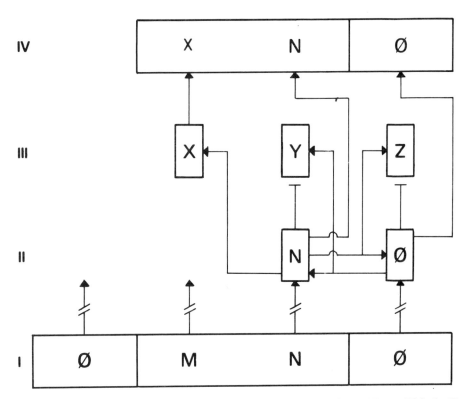

Figure 2–3. Dysfunction underlying unilateral misrepresentation. (From Bisiach, E., and Berti, A. Dyschiria: an attempt at its systemic explanation. In M. Jeannerod, ed: *Neurophysiological and Neuropsychological Aspects of Spatial Neglect.* Amsterdam: Elsevier, 1987, pp. 183–201. With permission.)

IMPLICATIONS OF ANOSOGNOSIA AND RELATED DISORDERS FOR THEORIES OF HIGHER BRAIN FUNCTIONS

From the beginning of this chapter it has been intimated that the study of anosognosia—more exactly, study of the manifold symptomatology in which anosognosia is embedded—has preeminent relevance for the understanding of human cognitive processes. This remark may appear self-evident, and indeed it *should be,* notwithstanding the amazing paucity of psychological speculation on this subject in the clinical literature and the almost ubiquitous disregard of anosognosia and related disorders in the extensive literature that other disciplines have accumulated on cognition. Contemporary functionalism is in part responsible for this gap between cognitive science and clinical neurology. Until recently, paradigmatic disregard of the physical instantiation of mind has influenced much of postbehaviorist psychology, delaying its development in a promising direction. A reversal in trend is well under way, however—witness the conference that occasioned this chapter. Except for the last subsection, what follows is a concise overview of arguments that have been developed more extensively elsewhere (see below), where further details can be found.

Structure of Cognitive Representations

The initial, perhaps basic, implication of clinical phenomena such as unilateral neglect and some forms of anosognosia concerns the structure of cognitive representations. It has long been debated whether the latter is analogue, sensory-like as suggested by the well known investigations of the groups led by Shepard and Kosslyn (e.g., Shepard, 1975; Kosslyn, 1980), or more abstract and more similar to the structure of language than to the structure of perceptual processes (e.g., Pylyshyn, 1984). It has been argued that the controversy may not find a solution unless it is with reference to the physical medium in which cognitive representations are instantiated (Anderson, 1978). The occurrence of representational lacunae or pathological representations confined to one side of space as a consequence of focal damage to the opposite hemisphere seems to offer that kind of solution (Bisiach and Berti, 1987). An objection to the effect that such disorders might be due to local impairment of an analogue wired-in device, subserving cognitive processes but not itself endowed with authentic cognitive competence, is contradicted by the fact that no superordinate cognitive mechanism detects, and compensates for, these disorders; on the contrary, cognitive processes not directly involved by the latter may be entrapped by them. Indeed it has been shown experimentally that hemineglect may indirectly contaminate cognitive processes related to the unimpaired side of space (Bisiach, Berti, and Vallar, 1985). In the clinical setting, the same is demonstrated by the logical misconduct of anosognosic patients trying to rationalize absurd beliefs concerning a single side of their body *(vide infra).*

Thought and Language

A second implication, deriving directly from the first, concerns the role of language in thought processes. Language, by itself, is unable to compensate for the representational lacuna that hemineglect patients may reveal in the mental description of familiar surroundings. It is passively caught in the tangle of spatially circumscribed misrepresentation and wild reasoning of anosognosic patients. This fact suggests that it is not an autonomous representational system but a means for communicating contents supplied by nonlinguistic thought processes occurring on the basis of an analogue representational medium (Bisiach, 1988a; see also Arbib, Conklin, and Hill, 1987, for a comparable position argued on different grounds).

Consciousness

The third implication is much more problematic insofar as it relates to a concept that is still under laborious scrutiny (see the volume edited by Marcel and Bisiach, 1988, for a collection of disparate views). At any rate, there are at least two aspects under which the relevance of anosognosia and related phenomena are self-evident; both concern the fractionability of consciousness.

One aspect relates to clinical observations in which contradictory inferences about awareness of neurological disorders could be drawn from verbal and nonverbal behavior. As we have seen, a patient may verbally admit his hemiplegia while acting, or appearing disposed to act, as if he were healthy. Conversely, there are hemiplegic patients who resolutely deny illness but nonetheless lie still in bed, never initiating spontaneous activities, wherever situated in the automatic/nonautomatic continuum, that require the coordinate use of the limbs of both sides. This *double* dissociation cannot be conceptualized in terms of overt versus tacit knowledge unless such a distinction is operationalized in terms of verbal versus nonverbal indicators of knowledge (which would beg the question). It raises the issue of the choice among criteria of consciousness. More precisely, it shows that, regardless of the criteria one decides to adopt, they are primarily related to the monitoring of the result of computations (concerning, in the specific instance, knowledge of illness) performed by a component of the central nervous system to other components of the same system. Impairment of this kind of internal monitoring can therefore be expected to occur according to differing, sometimes selective, patterns. This double dissociation also contributes to showing how deceptive it would be to assume the possibility of outside knowledge of phenomenal, subjective qualities of conscious mental states of the "person" under observation (Bisiach, 1988b).

The other aspect relates to the extensional qualities of consciousness. Consciousness is sometimes regarded as a property of a unitary, hierarchically superordinate control device (Johnson-Laird, 1988; Umiltà, 1988). The syndrome of unilateral neglect-misrepresentation suggests a different view, according to which consciousness—in both information-processing and phenomenal terms—is a property that characterizes different kinds of brain activity. Among these activities are conative processes that organize and control the stream of thought. Awareness of such processes has been termed by Oatley (1988) "Vygotskyan consciousness." This aspect of consciousness, in computer-metaphorical terms, may be compared to the operations of a central processing unit. Following Luria (1966), many are inclined to localize these functions in the frontal lobes. A different aspect of consciousness relates to modality-specific representations that, aroused by sensory processes or internally generated, impinge on a network (of which a model was described in the preceding section). This aspect, to which Kinsbourne (1988) applied the term "panoramic consciousness," relates to parallel, spatially distributed processes; it may be held to be inherent in analogue neural activities from a certain level, e.g., the level the impairment of which results in phenomena of blindsight (Weiskrantz, 1986) up to levels the impairment of which results in unilateral representational disorders. Damage to lower levels abolishes consciousness relative to stimuli that prove still able to bypass the lesion and generate highly integrated behavior. It abolishes those earliest states of sensory awareness that Oatley (1988) collectively termed "Helmholtzian consciousness" but not the nervous system's ability to monitor the lack of awareness in the form of a sensory scotoma. Damage to higher levels, in contrast, abolishes this ability, and the patient is unaware of his hemianopia or hemiplegia. No hierarchically superordinate apparatus exists that is capable of obviating failures in the detection and monitoring of the disorder.

Propositional Attitudes

A further complex of implications is specifically related to anosognosia: It concerns inferences that may be drawn about "propositional attitudes," such as beliefs and desires, from phenomena of local loss or distortion of the latter after focal brain damage. What follows is meant only to be an outline of some aspects of the issue and to offer incentive for discussion, rather than belabored conclusions touching on problems that have so far been dealt with mainly in philosophical writings. Moreover, terms such as "beliefs" and "desires" are here used almost as passe-partout words, though it is apparent from what has already been set forth and what follows that a conceptual analysis of such words in neurological terms—assuming this enterprise were to some (present or future) extent possible—would imply a great deal of refining of the commonsense notions they express, if not their abandonment by a mature cognitive science, as foreshadowed by some philosophers (e.g., Stich, 1983) on a different ground. Given these premises, a convenient way in which to proceed is to present a typical case where crude facts are sufficiently eloquent to bring into focus the most salient points to be considered.

> Patient L.A.-O. (clinical record NA 472, 1980) was a 65-year-old, right-handed woman who was admitted to the emergency department of our hospital on the evening of 2 July 1980. Shortly before admission she had suddenly developed left hemiplegia without loss of consciousness. Alert and cooperative, she claimed that the reason for her hospitalization was sudden weakness and annoying paresthesia of the *right* limbs; her narrative, supplied in a mild state of anxiety, was indeed accompanied by sustained massage of the allegedly hyposthenic right inferior limb. She also claimed that the left hand did not belong to her but had been forgotten in the ambulance by another patient. On request, she admitted without hesitation that her left shoulder was part of her body and *inferentially* came to the same conclusion as regards her left arm and elbow, given, as she remarked, the evident continuity of those members. She was elusive about the forearm but insisted in denying ownership of the left hand, even when it had been passively placed on the right side of her trunk.

She could not explain why her rings happened to be worn by the fingers of the alien hand. A dense left hemianopia was found on the confrontation test. On double simultaneous stimulation of the *right* visual field she showed consistent extinction of the left stimulus. Acoustic stimuli (finger-snapping) delivered near the left ear were referred to either the symmetrical position in the right hemispace or the vertex. She showed a severe somatosensory deficit on the left side of the body, including the face; intense tactile stimuli were perceived but were referred to symmetrical points on the right half of the body. The patient also showed marked hemineglect on a cancellation task. She did not object to being bedridden; and although she used her right upper limb for a variety of purposes, she never engaged in activities that required the use of both hands.

Two days later the symptoms had partially faded. At the beginning of the examination she still maintained that she had been taken to the hospital because of weakness of her right limbs and was totally anosognosic as regards the paralysis of her left hand. At the end of the examination, however, she appeared genuinely convinced that her left limbs were defective. She volunteered the information that only on that very morning she had begun to recognize her left hand as her own while being perfectly reminiscent of her past denial. The visual field defect had cleared considerably; she still showed left visual extinction on double stimulation if one of the two stimuli was delivered to the left hemifield but not if both stimuli were presented within the right hemifield. Hemineglect was absent on the cancellation tasks; however, requested to pick up a series of small cubes aligned from left to right in front of her, she collected them, using her right hand and starting from the rightmost cube, until she arrived to the sagittal midplane of her trunk. At this point, she pushed the remainder leftwards and said *"There aren't any more."* A CT scan performed on 15 July 1980 revealed an area of reduced density, in all likelihood a softening, in the corona radiata of the right hemisphere.

The case of patient L.A.-O. is paradigmatic; it contains in a nutshell all the challenges to cognitive science in its effort to explain "propositional attitudes," i.e., the various types of relation that are held by many authors to exist between a mental representation (sometimes conceived as a "proposition" or, more explicitly, as a "sentence in the head") and the "attitude" (e.g., belief, desire, fear) an organism has toward that representation.[3]

It would be inappropriate here to embark on a discussion of how specious this distinction between a mental representation and an attitude toward that representation—or, more generally, the dichotomy between mental representations and processes operating on them—might prove to be. Rather, let us begin by noting, in patient L.A.-O., the spatially ordered transition from a "true" belief relative to her shoulder to a "false" belief relative to her hand, through the intermediate attitude of doubt or suspicion concerning her elbow and forearm. The first, self-suggesting move in trying to explain the patient's behavior is in terms of a proximal-to-distal decreasing degree of bilateral cortical representation of the upper limb. However plausible, this explanation fails to account for the most astonishing fact: the denial of ownership of a limb, which flies in the face of all visual evidence. The negative (as opposed to assertive) aspects of somatopara-

---

[3]It is not possible here to elucidate further the concept of "propositional attitude." The interested reader is referred to a discussion of propositional attitudes in Dennett (1986).

phrenia are something that the simplistic model outlined in the preceding section is insufficiently detailed to accommodate. Indeed, to deny something entails having a mental representation of what is being denied. If so, contrary to Zingerle's (1913) early interpretation, statements such as those made by patient L.A.-O. are not made by default; they must in fact originate in a parasitic representation rather than in a lack of representation of one's hand. The overwhelming strength of the parasitic representation suggests that the corresponding neural activity is probably different from the activity that constitutes the unbridled thought processes occurring in the absence of the controlling influence of sensory information flow (as in dreams and in states of sensory deprivation) and is perhaps attributable to a focus of irritation consequent to the lesion of the right hemisphere. If true, this hypothesis supports the contention that the delusions of somatoparaphrenia do not originate in a disordered activity of language centers disconnected from other brain areas, as suggested by Geschwind (1965), but in other structures (possibly located in the damaged hemisphere itself) of which language is but the passive spokesman (Bisiach, 1988a). Most amazingly, despite the exceptional strain, such delusions find no relaxation within the whole network of beliefs held by the patient, a network of which they may constitute the only, infinitesimal flaw. On the contrary, urged by the clinician's cross-examination, they may further vitiate the patient's thought processes, as in patient P.R., another case of ours (Bisiach, 1988a).

> As a consequence of a right-hemisphere stroke, P.R. had a severe left hemiplegia and hemineglect anosognosia and obstinately refused to admit that his left arm belonged to him, unshakenly maintaining that it was the examiner's arm. Because he was an educated man, he could maintain relatively fluent conversation on a variety of topics without disclosing any sign of intellectual impairment. Indeed, he had himself supplied a detailed and exact anamnesis, except for one probably revealing particular: He had left out the report of a surgical operation he had undergone a few years before for removal of a *left* inguinal herniation. On one occasion, the examiner placed P.R.'s left hand on the bedclothes, between his own hands and asked the patient whose hands they were: Unhesitatingly, P.R. replied that they were the examiner's hands. Questioned as to whether he had ever met a three-handed man, P.R., pointing to the three arms in front of him, answered that because the examiner had three arms he also must have three hands. Although one day P.R. spontaneously commented on the apparent singularity of some of his statements, he never questioned their soundness. Notwithstanding his expressed conviction, he too manifested no desire to leave his bed or to do anything that presupposed use of his left limbs.

The irreducibility of dogmatic beliefs such as those entertained by L.A.-O. and P.R. is vividly evident in a patient mentioned by Hécaen (1972) who had spontaneously declared that she could not believe the evidence provided by her own sight about the ownership of a limb that she could not help believing was not hers.

Three conclusions may be drawn from the data that have been collected during the last century by observing the behavior of anosognosic patients.

1. These data question the isotropic-Quinean conception of cognitive processes (Fodor, 1983), where "isotropic" is used to mean the homogeneous interconnection of such processes and "Quinean" their interdependence (in the sense that, for

example, any belief has access to, and is conditioned by, all other beliefs, occurrent or dispositional, held by the subject). At least, these data show that the dynamics of beliefs may be viewed differently by the cognitive biologist and the logician. More precisely, they show that certain (wholly irrational) beliefs, rather than being inferred from other beliefs, may settle down and subsist decontextualized in a subject's mind; they also suggest that a check for coherence is a secondary process that may or may not take place, even in cases in which the network of all other beliefs is intact.

2. It seems likely that, especially in the most severe form of misoplegia (i.e., hatred for the limbs contralateral to the brain lesion), the mechanisms that determine the dominance of a devious belief actively inhibit negotiation between the latter and any other belief held by the patient.

3. Finally, the selective, modality-specific character of anosognosic beliefs and, in the specific case of denial of unilateral motor impairment, the segregation in space of such beliefs suggest that the belief system, whatever it might turn out to be in neural terms, is mapped on the analogue medium of sensory-specific representations.

These conclusions seem to apply also to other propositional attitudes, such as desires, which points to the fact that the involvement of propositional attitudes in anosognosia is secondary to the pathology of the representational system. In the case of desires, the issue is more perplexing. There are desires in anosognosia that, although absurd, have all the marks of coherence with the underlying delusional belief, e.g., the desire to rid oneself of a limb that is perceived as being extraneous to the patient. Nonetheless, the same patient may seem to have lost any desire to use the limb contralateral to the brain lesion. As previously argued, if a patient denies that the left, paralyzed hand he can see attached to his body is his own and maintains that he is free to move "his" left hand, such a patient must have the concept of his left hand; the absence of any desires related to that hand then seems paradoxical.

One way to solve this paradox might be by assuming that in the area of cognition, where a pathological representation coexists with the vestiges of a previous (normal) representation, the latter cannot, for some reason, be accessed in order to shape desires, however pressing might be adaptational needs vis-à-vis the constitution of those desires (remember Seneca on the recovery of functions in anosognosic subjects).

Another possibility is that devious "conscious" beliefs—conscious in the questionable sense that they are verbally expressed and some aspects of nonverbal behavior, e.g., misoplegic outbursts, are consistent with their verbal expression—are shadowed, as it were, by "nonconscious" true beliefs about illness and parts of the body. Absence of desires to move the paralyzed limbs would thus be congruous with such "nonconscious" beliefs about those limbs. This view is consistent with the idea of a fractionability of consciousness argued above.

The matter, however, is more complex. On the one hand, there are patients who acknowledge hemiplegia in words and nonetheless conceive and try to satisfy desires (e.g., knitting, walking) that are utterly incompatible with the expressed beliefs about illness. On the other hand, as we have just noted, patients who firmly deny hemiplegia and refuse to believe the paralyzed limbs to be theirs may not manifest such desires or spontaneously initiate activities that are precluded by their motor impairment.

Here we have two kinds of anosognosic behavior, one of which is the converse of the other. Taken together, they raise the question of why desires and attempts to satisfy them might be *inconsistent* with the *expressed* beliefs (which are *true* in the first and *false* in the second type of behavior) while appearing *consistent* with *unexpressed* beliefs (which happen to be *false* in the case of the first and *true* in the case of the second type of behavior). Up to a certain point, an interesting parallel can be drawn with some studies on normal people, surveyed by Stich (1983, Chapter 11), suggesting the existence of two, relatively independent cognitive systems underlying beliefs. According to Wilson (unpublished material cited by Stich, p. 236), one of these systems "mediates behavior (especially unregulated behavior), is largely unconscious, and is, perhaps, the older of the two systems in evolutionary terms. The other, perhaps newer, system is largely conscious, and its function is to attempt to verbalize, explain, and communicate what is occurring in the unconscious system." These two systems can be experimentally manipulated independently. The second, called by Wilson the "verbal explanatory system," is reminiscent of the "interpreter," which was identified and localized in the left hemisphere by Gazzaniga (1988) on the basis of split-brain studies.

In cases of anosognosia such as those just considered, desires concerning the affected limbs (or the absence of any such desires) might depend on the nonconscious cognitive system. Perhaps a demonstration of the struggle between conscious and nonconscious cognitive systems is the extreme form of allochiria shown by patient L.A.-O. when referring her motor impairment to the right, unaffected limbs.

It is difficult to explain on this basis the nonverbal behavior of misoplegic subjects. However, further reflection grounded on what is still anecdotal clinical evidence, easily leads to unwarranted speculation. For the moment, it seems sufficient to have found a bridge toward another field of inquiry and to have identified a promising point for future research on anosognosia.

The last issue to be considered concerns a particular type of self-related beliefs: the belief that a certain activity performed by the organism is an activity *willed* by the subject himself. In anosognosic hemiplegics, a belief of this kind may be expressed regarding actions that the patients claim to have performed with their paralyzed limbs. It does not happen in patients in whom movement is precluded by failure of the motor transducer rather than by a lesion apt to cause concomitant anosognosia. Whatever the neural basis for the anosognosic belief of having moved the paralyzed limb (we still do not know which premotor events take place in these circumstances), we must take note of the fact that this belief subsists independent of any feedback, even when the pathways that would carry kinesthetic information are spared and the patient can perceive passive movements.

On the other hand, and even more surprisingly, the belief of having *deliberately* moved a limb may subsist in the absence of the causal chain (whatever it may be) that normally leads to a "willed" movement. This issue is a most intriguing one that studies on anosognosia have thus far disregarded. Data relevant to this point have been published in a different context by Hécaen, Talairach, David, and Dell (1949). Prior to the execution of thalamic coagulation for the relief of severe pain in patients suffering from thalamic syndrome, Hécaen et al. stimulated the central nucleus electrically, which caused clenching and unclenching of the patients' fists or pill-rolling movements contralateral to the stimulated thalamus. The patients asserted the *willful* character of such induced movements but were unable to tell why they had made them. The authors emphasized that the patients denied any kind of paresthesia, the occurrence of which had been suggested to them by the examiners as a possible explanation of their movements. Once again we are in the presence of apparently noninferred beliefs that crop up through mechanisms that might be understood at some point in the future.

CONCLUSION

These findings, and probably many others, are the implications of anosognosia and related phenomena for cognitive science. Their weight derives from their relevance to foundational themes currently debated under the intersecting viewpoints of different disciplines and persuasions. Though not subtended by an explicit theoretical commitment, the authors' treatment of categories such as propositional attitudes in a neurological framework might be welcomed by some reader for the wrong reason: Nothing in this chapter is intended to advocate a neurological reduction of the psychological categories it has dealt with—and least of all their principled elimination.

REFERENCES

Anderson, J. R. (1978). Arguments concerning representations for mental imagery. *Psychol. Rev.* 85:249–277.

Angelergues, R., de Ajuriaguerra, J., and Hécaen, H. (1960). La négation de la cécité au cours des lésions cérébrales. *J. Psychol.* 4:381–404.

Anton, G. (1893). Beitrage zur klinischen Beurtheilung und zur Localisation der Muskelsinnstoerungen im Grosshirne. *Z. Heilk.* 14:313–348.

Anton, G. (1899). Ueber die Selbstwahrnehmung der Herderkrankungen des Gehirns durch den Kranken bei Rindenblindheit und Rindentaubheit. *Arch. Psychiatr. Nervenkr.* 32:86–127.

Arbib, M. A., Conklin, E. J., and Hill, J. (1987). *From Schema Theory to Language.* New York: Oxford University Press.

Babinski, J. (1914). Contribution à l'étude des troubles mentaux dans l'hémiplégie organique cérébrale (anosognosie). *Rev. Neurol. (Paris)* 27:845–848.

Babinski, J. (1918). Anosognosie. *Rev. Neurol. (Paris)* 31:365–367.

Battersby, W. S., Bender, M. B., Pollack, M., and Kahn, R. L. (1956). Unilateral "spatial agnosia" (inattention) in patients with cerebral lesions. *Brain* 79:68–93.

Bisiach, E. (1988a). Language without thought. In L. Weiskrantz (ed.), *Thought Without Language.* New York: Oxford University Press, pp. 464–484.

Bisiach, E. (1988b). The (haunted) brain and consciousness. In A. J. Marcel and E. Bisiach (eds.), *Consciousness in Contemporary Science.* New York: Oxford University Press, pp. 101–120.

Bisiach, E., and Berti, A. (1987). Dyschiria: an attempt at its systemic explanation. In M. Jeannerod (ed.), *Neurophysiological and Neuropsychological Aspects of Spatial Neglect.* Amsterdam: Elsevier, pp. 183–201.

Bisiach, E., and Vallar, G. (1988). Hemineglect in humans. In F. Boller and J. Grafman (eds.), *Handbook of Neuropsychology,* Vol. 1. Amsterdam: Elsevier, pp. 195–222.

Bisiach, E., Berti, A., and Vallar, G. (1985). Analogical and logical disorders underlying unilateral neglect of space. In M. I. Posner and O. S. M. Marin (eds.), *Attention and Performance XI.* Hillsdale, N.J.: Lawrence Erlbaum Ass., pp. 239–249.

Bisiach, E., Luzzatti, C., and Perani, D. (1979). Unilateral neglect, representational schema and consciousness. *Brain* 102:609–618.

Bisiach, E., Vallar, G., Perani, D., Papagno, C., and Berti, A. (1986). Unawareness of disease following lesions of the right hemisphere: anosognosia for hemiplegia and anosognosia for hemianopia. *Neuropsychologia* 24:471–482.

Black, S. E., and Kertesz, A. (1984). A case of reduplicative paramnesia and neglect due to a right hemisphere lesion studied by nuclear magnetic resonance. Presented at the 7th European Conference of the International Neuropsychological Society. Aachen, 13–15 June 1984.

Cappa, S., Sterzi, R., Vallar, G., and Bisiach, E. (1987). Remission of hemineglect during vestibular stimulation. *Neuropsychologia* 25:775–782.

Critchley, M. (1953). *The Parietal Lobes.* London: Hafner Press.

Critchley, M. (1955). Personification of paralyzed limbs in hemiplegics. *Br. Med. J.* 2:284–286.

Critchley, M. (1974). Misoplegia or hatred of hemiplegia. *Mt. Sinai J. Med.* 41:82–87.

Cutting, J. (1978). Study of anosognosia. *J. Neurol. Neurosurg. Psychiatry* 41:548–565.

Dennett, D. C. (1986). *The Intentional Stance.* Cambridge, MA: MIT Press.

Finke, R. A. (1985). Theories relating mental imagery to perception. *Psychol. Bull.* 98:236–259.

Fodor, J. A. (1983). *The Modularity of Mind.* Cambridge, MA: MIT Press.

Friedland, R. P., and Weinstein, E. A. (1977). Hemi-inattention and hemisphere specialization: introduction and historical review. *Adv. Neurol.* 18:1–31.

Gainotti, G. (1972). Emotional behavior and hemispheric side of the lesion. *Cortex* 8:41–55.

Gazzaniga, M. S. (1988). Brain modularity: towards a philosophy of conscious experience. In A. J. Marcel and E. Bisiach (eds.), *Consciousness in Contemporary Science.* New York: Oxford University Press, pp. 218–238.

Gerstmann, J. (1942). Problems of imperception of disease and of impaired body territories with organic lesions. *Arch. Neurol. Psychiatry* 48:890–913.

Geschwind, N. (1965). Disconnexion syndromes in animals and man. *Brain* 88:237–294, 585–644.

Goldstein, K. (1939). *The Organism, A Holistic Approach to Biology Derived from Pathological Data in Man.* New York: American Book Company.

Gross, H., and Kaltenbäck, E. (1955). Die agnosie. *Wien. Z. Nervenheilk.* 11:374–418.

Healton, E. B., Navarro, C., Bressman, S., and Brust, J. C. M. (1982). Subcortical neglect. *Neurology* 32:776–778.

Hécaen, H. (1972). *Introduction à la Neuropsychologie.* Paris: Larousse.

Hécaen, H., Talairach, J., David, M., and Dell, M. B. (1949). Coagulations limitées du thalamus dans les algies du syndrome thalamique: résultats thérapeutiques et physiologiques. *Rev. Neurol. (Paris)* 81:917–931.

Jones, E. (1910). Die Pathologie der Dyschirie. *J. Psychol. Neurol.* 15:145–183.

Johnson-Laird, P. N. (1988). A computational analysis of consciousness. In A. J. Marcel and E. Bisiach (eds.), *Consciousness in Contemporary Science.* New York: Oxford University Press, pp. 357–368.

Kinsbourne, M. (1980). Brain-based limitations on mind. In R. W. Rieber (ed.), *Body and Mind.* New York: Academic Press, pp. 155–175.

Kinsbourne, M. (1987). Mechanisms of unilateral neglect. In M. Jeannerod (ed.), *Neu-*

rophysiological and Neuropsychological Aspects of Spatial Neglect. Amsterdam: Elsevier, pp. 69–86.

Kinsbourne, M. (1988). Integrated field theory of consciousness. In A. J. Marcel and E. Bisiach (eds.), *Consciousness in Contemporary Science.* New York: Oxford University Press, pp. 239–256.

Kinsbourne, M., and Warrington, E. K. (1962). A variety of reading disability associated with right hemisphere lesions. *J. Neurol. Neurosurg. Psychiatry* 25:339–344.

Kinsbourne, M., and Warrington, E. K. (1963). Jargon aphasia. *Neuropsychologia* 1:27–38.

Kosslyn, S. M. (1980). *Image and Mind.* Cambridge, MA: Harvard University Press.

Luria, A. R. (1966). *Higher Cortical Functions in Man.* Hants: Tavistock Publications.

Marcel, A. J., and Bisiach, E. (eds.) (1988). *Consciousness in Contemporary Science.* New York: Oxford University Press.

McGlynn, S. M., and Schacter, D. L. (1989). Unawareness of deficits in neuropsychological syndromes. *J. Clin. Exp. Neuropsychol.* 11:143–205.

Merzenich, M. M., and Kaas, J. H. (1980). Principles of organization of sensori-perceptual systems in mammals. *Prog. Psychobiol. Physiol. Psychol.* 9:1–41.

Oatley, K. (1988). On changing one's mind: a possible function of consciousness. In A. J. Marcel and E. Bisiach (eds.)., *Consciousness in Contermporary Science.* New York: Oxford University Press, pp. 369–389.

Pick, A. (1898). *Beiträge zur Pathologie und Pathologische Anatomie des Zentralnervensystems mit Bemerkungen zur normalen Anatomie desselben.* Berlin: Karger, pp. 168–185.

Pylyshyn, Z. W. (1984). *Computation and Cognition.* Cambridge, MA: MIT Press.

Sandifer, P. H. (1946). Anosognosia and disorders of body scheme. *Brain* 69:122–137.

Schilder, P. (1935). *The Image and Appearance of the Human Body.* London: Kegan, Paul, Trench, Trubner, and Co.

Shepard, R. N. (1975). Form, formation and transformation of internal representations. In R. L. Solso (ed.), *Information Processing and Cognition: The Loyola Symposium.* Hillsdale, NJ: Lawrence Erlbaum Associates, pp. 87–122.

Sprague, J. M., Chambers, W. W., and Stellar, E. (1961). Attentive, affective, and adaptive behavior in the cat. *Science* 133:165–173.

Stich, S. P. (1983). *From Folk Psychology to Cognitive Science. The Case Against Beliefs.* Cambridge, MA: MIT Press.

Umiltà, C. (1988). The control operations of consciousness. In A. J. Marcel and E. Bisiach (eds.), *Consciousness in Contemporary Science.* New York: Oxford University Press, pp. 334–356.

Vallar, G., and Perani, D. (1987). The anatomy of spatial neglect in humans. In M. Jeannerod (ed.), *Neurophysiological and Neuropsychological Aspects of Spatial Neglect.* Amsterdam: Elsevier, pp. 235–258.

Von Hagen, K. O., and Ives, E. R. (1937). Anosognosia (Babinski), imperception of hemiplegia. *Bull. Los Angeles Neurol. Soc.* 95–103.

Warrington, E. K. (1962). The completion of visual forms across hemianopic visual field defects. *J. Neurol. Neurosurg. Psychiatry* 25:208–217.

Watson, R. T., and Heilman, K. M. (1979). Thalamic neglect. *Neurology* 29:690–694.

Weinstein, E. A., and Kahn, R. L. (1955). *Denial of Illness. Symbolic and Physiological Aspects.* Springfield, IL: Charles C Thomas.

Weiskrantz, L. (1986). *Blindsight.* Oxford: Clarendon Press.

Zingerle, H. (1913). Ueber Stoerungen der Wahrnehmung des eigenen Koerpers bei organischen Gehirnerkrankungen. *Monatsschr. Psychiatr. Neurol.* 34:13–36.

Zubec, P. (1969). *Sensory Deprivation: 15 Years of Research.* New York: Meredith.

3

Anosognosia of Linguistic Deficits in Patients with Neurological Deficits

ALAN B. RUBENS
AND MERRILL F. GARRETT

The extreme character of many of the departures from coherent, well-formed speech in aphasia makes any apparent unawareness of the deviant performance impressive, as our normal subjective experience suggests a ready sensitivity to errors in our own speech and that of others. The phenomenon of anosognosia for aphasia presents a particularly striking failure of that sensitivity. In this chapter, we concentrate on the most discussed of such failures—jargon aphasia. We consider the extent to which these and related instances of anosognosia may be understood as a compromise of the normal monitoring functions for speech, or if some cases may require the postulation of a more fundamental alteration of consciousness or of language processing systems.

Observational and experimental evidence strongly attest to significant monitoring functions in the normal course of speaking. We constantly interrupt our own conversational efforts and reformulate or correct initial (sometimes barely initiated) trains of utterance. Several sorts of monitoring processes have been suggested (Levelt, 1989), including those internal to the production system itself and those that depend on the comprehension system to interpret either a prearticulatory or an acoustic code. There is good evidence for the existence of both of the latter monitoring systems (Baars, Motley, and McKay, 1975; Lackner and Tuller, 1979; Levelt, 1989).

Despite the robust evidence for monitoring, it is also clear that normal speakers and listeners are often "unaware" of their language errors. Sharply focused attention may be necessary to pick up certain phonological and syntactic deviations (Cutler, 1982). Even gross lexical substitutions that may bedazzle a listener can go unnoticed by the speaker who produces them—until, that is, their attention is drawn to the error. At that point, if the intervention is immediate, normal speakers are able to note the error; but a delay of even a few seconds with interpolated material makes recovery of the details of the error unlikely, though awareness of the occurrence of an error may persist.

These aspects of normal performance must affect our assessment of aphasic performance, and they provide perspectives for the discussion of anosognosia in aphasia. Two factors are immediately suggested as relevant: (1) attentional focus in production, and (2) perceptual reconstruction in comprehension. As speakers, we can selectively attend to various aspects of the constructive process. Depending on the demands of the communicative situation, one may, for example, attend to the sense of the message, to the lexical selections that are most apposite for the audience, or to precision of accent and articulation. Perceptual reconstruction, by contrast, is the result of mechanisms that are a normal feature of language comprehension—what one might term "perceptual correction mechanisms." One of the things that listeners do automatically is penetrate the haze of false starts, repetitions, infelicities, and occasional ungrammaticality that are the surface results of a speaker's pursuit of an underlying, well-formed target of expression. As listeners, we normally ignore or correct those deviances in order to reconstruct the intended message (Forster, 1979). To the extent that production monitoring relies on comprehension processes, such mechanisms of correction clearly contribute to the potential for failure to detect language error at the level of conscious report.

The general point to bear in mind is that insensitivity to language error is not an exotic behavior. Much depends on the circumstances and priorities of the speaker. The real-time flow of spoken language can readily conceal significant deviance from a speaker who, it must be borne in mind, often *knows* precisely what he or she is intending to say. Evaluating these contingencies in the analyses of reports of anosognosia is not always straightforward.

ANOSOGNOSIA IN APHASIA

Monitoring Behavior in Aphasics

Anosognosic behavior is presented when a speaker does not attempt to correct an error and, confronted with that error, denies its occurrence. Such apparent unawareness of language error is common with certain types of aphasia, most notably jargon aphasia. Before discussing jargon aphasia, however, we consider some general findings concerning self-monitoring by aphasic patients. Such evidence indicates that most types of aphasic speakers retain the impulse, if not the effective capacity, to monitor and correct their language output. Attempts at self-correction are commonly observed clinically (e.g., Wepman, 1958) with varying degrees of success related to the severity and type of aphasia. Wepman reported that patients whose ability to recognize or correct their errors was impaired were aware of this difficulty; their complaint of this disability thus indicates that a global awareness of error can accompany impaired responses to specific instances of language deviance.

A systematic study by Marshall and Tompkins (1982) investigated the use of six explicitly defined verbal self-correction patterns in the speech of fluent and nonfluent aphasic patients, cross-classified by high and low verbal expressive ability, and by six types of aphasia, including Broca's, anomic, Wernicke's, and transcortical aphasia. Most nonfluent and fluent patients, regardless of verbal expression level, severity level, or type of aphasia, generated a substantial amount of self-correction: All groups attempted self-correction on at least one-half of their erroneous responses. Note that it was true for grouping by classic aphasia type as well; the groups did not differ significantly in the proportion of self-correction efforts. However, when measured by their success at self-correction, the high level verbal expression patients (of both high and low fluency) were significantly superior to those with lower level performances in verbal expression. Otherwise, there was no essential difference between the fluent and the nonfluent groups in terms of success of self-correction. Thus the less impaired subjects (both Broca's and anomic aphasics) had the highest proportion of self-correction success, whereas the Wernicke's and severe Broca's aphasics had less success. It therefore appears that error detection occurs with equal frequency in Broca's and Wernicke's aphasia despite the general impression that Wernicke's aphasics are less concerned with monitoring their speech.

A more detailed contrast of monitoring style appears in a report by Schlenck, Huber, and Willmes (1987). These authors identified two types of speech behavior, repairs, and anticipatory adjustments ("prepairs" in their terminology). Repairs are focused on the correction of errors in a just-preceding utterance; by contrast, attempts at coping with anticipated difficulty with an upcoming utterance include pauses, repetition of the immediately preceding utterance, phonemic approximations, and circumlocutions. The contrast between these types was aimed at determining whether monitoring in aphasic patients was based on a prearticulatory stage or on a post-utterance, comprehension-based system on the assumption that repairs are characteristic of the comprehension-based monitor and that "prepairs" reflect anticipatory monitoring at a prearticulatory stage. When Schlenck and his colleagues counted the two types of monitoring patterns in a group of aphasic patients, they found that anticipatory adjustments were far more common than repairs in all their patients; in particular, Broca's and Wernicke's aphasics did not differ in terms of the frequency of prepairs. Although this finding suggests a prearticulatory stage of monitoring, it does not tell us what that stage is (e.g., conceptual or linguistic) or how it relates to comprehension because there is no bar to the routing of a prearticulatory representation to the comprehension system for monitoring. However, they did find that patients with low auditory comprehension scores were less likely to make prepairs than those with high auditory comprehension scores, which indicates that comprehension ability may be related to successful anticipation of production difficulties. The relatively low frequency of repairs in both Broca's and Wernicke's aphasics may also point to poor functioning of comprehension-based monitoring. These findings increase the plausibility of accounts of anosognosic behavior that arise from interference with monitoring that relies on comprehension abilities.

It would be useful to know the relation that would hold between monitoring and anosognosic behavior in self-monitoring groups of this kind. It is conceivable that errors detected by a patient would be acknowledged, though many others of similar character that are not detected by the patient would be denied. The evidence for existence of monitoring activity is not prima facie evidence against anosognosic behavior, though, by contrast, evidence that monitoring is largely absent may suggest anosognosic behavior. The latter condition is precisely the clinical impression given by jargon aphasics in particular, who appear indifferent to errors in their speech.

Anosognosia in Jargon Aphasics

The literature on anosognosia focuses largely on the general lack of awareness of their language deficit in patients with jargon aphasia, a disturbance viewed by Alajouanine (1964) as an "anosognosic disintegration of the semantic values of language" and called by Critchley (1964) "anosognosic aphasia." Alajouanine (1956) emphasized that anosognosia and severe comprehension deficits routinely accompany jargon aphasia.

Jargon aphasia is usually associated with Wernicke's aphasia but may be found in transcortical sensory aphasia and in some of the repeated stereotyped utterances associated with global aphasia. It is characterized by copious amounts of meaningless utterances, phonemic or semantic paraphasia, or in some instances what may be a combination of the two—neologistic paraphasia. Typically, patients with jargon aphasia do not appear to monitor their own utterances: There are few of the hesitations, pauses, and self-corrections found in most of the other aphasic syndromes. These patients' behavior generally suggests that they are unaware that listeners do not understand them and that they themselves do not comprehend what is said to them.

What does this general impression of anosognosic behavior mean? Several explanations are available. The failure to respond to or correct production error may be a consequence of a breakdown in normal monitoring functions that stems from the comprehension limitations associated with the aphasia, it may be a form of attentional limitation that prevents focusing on relevant levels of speech representation, or it may be a consequence of both. Alternatively, one might seek to attribute these patients' anosognosic behavior to a more fundamental compromise of conceptual capability, i.e., a problem not specific to the language limitations at all. Finally, it has been suggested that the jargon emerges as a consequence of anosognosia—that it represents an adaptive response on the part of the jargon aphasics. We consider these possibilities in light of various forms of evidence that have been offered.

According to Alajouanine and to Weinstein and his group, anosognosia is central to the deficit of jargon aphasia. Weinstein, Cole, Mitchell, and Lyerly (1964) stated that jargon occurs when aphasia and anosognosia coexist. They proposed that jargon aphasia is adaptive in nature and is one of a series of strategies the aphasic patient uses to deal with the stress of his deficit. They argued that jargon aphasia is the result of an attempt to communicate metaphorically, and as a consequence the speech consists of idiosyncratic, incomprehensible jargon. In their study of 28 patients with right-sided, sensorimotor deficits, they found a dissociation between anosognosia and aphasia: Most of their patients with severe anosognosia had little if any aphasia, and most of those who exhibited aphasia did so without anosognosia. None of four patients with only mild anosognosia showed jargon. However, four of the patients did have jargon with verbal stereotypes, and these patients showed severe anosognosia for their aphasia. Importantly, in three of these patients, the jargon occurred mostly when they responded to questions relating to their disability. The picture Weinstein et al. invited is one of a psychodynamic relation between the anosognosia and language limitations that gives rise to jargon.

Weinstein and Lyerly (1976) reported that the premorbid personalities of jargon aphasic patients were characterized by compulsiveness, excessive drive, high standards, excessive work orientation, and dread and denial of illness. These patients previously had tended to ignore and rationalize illness and to be frightened of disability in general. On these and related grounds, Weinstein et al. (1964 and 1966) characterized jargon aphasia as a disturbance not only of language but of consciousness and social interaction.

Brown (1981) has argued against Weinstein's adaptive interpretation of anosognosia and jargon aphasia, noting that lack of awareness in many patients is often not general but specific to aphasia, and even to language error-type. Lack of awareness sometimes involves the language deficit but not the accompanying motor or neurological deficit. Brown described a patient who had fluent aphasia due to a lesion of the left temporal lobe and who, when fatigued during testing, progressed through several stages of affective tone and types of abnormal language behavior. "He begins a conversation as an anomic with frustration, self-correction and word-search. Over a few minutes this passes to a stage where neologisms fill the anomic gaps and then to fluent neologistic jargon, with euphoria, logorrhea, and hyperfluency and lack of error awareness." Brown contended that this rapid evolution could not be explained psychodynamically. Several difficulties with motivational accounts of anosognosia were summarized by McGlynn and Schacter (1989), the most telling of which is the selective nature of anosognosia—present for certain aspects of a patient's symptoms, absent for others. This feature is of considerable interest, and we return to it later.

Another factor in Weinstein and colleagues' position on anosognosia is the claim that jargon ensues as a result of more extensive neurological damage than that to the areas responsible for language. Weinstein, Lyerly, Cole, and Ozer (1966) compared jargon aphasics to 24 aphasics without jargon or verbal stereotypy. All of the jargon aphasics had bilateral damage, whereas the other aphasics had mostly unilateral brain lesions. The jargon aphasics tended to deny their other deficits, such as hemiparesis or hemianopia. They appeared cheerful and did not become upset when speaking paraphasically. The authors concluded that jargon aphasia requires that a left hemisphere lesion be accompanied by further neurological damage, which adds the anosognosic component.

Along the same lines, Brown (1981) reported four patients with severe semantic jargon, all with bilateral lesions and, interestingly, all polyglots. In these patients semantic jargon was accompanied by confusion, impaired verbal memory, and moderate comprehension impairment. These observations show a relatively high incidence of bihemispheric lesions in aphasia with anosognosia and lend support to the contention that additional brain pathology is a factor in anosognosia. Weinstein and colleagues argued that such damage, when added to the specific left posterior temporal lesion, produces a further disturbance of consciousness that is required for the production of jargon aphasia and anosognosia. A compatible observation is that most patients with Wernicke's aphasia and single left hemisphere lesions, except during the acute period, do not have conspicuous anosognosia.

The findings of Gainotti (1972) are also relevant. He reported anosognosia in only 5 of 16 Wernicke's aphasics with left hemisphere damage. At the same time, however, we note that these five cases amount to 30 percent of Gainotti's left-hemisphere patients, and they were anosognosic, indicating that although bilateral involvement may be conducive to anosognosia it is not necessary.

Kertesz' views (1979) bear on the latter point. After a thorough review of the literature and his own patient material, Kertesz reached the following conclusions about the anatomical location of lesions responsible for jargon aphasia: Lesions of severe or persisting neologistic jargon aphasia involve the posterior end of the first temporal gyrus and the supramarginal region. Less severely affected patients with semantic jargon have lesions located more posteriorly in the temporo-parieto-occipital junction, an area commonly damaged in transcortical sensory aphasia. Semantic jargon is commonly seen with dementia, particularly Alzheimer's disease. In these patients, semantic jargon appears in the context of transcortical sensory aphasia with relatively intact repetition but poor comprehension. It is well known that Alzheimer's disease preferentially involves the parieto-temporo-occipital association area in its early stages.

Exceptions to the General View About Awareness

There is considerable variability in the degree of awareness of aphasia in published cases of jargon aphasia. This variability includes not only the level of severity of anosognosia but also selective lack of awareness of some language deficits, though not of other existing language or neurological deficits. Such awareness argues against an essential connection between anosognosia and jargon symptoms.

There have been a number of reports of patients with a severe auditory comprehension deficit and blatant jargon aphasia who seem acutely aware that they are aphasic. Lecours et al. (1980) described a 66-year-old woman whose neurological examination indicated an infarct of the left temporal lobe. She had severely impaired auditory comprehension, more mildly impaired reading comprehension, and a severe naming and repetition deficit; she was classified as having Wernicke's aphasia. She complained paraphasically and at great length about her aphasia, even to the point of noticing that her reading comprehension was superior to her auditory comprehension. Thus she manifested a full-blown jargon aphasia with severely impaired auditory comprehension, yet showed no anosognosia.

A 72-year-old male patient of ours clinically displayed a similar clinical picture. His speech consisted of logorrheic, paraphasic jargon in which he constantly bemoaned the fact that his speech was "not right" and tried to describe his speech problems. Because of the severe phonemic and semantic paraphasia, it took several replays of taped interviews to decipher his meaning: the predilection phrases "I can't speak it" and "I can't say it" were enmeshed in his unceasing outpouring of uncorrected jargon. These two cases demonstrate that paraphasic logorrheic speech can flow on at great length even though the patient has a global awareness that there is a linguistic deficit.

The introspections of patients who have recovered from a period of aphasia in which they manifested uncorrected, meaningless speech and poor comprehension can also provide insight into the awareness of such patients for their deficit. Lecours and Joanette (1980) described a patient with epileptic episodes of aphasia during which there was a phase of logorrheic jargon with poor comprehension. Between episodes the patient said that when he was aphasic he knew that his speech was not normal but that he could not identify specific errors. He was unaware, for example, that he sometimes inserted an English cliché into his French jargon. In other words, he was globally aware of his aphasia at a time when he was unable to detect and identify specific aphasic errors.

The preceding examples of awareness in jargon cases fit the view of Cohn and Neuman (1958), who concluded that nearly all patients with jargon aphasia have some degree of awareness of their speech disorder. They also concur with the report of Wepman (1958), who stressed that although most patients with aphasia are impaired to some extent in their ability to monitor and correct their speech errors the overwhelming majority have some awareness of their deficit.

Such observations indicate that simple monitoring failure does not provide a general account of anosognosia in jargon cases, though it is unclear what aspects of the monitoring functions may be preserved. Some additional evidence from the work by Peuser and Temp (1981) is relevant. They tested self-monitoring by examining the effect of delayed auditory feedback on speech flow in aphasics. Their patient with neologistic jargon showed no interruption or change in speech flow whatsoever. Their patient with semantic jargon, however, demonstrated relatively intact external feedback by interrupting his speech flow, speaking more slowly, and increasing the loudness of his utterances. Alajouanine, Lhermitte, Ledoux, Renaud, and Vignolo (1964) had previously reported that jargon aphasics showed minimal changes in their speech patterns in the delayed auditory feedback setting. Boller, Vrtunski, Kim, and Mack (1978) also reported that delayed auditory feedback affected nonfluent aphasics more than fluent aphasics. According to Peuser and Temp, faulty feedback and not necessarily a complete lack of awareness of the speech disorder, is the essential factor in jargon aphasia. These observations support the claim that the external feedback system is faulty in jargon aphasia and, furthermore, that it may implicate a contrast between semantic functions and other language functions.

The general view that jargon patients believe they are communicating well and hence do not show the halts, hesitations, and corrections of normal speech also needs more specific treatment. For example, we note Butterworth's finding (1979) concerning hesitations in jargon aphasia. He measured hesitation pauses in the speech of a jargon aphasic and found a greatly increased likelihood of hesitation just prior to the production of neologisms (22% for normal nouns versus 54% for neologistic words in noun environments). This finding indicates that at some level of monitoring lexical retrieval failures are registered. Butterworth thus argued that jargon is inserted by a component of the morphophonological system as a means of maintaining continuous speech output, but that such monitoring need not be a consciously mediated process.

Several interesting observations of jargon aphasics' response to their own recorded speech or variants of it bear on this issue. It has been reported that the anosognosic aphasic patient, although apparently unaware of his own speech errors, is able to reject jargon and foreign languages produced by others. Kinsbourne and Warrington (1963) described a patient with jargon aphasia and anosognosia due to a left hemisphere stroke and accompanied by right hemiplegia, blindness of the left eye, and a right hemianopia. He appeared unaware of his hemianopia and denied his speech deficit. However, he was aware of his hemiplegia and blindness in the left eye. He was satisfied with his own speech output when hearing it played back on a tape recorder, but he rejected the identical utterance when it was recorded by another speaker. A second patient with jargon aphasia was similarly pleased with his own tape-recorded speech. Both patients were satisfied with their own written sentences but rejected them as meaningless when transcribed by one of the examiners. Alajouanine had previously commented on the fact that patients, when hearing their own errors mimicked by the physician, rejected them as meaningless. These patients also are aware of when they are being spoken to in a foreign language (Weinstein et al., 1964 and 1966). As a group, patients with severe impairment of auditory comprehension, including those without jargon aphasia, are able to distinguish between their native language and a foreign language or phonemic jargon, but they have difficulty distinguishing normal language from semantic jargon (Boller and Green, 1972; Green and Boller, 1974).

Selective Awareness of Symptoms

Modality of language exercise can determine awareness of aphasic disturbance. For example, one of two patients reported by Peuser and Temp (1981) who showed such evidence for awareness was a woman with neologistic jargon. She spoke fluently and without hesitation, rarely correcting her errors, but was reluctant to write and behaved as though aware of her writing disturbance. Both their patients, in fact, appeared to recognize their impairment in writing more than that in their spoken language.

The pattern of recovery in jargon cases also suggests a selective awareness of error. It is generally agreed that the most common pattern of recovery from jargon aphasia progresses through an initial severe stage where speech is neologistic, to semantic jargon, where most words, although inappropriate, are recognizable, and finally to a stage of anomic circumlocutory speech deficient in information-bearing words (Kertesz and Benson, 1970). According to Buckingham and Kertesz (1974), one of the common final outcomes of jargon aphasia is idiomatic speech that includes clichés, puns, and malapropisms. They, along with Weinstein and Puig-Antich (1974), believed that these speech forms represent analogues of jargon that are most often elicited in answers to the same class of questions that generated jargon in the more acute stage of the aphasia. (Their emergence may reflect awareness of the underlying language problem and constitute a partial attempt at control or correction.) Most importantly, throughout this period of evolution, neologistic errors are more often corrected, whereas uncorrected semantic errors persist.

We previously noted other evidence for a dissociation of sensitivity to semantic and phonological processes: Jargon aphasics' responses to deviance in their own and others' tape-recorded speech showed that semantic jargon is more likely to be accepted than neologistic jargon. A striking example of the same sort of distinction comes from Marshall, Rappoport, and Garcia-Bunel (1985). They reported the unusual case of a 62-year-old woman with Wernicke's aphasia and auditory sound agnosia due to bilateral temporal lobe strokes, who nonetheless attempted to correct her phonemic paraphasias but appeared unaware of most of her semantic paraphasias. Her auditory comprehension was severely impaired, and speech was fluent, consisting mostly of neologistic jargon. Attempts at self-corrections often led to even more aberrant phonemic combinations. Writing was only minimally affected and demonstrated an excellent naming ability. Reading comprehension was also far superior to auditory comprehension. The relative sparing of writing, written naming, and reading comprehension suggested a mild aphasia in the presence of severe auditory agnosia. Intact self-monitoring was demonstrated by the fact that she refused to continue with delayed auditory feedback testing because it made her uncomfortable. This case is informative not only for the evidence it provides against motivational accounts of jargon but also for the indication that anosognosia for spoken language can be present in patients whose basic language comprehension capacities are intact. This point suggests that the locus of the anosognosia lies in the process of associating the spoken output with the comprehension system.

The dissociation of awareness for semantic and phonological error in the case of Marshall et al. and the similar dissociation in the usual recovery sequence for jargon imply that semantic processes and form-based language processes interact with awareness mechanisms in different ways, with semantic errors remaining opaque to consciousness at a stage when form errors are responded to. This pattern may be linked to several independent observations. It fits experimentally supported dissociations of semantic and form-based processes in normal lexical and sentence processing (Forster, 1979; Garrett, 1982) and with event-related potential (ERP) studies of lexical processes. The latter show ERP responses specific to semantic expectancy, i.e., violations of semantic constraint produce modulation of late ERP components (N400), though violations of form expectation do not (e.g., Kutas and Hillyard, 1980).

Studies of aphasics' abilities to make accurate grammaticality judgments also offer a useful comparison. Accounts of the comprehension deficit in agrammatism (Schwartz, Linebarger, Saffran, and Pate, 1987) illustrate the line of possibility. Agrammatics who show a significant comprehension limitation in semantic interpretation tasks are able to make correct well formedness judgments for the very same sentences they systematically misinterpret. The account offered by Schwartz et al. stressed the presence of intact syntactic and phonological representations and placed the loss in the processes that use such representations to constrain semantic interpretation. Correspondingly, if one assumes that comprehension failure in cases such as that of Marshall et al. arises at the mapping from phonologically and syntactically specified form representations to interpreted semantic representations, the anosognosic pattern would follow. Mismatches at the semantic level would suffer the auditory comprehension deficit and be imperfectly responded to if at all, but the representation of phonological word and phrasal form might nonetheless be intact and capable of supporting a response in patients whose general monitoring abilities seem to be preserved, as was the case with the patient of Marshall et al.

DISCUSSION

It is clear that as they are speaking most patients with jargon aphasia are unaware of their errors and of the fact that others fail to understand them. This fact may reflect a general lack of awareness of aphasia or some more specific deficit of monitoring speech, because of either the constraints of real-time performance (e.g., a processing capacity or attentional limitation) or some particular loss for given types of language structure (semantic, syntactic, phonological). Some patients seem totally unaware of a language disturbance of any kind, but most show varying degrees of awareness that some problem relating to their communicative skills exists. Even in the case of severe neglect of left hemiparesis, patients often indicate some level of awareness of the deficit depending on how they are questioned. They often admit that their left side is paralyzed when it is demonstrated by the examiner but a moment later deny the deficit. Their deficit would nonetheless be classified as anosognosia. Similarly, less than total lack of awareness of aphasia does not make the diagnosis of anosognosia untenable. The timing and nature of the questioning are clearly important factors for establishing the limits of the anosognosia. In this respect, the investigation of anosognosia does not differ from the similar investigation of awareness in normal listeners. [See, for example, Norman's (1969) discussion of immediate and delayed dichotic listening reports.]

It is clear that most jargon aphasics have difficulty speaking and monitoring their own speech simultaneously. However, lack of awareness of speech deficit seems to go beyond the immediate monitoring of their own speech. The examples of anosognosic aphasic patients accepting their own tape-recorded speech as correct but rejecting the same productions when spoken by others is puzzling. It is possible that they are simply acknowledging the familiarity of their own voice and rejecting the unfamiliar voice of others, regardless of content. More studies of such phenomena are needed to confirm this effect. It is also clear that systematic studies of the aphasic population at large and their response to their own recorded speech errors would be of great value for understanding awareness in aphasia. The possibility that listening capacity in general and the ability for flexible attentional focus in particular decline during the act of speaking seems strong. This area might be explored with the use of auditory evoked potentials, comparing auditory cortical evoked changes before and during the speech act in anosognosic aphasic patients and normal controls.

A role of the right hemisphere in jargon aphasics' awareness of their speaking errors is suggested by the relatively high proportion of jargon aphasics who manifest bilateral lesions. It is not possible, however, to determine based on current evidence what that role might be, though it is tempting to suppose that it may be clarified when we have a better understanding of the differences among such patients with respect to the detailed character of their anosognosic behavior. More information on the monitoring capabilities of these patients could contribute to our understanding. Testing these patients using delayed auditory feedback while carefully controlling the parameters of feedback delay, pitch alteration, and loudness alteration, for example, could establish the intactness of basic attentional and auditory monitoring mechanisms that would be required for such patients to be responsive to higher-order language structures. Knowing their response to semantic, phonological, and syntactic deviance types could also be helpful.

The just-mentioned issues are related to the final general point we wish to emphasize. The evidence for selective loss of awareness for various aphasia symptoms is of several sorts: the typical recovery sequence for jargon aphasics, their differential sensitivity to deviance when monitoring tape-recorded speech or transcripts of jargon, and case studies showing modality-specific awareness as well as differential awareness of specific types of language information. This point indicates the need to develop an account of monitoring processes that treat different classes of language structure as having distinct access to conscious report. In particular, the jargon aphasics' selective loss of awareness for their deficit shows that semantic jargon is less likely to be attended/recovered than neologistic jargon. This fact, coupled with their impaired auditory comprehension performance, suggests a breakdown in the specific mechanisms that relate lexical and sentence form to semantic interpretation. The modular functions of language processing may thus have a more direct connection to awareness phenomena than might initially be supposed. Schacter (1989) reviewed several types of evidence concerning awareness phenomena and suggested the outline of a system responsible for awareness that consists of two components: a posterior component (CAS, or conscious awareness system), which receives multiple inputs from modular perceptual and memory systems, and a frontal executive component. CAS computes a single output that it relays to the frontal executive system. Depending on the nature of the injury—whether to CAS, to the modules that feed it, to the link between it and the executive system, or to the executive system itself—different patterns of global or specific awareness of deficit would ensue. Something of this order of complexity appears to be required for a description of the patterns of anosognosia in aphasia.

REFERENCES

Alajouanine, Th. (1956). Verbal realization in aphasia. *Brain* 79:1–28.

Alajouanine, Th., Lhermitte, F., Ledoux, M., Renaud, D., and Vegnolo, L. A. (1964). Les composantes phonemiques et semantiques de la jargonaphasie. *Rev. Neurol. (Paris)* 110:1–20.

Baars, B., Motley, M., and McKay, D. G. (1975). Output editing for lexical status from artificially elicited slips of the tongue. *J. Verbal Learn. Verbal Behav.* 14:382–391.

Boller, F., and Green, E. (1972). Comprehension in severe aphasia. *Cortex* 9:382–394.

Boller, F., Vrtunski, P. B., Kim, Y., and Mack, J. L. (1978). Delayed auditory feedback and aphasia. *Cortex* 14:212–226.

Brown, J. (1981). Introduction. In Brown, J. (ed.), *Jargon Aphasia.* Orlando: Academic Press.

Buckingham, H. W., and Kertesz, A. (1974). A linguistic analysis of fluent aphasia. *Brain Lang.* 1:43–61.

Butterworth, B. (1979). Hesitation and the production of neologisms in jargon aphasia. *Brain Lang.* 8:131–161.

Cohn, R., and Neuman, M. A. (1958). Jargon aphasia. *J. Nerv. Ment. Disord.* 127:381–399.

Critchley, M. (1964). The neurology of psychotic speech. *Br. J. Psychiatry* 110:353–364.

Cutler, A. (1982). The reliability of speech error data. In Cutler, A. (ed.), *Slips of the Tongue.* The Hague: Mouton.

Forster, K. I. (1979). Levels of processing and the structure of the language processor. In W. Cooper and E. Walker (eds.), *Sentence Processing.* Hillsdale, N.J.: Lawrence Erlbaum Associates.

Gainotti, G. (1972). Emotional behavior and hemispheric side of lesion. *Cortex* 8:41–55.

Garrett, M. F. (1982). Production of speech: observations from normal and pathological language use. In A. Ellis (ed.), *Normality and Pathology in Cognitive Functions.* London: Academic Press.

Green, E., and Boller, F. (1974). Features of auditory comprehension in severely impaired aphasics. *Cortex* 10:133–141.

Kinsbourne, M., and Warrington, E. K. (1963). Jargon aphasia. *Neuropsychologia* 1:27–37.

Kertesz, A. (1979). *Aphasia and Associated Disorders,* New York: Grune & Stratton.

Kertesz, A., and Benson, D. F. (1970). Neologistic jargon: a clinico-pathological study. *Cortex* 6:362–386.

Kutas, M., and Hillyard, S. (1980). Reading senseless sentences: Potentials reflect semantic incongruity. *Science* 207:203–205.

Lackner, J., and Tuller, B. (1979). The role of efference monitoring in the detection of self-produced speech errors. In W. Cooper and W. Walker (eds.), *Sentence Processing.* Hillsdale, N.J.: Lawrence Erlbaum Associates.

Levelt, W. J. M. (1989). *Speaking.* Cambridge, MA.: MIT Press.

Lecours, A., and Joanette, Y. (1980). Linguistic and other psychological aspects of paroxysmal aphasia. *Brain and Language* 10:1–23.

Lecours, A., Travis, L., Nespoulous, J. (1980). Neologismes et anosognosie. *Grammatic* 7:101–114.

Marshall, R. C., and Tompkins, C. A. (1982). Verbal self-correction behaviours of fluent and nonfluent aphasic subjects. *Brain Lang.* 15:292–306.

Marshall, R. C., Rappoport, B. Z., and Garcia Bunel, L. (1985). Self monitoring behavior in a case of severe auditory agnosia and aphasia. *Brain Lang.* 24:297–313.

McGlynn, S., and Schacter, D. (1989). Unawareness of deficits in neuropsychological syndromes. *J. Clin. Exp. Neuropsychol.* 11:143–205.

Norman, D. A. (1969). Memory while shadowing. *Q. J. Exp. Psychol.* 21:85–93.

Peuser, B., and Temp, K. (1981). The evolution of jargon aphasia. In Brown, J. (ed.), *Jargon Aphasia.* Orlando: Academic Press, pp. 259–293.

Schacter, D. (1989) On the relation between memory and consciousness In Roediger, H., and Craik, F. (eds.), *Varieties of Memory and Consciousness.* Hillsdale, N.J.: Lawrence Erlbaum Associates. pp. 355–389.

Schlenck, K. J., Huber, W., Willmes, K. (1987). Prepairs and Repairs: Different monitoring functions in aphasic language production. *Brain and Language* 30:224–226.

Schwartz, M., Linebarger, M., Saffran, E., and Pate, D. (1987). Syntactic transparency and sentence interpretation in aphasia. *Lang. Cogn. Processes* 2:85–113.

Weinstein, E. A., and Cole, M. Concepts of anosognosia. In Halpern, L. (ed.), *Problems of Dynamic Neurology: Functions of the Human Nervous System.* Jerusalem: Jerusalem Post Press.

Weinstein, E. A., and Lyerly, O. G. (1976). Personality factors in jargon aphasia. *Cortex* 12:122–133.

Weinstein, E. A., Cole, M., Mitchell, M. S., and Lyerly, O. G. (1964). Anosognosia and aphasia. *Arch. Neurol.* 10:376–386.

Weinstein, E. A., and Puig-Antich, J. (1974). Jargon and its analogues. *Cortex* 10:75–83.

Weinstein, E. A., Lyerly, O. G., Cole, M., and Ozer, M. S. (1966). Meaning in jargon aphasia. *Cortex* 2:165–187.

Wepman, J. M. (1958). The relationship between self-correction and recovery from aphasia. *Journal of Speech & Hearing Disorders* 23:302–305.

4
Anosognosia: Possible Neuropsychological Mechanisms

KENNETH M. HEILMAN

Anosognosia is the denial of illness that may be seen in brain-injured patients. In general, denial of illness takes two forms. There may be verbal, explicit denial of illness, or there may be a lack of genuine concern about the deficit. The verbal explicit denial is termed *anosognosia,* and indifference has been termed *anoso-diaphoria* (Critchley, 1953).

Anosognosia was first described by Von Monakow (1885) and Anton (1896). However, it was Babinski (1914) who first coined this term. Whereas subsequently anosognosia has been noted by many other authors, these important signs have not been the prime target of intensive investigation as has been the case with aphasia, alexia, and amnesia. Despite the lack of interest, these behavioral aberrations are not trivial. Not only may anosognosia impair a patient's desire to seek medical aid, it may also impair his desire to seek rehabilitation or to benefit from rehabilitation programs. Perhaps equally important, neuropsychological studies of anosognosia may help us understand not only why patients deny their illness but also myriad other behavioral anomalies such as hypochondriasis, where a physically healthy person is convinced that he is ill. Hypochondriasis may be the mirror of anosognosia.

This article is not an extensive review of anosognosia, rather it is a discussion focusing on the neuropsychological mechanism that may be responsible for the various forms of anosognosia. The reader must be forewarned, however, that there are many unanswered questions and that much of what is discussed is speculative. The basic postulate that I will pursue is that anosognosia is a failure of monitoring and may be related to (1) an impaired monitor, (2) the absence of feedback, (3) false feedback, and (4) the improper setting of the monitor.

Anosognosia is seen with many behavioral syndromes. I discuss the following three: Wernicke's aphasia, Anton's syndrome, and left hemiplegia (denial of hemiplegia). These three syndromes are discussed because they allow examination of the four basic mechanisms that may underly anosognosia.

WERNICKE'S APHASIA

Wernicke's aphasia is a well known language disorder where patients have fluent speech with neologisms and phonemic and semantic paraphasic errors (jargon aphasia). Comprehension is severely impaired, as is naming and repetition. Patients with Wernicke's aphasia frequently also have difficulty reading and writing. Because patients with Wernicke's aphasia cannot always adequately express themselves they often do not demonstrate a verbal explicit denial of illness; however, there are two observations suggesting that many of these patients have an anosognosia. Unlike the conduction aphasic who makes phonemic errors and attempts to correct his errors, patients with Wernicke's aphasia make no attempt at correction. Second, when the patient speaks in incomprehensible jargon, he often shows anger or disappointment with the person to whom he is speaking because that person does not understand him. (Alajouanine, 1956)

Wernicke's aphasia is most often seen with lesions that destroy the posterior portion of the superior temporal gyrus of the left temporal lobe (Benson, 1985). Commonly, the left inferior parietal lobe, including the supramarginal and the angular gyri, are also injured.

The anosognosia associated with Wernicke's aphasia may be related to defective monitoring (Fig. 4–1). Wernicke proposed that the posterior portion of the superior temporal gyrus contained auditory word representations (or images of word sounds). If the neural representations of word sounds are destroyed, not only can the Wernicke's aphasic not correctly express himself, he also cannot monitor his own errors.

To be able to monitor one's errors, one needs both an accurate neural representation and feedback access to that representation. One then can match behavioral output to the intact representation. Because Wernicke's aphasics have lost their representations of word sounds they do not correct their errors.

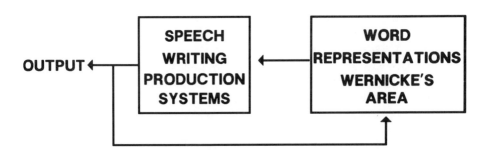

Figure 4–1. Feedback system used to monitor speech.   In Wernicke's aphasia the system is impaired because of destruction of word representations.

They do not understand why others cannot understand them because they are unable to match this feedback to an intact representation. Marshal and Tompkins (1982) studied the relations between self corrections and comprehension, and found that as comprehension improved, self corrections increased, providing support for the postulate that the anosognosia associated with Wernicke's aphasia is related to a defective monitor.

ANTON'S SYNDROME

Patients with Anton's syndrome (1896) deny cortical blindness. That is, although the patient's pupils respond to light, the patient is unable to demonstrate functional sight (e.g., the patient cannot count fingers or discriminate objects, shapes, or colors). Some patients with Anton's syndrome cannot even correctly tell if the room lights are on or off. Despite being profoundly cortically blind, patients typically deny having any visual difficulty. They confabulate responses such that they guess how many fingers the examiner is holding up or whether the lights are on or off. When confronted with their errors, they often make excused such as "The lights are too dim" or "I don't have my glasses."

Patients with Anton's syndrome often have visual hallucinations (that can be either simple or complex). They may have a loss of memory and a confusional state (Hécean and Albert, 1978). Frequently, after weeks to months the anosognosia abates. Anton's syndrome is usually associated with bilateral cerebral infarcts in the distribution of the posterior cerebral arteries. These infarcts usually involve both the primary visual areas of the calcarine cortex (Brodmann's area 17) and visual association areas such as Brodmann's areas 18 and 19. Not infrequently the parietal and temporal lobes are injured as well.

There have been many attempts to explain why patients with Anton's syndrome deny their blindness. The memory loss associated with Anton's syndrome may be related to damage outside the occipital lobes. The posterior cerebral arteries serve not only the occipital lobe but also the medial temporal lobe, and memory loss may be related to injury of the medial temporal lobes (Caplan and Hedley-White, 1974). The basilar system also serves the medial thalamus, and memory loss has been described with infarctions of the thalamus (Speedie and Heilman, 1982). Similarly, confusional states have been associated with lesions in the region of the fusiform and lingual gyri, especially on the left side, which are also served by the posterior cerebral arteries (Devinsky, Bear, and Volpe, 1988). Although Hécean and Albert suggested that confusion and memory loss may play a role in the anosognosia associated with Anton's syndrome, one sees patients who have left posterior cerebral artery infarctions who are amnestic and alexic but who do not have anosognosia. One also sees Anton's syndrome even in the absence of a confusional state. We therefore cannot conclude that the denial of illness seen with Anton's syndrome is related to either memory loss or confusion.

The second explanation is similar to that proposed to explain the anosognosia associated with Wernicke's aphasia, i.e., that the monitor has been destroyed. However, unlike Wernicke's aphasia, it is not clear what brain areas monitor visual input. Perhaps it is a part of the visual association cortex that is often damaged in this syndrome. Alternatively, as suggested by Anton, the damaged visual areas are disconnected from other areas of the brain, including speech-language areas. It has been well established that the speech areas in the absence of input often confabulate a response. For example, when Gazzaniga (1970) flashed sexual pictures to the left visual field, which projects to the right hemisphere of a patient with a callosal disconnection, the patient giggled. Gazzaniga asked her why she was giggling, and the patient confabulated a response. It appears that her right hemisphere saw the picture and mediated an emotional response, but because of callosal disconnection her left hemisphere, which mediates speech and language, was not privy to the visual information that was projected to the right hemisphere, and the left hemisphere appeared to confabulate a response. Normally, the hypothetical visual monitor (which may be in one of the visual association areas) assesses input and provides other parts of the brain with information as to visual input. If one closes one's eyes, there is a reduction of input, and the monitor lets the speech area know that it is receiving no input; but if the monitor is either destroyed or disconnected from the speech areas it cannot let the speech area know that there is no input. Under these circumstances the speech areas may confabulate a response (Fig. 4–2).

A third mechanism that may account for the anosognosia associated with Anton's syndrome is false feedback to the monitor. Monkeys who have had ablation or disconnection of their occipital lobes from the remaining cortex are still able to perform a wide variety of visual tasks (Pribram, Spinelli, and Reitz, 1969). Weiskrantz, Warrington, Sanders, and Marshall (1974) demonstrated that patients with a dense hemianopsia due to lesions in the geniculocalcarine system are still able to localize targets. These observations suggest that the geniculocalcarine system is complemented by another system. This second visual system appears to be mediated by the superior colliculus, pulvinar and temporoparietal regions. Although this system does not appear to function as well in man as it does in animals, it still may have input into either a visual monitor or into the speech or language systems. Therefore although patients with cortical blindness cannot make the discriminations required by the clinician, they are having visual input and therefore are denying blindness. However, this second visual system explanation cannot account for the observation that patients with cortical blindness confabulate and have hallucinations.

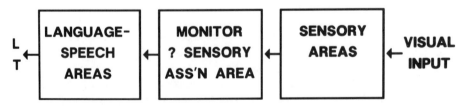

Figure 4–2. A failure to report sensory defects may be related to disconnection of sensory areas from a sensory monitor, destruction of the sensory monitor, or disconnection of the sensory monitor and/or sensory areas from the speech-language areas.

When a subject is asked to use visual imagery he often disengages from focusing visual attention and may even close his eyes to reduce visual input. Psychological studies have demonstrated that visual imagery and visual processing may be mutually inhibitory. This mutual inhibition suggests that both vision and visual imagery may compete for representations on a visual buffer. The visual buffer may be thought analogous to a television monitor, and visual input may be analogous to a television camera having input into a television monitor. Imagery then would be analogous to a videotape recorder having input into the same monitor. Patients with cortical blindness may still have visual imagery, and it is the visual imagery in the absence of visual input that may not only induce visual hallucinations but also may lead to anosognosia. It is possible that the speech area or the monitor receives information from the visual buffer rather than visual input systems. Because the buffer contains visual representations that come from imagery the confabulatory response may be based on this imagery. This false feedback postulate may also explain other forms of anosognosia. For example, amnesic patients with anosognosia may be more likely to retrieve memories (even though they are incorrect) than those amnesics who are without anosognosia.

DENIAL OF HEMIPLEGIA

Denial of hemiplegia is also most often seen with right hemisphere infarctions. Most often the lesion associated with denial of hemiplegia includes both frontal and parietal regions. Typically, on neurological examination the patient has a dense hemiplegia. However, when asked why he was brought to the hospital by his family he denies that there is anything wrong with him. When asked specifically about whether his left arm is impaired, he denies that anything is wrong with it. Depending on how aggressively the examiner demonstrates to the patient that he has lost control of the arm, the patient still denies any difficulty or minimizes it.

There have been many explanations of this dramatic behavioral aberration. I briefly discuss some of the major theories and then put forth new theories.

In one of the few systematic studies of anosognosia, Weinstein and Kahn (1953) studied the premorbid personalities of patients with anosognosia and found that, in general, even before they had their strokes they used denial mechanisms more frequently than did controls to deal with environmental stress. Whereas a premorbid personality may affect a patient's response to his own illness, this theory by itself could not account for the observation that denial of hemiplegia is more frequently associated with right than left hemisphere lesions. A corollary of Weinstein and Kahn's theory would have to be that those who use the denial mechanism would be more likely to have right than left hemisphere strokes, which seems unlikely.

In our discussion of the anosognosia associated with Anton's syndrome, we discussed the disconnection hypothesis. Geschwind (1965) posited a similar disconnection hypothesis to explain the anosognosia associated with right hemisphere disease. Lesions of the right hemisphere theoretically could not only destroy the sensory monitor but also disconnect this monitor from the left hemisphere, which mediates language and speech. There are two sensory feedback systems by which one may learn that a limb is not working: somatosensory (proprioceptive) and visual. A large right hemisphere lesion may not only disconnect these inputs and destroy the areas that monitor the inputs, it may also disconnect the monitor from the left hemisphere. However, if the hand is brought from the left side to the right side so it can be seen in the right visual field, the left hemisphere should then be able to gain the information that the hand is not working. In many cases of denial of hemiplegia, however, moving the paralyzed left arm into the right visual field does not seem to influence the anosognosia, suggesting that the disconnection from speech-language areas cannot entirely explain this form of anosognosia.

Patients with right hemisphere infarctions often demonstrate flattening of affect (see Heilman and Valenstein, 1985, for a review). In part, this flattening of affect appears to be related to a reduced ability to communicate emotion. For example, it has been demonstrated that patients with right hemisphere damage are impaired in terms of making emotional faces and emotional inflections of their voice. In addition, studies of autonomic arousal following right hemisphere injury have also shown that these patients have a reduced autonomic activation. Whereas the indifference to a motor or a sensory disability (anosodiaphoria) may be related to an affective communicative disorder and defective arousal, these emotional disorders cannot account for the verbal explicit denial of illness termed anosognosia.

Neglect is a complex disorder that has both sensory (attentional) and motor (intentional) components. Even in the absence of sensory or motor loss, patients with neglect may fail to recognize, respond to, or orient to stimuli. Neglect may be spatial, personal, or both. Neglect is more commonly associated with right than left hemisphere lesions. If a patient has spatial neglect, he may be unaware of a right hemianopsia; and if he has personal neglect, he may be unaware of a hemiplegia. Although in certain cases anosognosia may be related to an impairment of awareness or neglect, Bisiach, Vallar, Perani, Papagno, and Berti (1986) demonstrated that neglect to the left side of the body or limbs was not always associated with denial of hemiplegia.

Head and Holmes (1911) proposed that a defect in the body schema was responsible for anosognosia. In many respects their proposal is similar to the neglect postulate (i.e., with damage to the body schema one loses awareness of a body part), and neglect of body parts has also been attributed to a defective body schema. The work of Bisiach et al. also refutes this explanation of anosognosia.

Mark and Heilman (1988) asked patients with right hemisphere lesions to place a mark on a line that was perpendicular to the midline of their body (and not to bisect the actual line). The lines were placed in a variety of horizontal spatial positions. There were two experimental conditions. With one condition, the patients were able to see their bodies, and in the other condition their bodies were hidden from view. Subjects were influenced by the line; that is, when the line was in right or left hemispace the subjects tended to err toward the spatial position of the line. Patients with right hemisphere lesions were influenced more by lines on the right than on the left. In addition, unlike controls, when patients with right hemisphere lesions were allowed to see their body, their performance did not improve. This study suggests that not only are right-hemisphere-damaged patients inattentive to the left (or attentionally biased toward the right) but also that they are in general inattentive toward their own body.

Most of the theories of anosognosia discussed so far are related to false feedback due to sensory defects, sensory disconnection, and inattention. Even though these sensory and cognitive theories may help explain the failure to recognize a hemianopia or even can explain unawareness of hemiplegia, they cannot explain denial of hemiplegia when the arm is brought into a normal visual and attentional field and the patient is explicitly asked to monitor the arm's function. Therefore, in contrast to these feedback hypotheses, I propose a "feed forward" or "intentional" theory of anosognosia.

The feed forward model deals with expectations. If you decide to entirely relax your arm and let it hang by your side, someone could see your relaxed arm and ask you if your arm was paralyzed. You might reply with confidence, "No, my arm is just relaxed." Theoretically, one's confidence that one's arm is voluntarily resting rather than paretic is based in part on comparator functions (Fig. 4–3). Because the arm is not moving there is no afferent input into the compar-

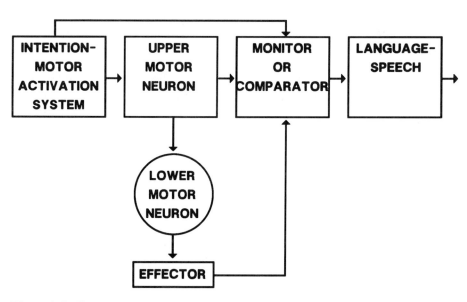

Figure 4–3. Comparator system used to detect passive movement and defects of active (intentional) movement. When there is a defect in the motor system or effector and one intends to make a movement, there is a mismatch in the comparator and one recognizes paralysis. However, if the intentional-preparatory systems are damaged along with the motor-effector system, there is no mismatch and one does not recognize paralysis.

ator that indicates movement. However, the intentional and premotor systems also have not fed into the comparator the "expectation" that movement should be felt, and hence there is no mismatch and you feel confident that your arm is not paralyzed. If during the time you are relaxing your arm you have an acute upper or lower motor neuron lesion and then attempt to move your arm, the intentional systems or premotor areas would feed the goal of the movement to the comparator; however, because you now have a motor lesion no sensory feedback indicating movement would reach the comparator. Hence there would be a mismatch in the comparator, and you would be aware that you were paralyzed. What would happen, however, if those brain areas responsible for activating the motor area were destroyed, impaired, or disconnected? Not only would you be unable to activate the motor neurons, but the comparator would not receive information that the arm was supposed to move. There would therefore be no mismatch, and you would not consider your arm paretic.

Whereas paralysis is caused by lesions of the upper and lower motor neurons, akinesia is thought to be related to an inability to activate these motor neurons. A full discussion of the mechanisms underlying akinesia is beyond the scope of this chapter; however, it has been demonstrated that limb akinesia can be caused by a variety of lesions including dorsolateral frontal lobe (Brodmann's area 6 and 8), inferior parietal lobes, basal ganglia (striatum and substantia nigra), thalamus (ventrolateral, anterior lateral, medial), and medial frontal lobes (supplementary motor area and cingulate gyrus). We believe that this network comprises an intention system (Watson, Valenstein, and Heilman, 1981). I propose that this intention system is responsible not only for activating motor systems but also for feeding information about motor expectations to comparator systems. Exactly what portion of this intention system feeds into the comparator is unknown, as is the site of the comparator.

This "feed forward" postulate cannot by itself explain why anosognosia of hemiplegia is more common after right than left hemisphere lesions. Studies in brain-damaged subjects, however, have demonstrated that contralateral akinesia is more frequently associated with right than left hemisphere lesions (Coslett and Heilman, 1989), suggesting that unilateral lesions of the right hemisphere are more likely to induce intentional deficits than are homologous lesions of the left hemisphere. As posited, these intentional deficits may lead not only to an akinesia but also to an anosognosia of hemiplegia.

CONCLUSIONS

In summary, it is proposed that anosognosia is induced by defects in monitoring or comparatory systems. I propose that the anosognosia associated with Wernicke's aphasia is related to a dysfunction in the monitor, and the denial of illness seen with cortical blindness is related to either a defect in the monitor, disconnection from speech-language areas, or misinterpreting internal images as coming through vision. Although denial of hemiplegia in some cases is also related to a feedback disorder, the feedback hypothesis cannot account for denial in all cases. As an alternative, a "feed-forward" mechanism is proposed. According to this hypothesis, the intention system does not set the monitor; hence when there is no movement feedback, there is no mismatch, and the person is not alerted to a motor failure. In their book, *Denial of Illness,* Weinstein and Kahn (1955) described a case of denial of hemiplegia who calls his arm "lazy." Laziness is not a defect of feedback systems but, rather, a defect of intentional "feed forward" systems.

REFERENCES

Alajouanine, T. (1956). Verbal realization in aphasia. *Brain,* 79:1–28.

Anton, G. (1896). Blindheit nach beiderseitiger Gehirnerkrankung mit Verlust der Orientierung in Raume. *Mittherl. Ver. Arzte Steiermark,* 33:41–46.

Babinski, J. (1914). Contribution à l'etude des troubles mentaux dans l'hémiplégie organique cérébrale (anosognosie). *Rev. Neurol. (Paris)* 27:845–847.

Benson, D. F. (1985). Aphasia. In: K.M. Heilman and E. Valenstein (eds.), Oxford; New York: *Clinical Neuropsychology.*

Bisiach, E., Vallar, G., Perani, D., Papagno, C., and Berti, A. (1986). Unawareness of disease following lesions of the right hemisphere: anosognosia for hemiplegia and anosognosia for hemianopsia. *Neuropsychologia* 24:471–482.

Caplan, L., and Hedley-White, T. (1974). Cueing and memory dysfunction in alexia without agraphia: a case report. *Brain* 97:251–262.

Coslett, H. B., and Heilman, K. M. (1989). Hemihypokinesia after right hemisphere strokes. *Brain Cogn.* 9:267–278.

Critchley, M. (1953). *The Parietal Lobes.* London: Edward Arnold.

Devinsky, O., Bear, D., and Volpe, B. T. (1988): Confusional states following posterior cerebral artery infarctions. *Arch. Neurol.* 45:160–163.

Gazzaniga, M. S. (1970). *The Bisected Brain.* New York: Appleton.

Geschwind, N. (1965). Disconnexion syndromes in animals and man. *Brain* 88:237–294, 585–644.

Head, H., and Holmes, G. (1911). Sensory disturbances from cerebral lesions. *Brain* 34:102–254.

Hécaen, H., and Albert, M. (1978): *Human Neuropsychology.* New York: Wiley.

Heilman, K. M., and Valenstein, E. (1985): *Clinical Neuropsychology.* New York: Oxford University Press.

Mark, V., and Heilman, K. M. (1988). Personal body neglect in hemispatial neglect. *Neurology* 38(suppl 1):171.

Marshall, R. C. and Tompkins, C. A. (1982). Verbal self-corrective behaviors of fluent and nonfluent aphasic subjects. *Brain and Language,* 15:292–306.

Pribram, K. H., Spinelli, D. N., and Reitz, S. L. (1969): Disconnection and visual behavior. *Brain* 92:301–312.

Speedie, L., and Heilman, K. M. (1982). Amnestic disturbance following infarctions of the left dorsomedial nucleus of the thalamus. *Neuropsychologia* 20:597–604.

Von Monakow, C. (1885). Cited by Weinstein E. A., and Kahn, R. L. (1955). *Denial of Illness.* Springfield, IL: Charles C Thomas.

Watson, R. T., Valenstein, E., Heilman, K. M. (1981). Thalamic neglect: Possible role of the medial thalamus and nucleus reticularis in behavior. *Archives of Neurology* 38:501–506.

Weinstein, E. A., and Kahn, R. L. (1953). Personality factors in denial of illness. *A.M.A. Arch. Neurol Psychiatry* 69:355–367.

Weinstein, E. A., and Kahn, R. L. (1955). *Denial of Illness.* Springfield, IL: Charles C Thomas.

Weiskrantz, L., Warrington, E. K., Sanders, M. D., and Marshall, J. (1974). Visual capacity in the hemianopic field following a restricted occipital ablation. *Brain* 97:709–728.

5
Disturbance of Self-Awareness After Frontal System Damage

DONALD T. STUSS

The clinical descriptions of frontal lobe unconcern and unawareness of deficit have been frequently documented and are widely accepted (Blumer and Benson, 1975). The characteristics of this disturbed awareness and the definition of terms, however, are more controversial. One problem has been the absence of a theoretical structure of self-awareness in which behavioral observations can be placed.

In this chapter, a brief review of disturbed awareness after frontal lobe pathology reported in earlier studies highlights the historical importance of the frontal systems to self-awareness and reality monitoring. Against this background, two frameworks are provided in an initial attempt to characterize more specifically the relation of the frontal lobes to the general concept of awareness. The first is a model that focuses on the anatomical organization of the brain as a means of understanding the clinical observations of alterations in behavior after frontal system damage (Stuss and Benson, 1986). The second is a psychological theory of self and consciousness that may provide insight for understanding disturbances of awareness after frontal lobe damage (James, 1890).

The core of the chapter presents three examples, one previously published case and two new case studies, that highlight key features of disturbance of awareness after frontal pathology. These observations are mapped onto the proposed theoretical structures in an attempt to extract the salient characteristics of disturbed awareness after frontal system brain damage. Finally, a schematic model differentiating disturbed awareness of fact from disturbed self-awareness is proposed.

HISTORICAL REVIEW

The history of disturbance of self-awareness after frontal lobe damage mirrors the problems of many modern investigations: inadequate documentation, inadequate or absent experimental design, variations in lesion size and etiologies, and pathologies frequently extending beyond the frontal lobes. Despite these problems, a delicate fabric related to the issues of unconcern, denial, and unawareness of deficit after damage to the frontal systems has been woven over the years.

The observations of altered behavior in animals with frontal pathology were phrased primarily in terms of activity, organization, and attention. Although obviously not interpretable as "self-awareness," certain descriptions dovetail with those made about human subjects. Bianchi (1895, 1922) reported that frontally damaged monkeys, in addition to not recognizing their owner and being impaired in inhibiting irrelevant reactions and deducing consequences, remained in a habitual state of indifference. Bekhterev (1907) proposed that such animals were unable to evaluate the consequences of their actions or relate new experiences to their past.

Even in early reports of human cases, the effects of damage to the frontal lobes were frequently described in terms relating to the "self," awareness, and concern about changes in behavior. Hoffman (1869) noted that patients with frontal lobe damage understood the nature of serious situations but seemed to take no real interest in the gravity of the situation. Similar descriptions have been heard over the years. Sachs (1927) noted that patients with frontal lobe tumors had a "peculiar indifference" to their problems. "When asked why they do not worry, they not infrequently shrug their shoulders" (Sachs, 1927). German and Fox's (1932) patient with a right frontal lobectomy and Brickner's (1936) stockbroker with both frontal lobes removed during treatment for a large cerebral meningioma displayed a lack of appreciation of the seriousness of their situation, a problem often out of proportion to other deficits they displayed. A patient with extensive mesial-orbital frontal damage secondary to a failed suicide attempt with a gun was totally blind yet unconcerned about his blindness (De Nobele, 1835).

Luria (1969) and Luria and Homskaya (1964) reviewed a series of early reports (mostly individual case studies; e.g., Harlow, 1868; Welt, 1888; Feuchtwanger, 1923; Kleist, 1934) and extracted two primary symptoms present in almost every patient with a mass lesion in the prefrontal regions: (1) a disturbance in complex active purposeful behavior; and (2) a deficient critical attitude toward their own impairment. Ackerly and Benton's (1947) comment about their patient who appeared to have bilateral congenital or early childhood frontal lobe deficit captures this second observation. Although objectively this patient's life was disordered, "in interviews he appeared quite satisfied with his adjustment. . . ."

Despite the possible influence of various premorbid abilities and psychopathologies in patients who underwent psychosurgery, the presence of lesions limited to the prefrontal cortex presented an opportunity for study of this cortical region. The observations repeatedly underlined some type of disturbance in concern about losses, self-awareness, and reality monitoring. Stengel (1952) reviewed the attitudes of hundreds of psychosurgery patients and reported that many denied having had the operation. Of those who recognized their postoperative impairments, few expressed resentment. They described their losses with a detached attitude, like some unbiased reporter. One purpose of lobotomy was to reduce the characteristics of self-concern: brooding, preoccupation, and self-consciousness (Freeman and Watts, 1942; Hutton, 1947; Greenblatt and Solomon, 1966). "They [postlobotomy patients] see their faults and weaknesses and vices clearly enough and recognize them for what they are, but far from privately brooding over them, they seem to regard them as interesting topics for comment" (Robinson and Freeman, 1954). Patients operated on for pain still admitted having pain yet were completely unconcerned (Fulton, 1948).

Other observations may be added. An absence of introspection or self-reflectiveness after frontal lobe damage was reported (Brickner, 1936; Ackerly and Benton, 1947). Second, the disturbance of self-awareness was not necessarily a total lack of interest or reaction. Goldstein (1944) noted that frontal patients may be interested in their environment.

Third, a dissociation between what the frontal patient knows or says, and how he or she behaves, appeared to be common. "He had an excellent sense of right and wrong when talking about it in an abstract manner, but showed no such sense in his actions" (Ackerly and Benton, 1947). Jarvie (1954) stated that five of six patients with frontal penetrating brain wounds were fully aware of their change in personality, which they were able to describe succinctly. This knowledge, however, had little impact on the control of their behavior. More recently, Milner (1965) described that, on a maze test, patients with frontal wounds made more errors and failed to self-correct, even though reporting an awareness of how they were to respond. "Awareness" in these examples obviously signifies knowledge rather than self-reflectiveness or awareness of the impact of behavior (Heath and Pool, 1948).

Denny-Brown (1951) rightfully urged caution, stating that the described deficits in self related to frontal lobe damage cannot be generalized to all aspects of consciousness or awareness. "Consciousness of person [*sic:* extrapersonal], or of surroundings, is more totally disordered by lesions of the parietal lobe."

Luria and Homskaya (1964) described the inability to correct erroneous behaviors as an inadequate evaluation by the patient of his or her action, a general disturbance in self-regulation. Konow and Pribram (1970), however, differentiated error knowledge or evaluation from error utilization. A patient with damaged frontal lobes can recognize errors easily in others and at least occasionally in himself. Error evaluation therefore appears to depend more on posterior brain functions. Error utilization, i.e., correction of inappropriate behaviors or erroneous responses in response to knowledge of errors, is disturbed primarily with anterior lesions, suggesting that frontal-limbic brain zones are relevant for this utilitarian function.

Several attempts were made over the years to provide more than a description of the disturbed awareness. Flechsig (1908) suggested that the fundamental role of prefrontal cortex was self-awareness or consciousness of the self *(selbstwusstsein)*. Freeman and Watts (1942, 1950), based on observations of their psychosurgery patients, first characterized the effects of prefrontal lobotomy as a disturbance in the capacity of foresight in relation to the self. This description was later elaborated into the concept of self-continuity. Robinson and Freeman (1954) defined self-continuity as recognition of a stable self that exists from the past through the present into the future, as well as a self that can change over time. Self-continuity is more intimate and personal than memory, as the facts of memory are not impaired after focal frontal lobe damage. Rather, the lobotomized patient has lost awareness of himself as a continuing and changing entity, with personal responsibility for such change. It was hypothesized that the lobotomized patient was freed from the tyranny of his own past because his or her self-continuity was now reduced.

A repeating theme in the history of disturbed awareness after frontal lobe damage concerns the role of time. Frontal-lobe-damaged patients respond only to concrete, present situations, having no thought or plans for the future; immediate concerns such as regard for one's family dissipate without an immediate presence (Goldstein, 1936, 1944). Ackerly and Benton's (1947) patient showed no concern in regard to the past or future. This temporal integration of experience, as phrased by Robinson and Freeman (1954), is the basis of self-continuity, allowing utilization of the past when interpreting the present and moving to the future: "It is an intimate awareness of the relatedness of what the self has done and experienced to what it will do and experience" (Robinson and Freeman, 1954, p. 84).

There has been only infrequent reference to the issue of localization of self-awareness and reality monitoring within the prefrontal cortex. Freeman and Watts (1948) postulated two levels of "consciousness." Accrued visceral consciousness of one's individual identity was hypothesized as being located in posterior prefrontal regions. Higher self-awareness was correlated with more progressively anterior localization, with religious self-consciousness coexisting with intact frontal polar regions. Luria (1969) suggested that the "disturbance of the critical attitude" was most clearly observed in patients with pathology in the basal portions of the frontal cortex. Blumer and Benson (1975), based on the ideas of Kleist (1934), postulated two basic types of personality change correlating with frontal convexity and orbital lesion location. In their descriptions, both types are described as exhibiting unconcern.

This brief review of early reports of the behavior of patients with frontal damage leaves little doubt that a disturbance in reality monitoring, unawareness, unconcern, and even denial of deficit, was a prominent observation. Initial attempts were made to construct a theoretical framework related to this disturbed self-awareness after frontal lobe damage. The remainder of this chapter attempts to extend these early postulates.

TWO FRAMEWORKS OF SELF

Hierarchy of Brain Functioning

Stuss and Benson (1986) proposed a hierarchical integrated organization of brain function in which self-awareness is considered the "highest" of brain activities.

Intimately related to the prefrontal regions, this theoretical construct of self-awareness (self-consciousness, self-reflectiveness) utilizes and interacts with other brain processes in the overall goal of developing an aware individual interacting with the environment in a personal and socially appropriate manner. This construct was postulated for at least two reasons. First, the history of frontal lobe studies strongly suggested that some type of disturbance of self-awareness was a prominent outcome; and, second, the experimental results and theoretical interpretation (following the work of many previous frontal lobe researchers), as well as the authors' philosophical bias, suggested that a human was not a reactive agent but an active and interactive entity developing one's future in light of past experience. In the original formulation of Stuss and Benson, the details of "self" had not been proposed. This chapter attempts to extend this concept in light of William James' psychological theory of self.

A brief description highlights the model (Fig. 5–1). Psychological processes such as attention, language, and memory are considered complex functional systems with their own inherent organization that works at an overlearned, automatic level. The systems are "fixed" in that they are relatively constant across the adult population, allowing scientific investigation. Such systems are also integrated in the sense that they involve various cortical and subcortical regions in both hemispheres in the working of one function, different regions participating in their own specialized way (Mesulam, 1981).

The frontal lobes interact with these posterior/basal brain regions, appearing to play a unique role. Although three "levels" have been described (Stuss and Benson, 1986, 1987), they must not be viewed as a tiered multilayered pyramid but as an interactive system. There are two frontal functional systems that provide the posterior/basal systems with the capacity to sequence and integrate

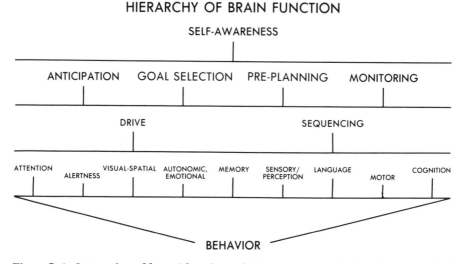

Figure 5–1. Interaction of frontal functions with the more posterior/basal systems related to behavior. (From Stuss, D. T., and Benson, D. F. *The Frontal Lobes.* New York: Raven Press, 1986. With permission.)

information; they also serve as an integral part of drive or motivation. Although certainly not only "frontal" in brain location, frontal damage does affect sequencing and drive, with some indication of specificity of localization. Sequencing may be more related to dorsolateral brain regions, and drive to more medial areas.

An executive or control function is also hypothesized as depending on frontal brain regions. This executive function provides conscious direction to the posterior/basal and frontal functional systems. The posterior/basal organized integrated fixed functional systems perform efficiently in routine, overlearned situations. In novel, complex, or nonroutine situations, however, conscious direction as provided by the frontal lobes is required. The frontal control system explores, monitors, fixates, selects, shifts, modifies, and judges all nervous system activities. The frontal lobes are necessary when a new activity is being learned and active control is required. After the activity has become routine, these activities can be handled by other brain (posterior/basal) regions, and full frontal participation is no longer demanded (Damasio, 1979; Shallice, 1982).

Self-awareness, consciousness, or self-reflectiveness is posited as the highest psychological attribute of the frontal lobes. In behavioral terms, it is revealed as unconcern, absent or deficient monitoring of behavior, and impaired self-regulation of behavior.

Several examples, scientific and metaphorical, help to understand this concept of brain organization. If positron emission tomography is used to monitor motor tasks, striking differences can be observed (Mazziotta and Phelps, 1986). An overlearned motor task such as writing one's signature appears to require primarily subcortical activity. If a new motor act of similar difficulty is demanded, frontal participation is observed.

Other examples are evident in everyday life. When learning to drive a car with a stick shift, each movement must be consciously controlled and commanded. With repetition, such movements become automatic. Indeed, much cognitive and motor learning is the translation of new acts into familiar and overlearned behaviors. Although this automaticity obviously has tremendous benefit, it frequently results in "capture errors" (Shallice, 1982). The differentiation between fast, overlearned, routine posterior/basal systems and the slower, deliberate, organizing role of the frontal lobes is mirrored in the food service industry. Fast food restaurants may be considered an example of a posterior/basal system, or perhaps a multiplicity of posterior/basal systems. Employees in good fast food establishments are efficient because they do not deviate from the norm. Indeed, they have been trained to be automatic (to become efficient posterior/basal systems). The efficiency due to reasonably fixed behaviors is one relevant factor in maintaining relatively constant, low prices and increased profit for the owners. The more the frontal lobes are required when preparing a meal, the slower the process, the more unique the outcome, and the greater the cost.

William James and the Self

In an attempt to provide a psychological structure that could be mapped onto the behavioral observations and behavioral-anatomical model summarized above, a decision was made to review the work of an early proponent of the importance of the self, William James (1890). William James, in discussions on self, consciousness, and personal identity, postulated that consciousness has certain characteristics. It is *personal*. "The universal conscious fact is not 'feelings and thoughts exist,' but 'I think' and 'I feel'" (p. 147). There is an individual "I" or "self" that is the core of each human being. There is as well a perceived *continuity,* providing a "community of self." Regardless of external variations, consciousness is continuous, one stream of thought, because it resides in one's memory, bridging gaps that may occur because of factors such as sleep. It is not, however, the recall of facts alone that provides the continuity. James presented an example of two individuals waking up in the same bed. Each reaches back to his or her own stream of thought at the moment of awakening and prior to falling asleep. Although one may have correct knowledge of the other's last drowsy state of mind, the knowledge is different because it is only conceived. What makes a personal memory different from mere conceptualization are the *feelings of warmth, intimacy, and immediacy.* Memories having these characteristics must be admitted as part of the "common self." Continuity and judgment of sameness are important for the sense of unity. The feelings of warmth and continuity are the bases by which this judgment is made. A direct corollary is that *knowledge* itself is *not sufficient* to provide the community of self.

The self has other characteristics important to the concept of awareness of deficit. The self is "cognitive," possessing the function of knowing. Indeed, we can become conscious of our own cognitive functioning. Humans not only know things; they know that they know them. James goes so far as to say that the *reflective* condition is more or less "our habitual adult state of mind" (p. 177). With these concepts, James appeared to herald the modern theory of metacognition.

Deliberate choice and *selective attention* are key characteristics of the stream of consciousness, present in many activities: ". . . all reasoning depends on the ability of the mind to break up the totality of the phenomenon reasoned about, into parts, and to pick out from among these the particular one which, in our given emergency, may lead to the proper conclusion. . . . Reasoning is but another form of the selective activity of the mind" (p. 186). Selective attention and consciousness are intimately interconnected: "Focalization, concentration, of consciousness are of its [attention's] essence" (p. 261). This statement selectivity emphasizes and unites. A corollary role is the ignoring of irrelevant information.

Time, both past and future, appears to be an essential component of James' theory of self. It has already been shown how memories are essential in achieving and maintaining the judged continuity of self. However, it is not a deterministic view. We are not bound by our past. "The problem with a man is less what act he shall now choose to do, than what being he shall now resolve to become" (p. 187). The aspects of future and will are important. It is through decisions that we slowly form our lives and selves.

In summary, James has provided us with another structure by which the matter of awareness of deficit can be judged. The self is a key factor in awareness. The self is characterized by concepts such as warmth, immediacy, and continuity of memories; choice and selectivity, particularly in relation to one's future; and self-reflectiveness. Knowledge by itself is insufficient. The parallel between James' concepts and the observations made by early researchers of frontal lobe dysfunction is obvious.

FRONTAL LOBES AND DISTURBED AWARENESS

Three examples from patients with frontal lobe disturbance are given. Based on this information and using the theoretical structures for assistance, characteristics of frontal lobe disturbance of awareness of deficit are summarized. The examples relate to specific patients, and so details of their lives are altered to retain confidentiality.

Reduplicative Paramnesia

Reduplicative paramnesia is a term used to describe an isolated disturbance (rather than loss) of memory, in which an individual is subjectively convinced that a familiar place or person has been duplicated (Pick, 1903). In the psychiatric literature the disorder referring to reduplication of persons is labeled the "Capgras syndrome" (Capgras and Reboul-Lachaux, 1923). If specifically sought, reduplication is relatively common (Weinstein and Kahn, 1955), with increasing reports suggesting a neurological base (e.g., Morrison and Tarter, 1984; Cummings, 1985; Lewis, 1987; Lipkin, 1988). In many of these studies, frontal lobe disturbance has been proposed as an explanation.

A review of a case previously published provides some insight into the characteristics of disturbance of awareness after frontal lobe damage (Alexander, Stuss, and Benson, 1979).

A 44-year-old man, patient R.B., who had been slowly developing obsessional concerns about financial matters, was involved in a motor vehicle accident with significant consequences. He suffered multiple physical injuries as well as a serious traumatic brain injury. A right frontal craniotomy revealed a large subdural hematoma and a necrotic right frontal lobe. His recovery course was stormy. He exhibited persistent serious neuropsychological deficits, particularly in memory and visuospatial functions, with altered behavior. These areas recovered slowly. Ten months after trauma, he was allowed a first weekend pass home. Upon his return to the hospital, a focal problem of disorientation was discovered. He was now convinced that he lived with a second, different family, virtually identical with his "first" family, both physically (general appearance) and in name. One exception was that his "present" children appeared to be approximately 1 year older than his first family. The new family also fortunately lived in the same house as had his previous family.

A complete neurological, radiological, and neuropsychological examination was completed on R.B. 3 years after trauma. Computed tomography (CT) scanning revealed atrophy of the right frontal and temporal regions, considerable patchy decrease in density of the left inferomedial frontal lobe, and generalized ventricular enlargement in the frontal horns that was greater on the right (Fig. 5–2). The neuropsychological assessment strongly suggested right hemisphere dysfunction, partic-

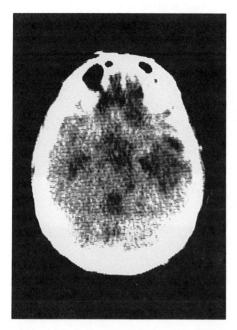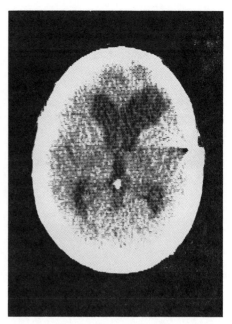

Figure 5–2. Left: CT scan showing bilateral inferior frontal and right temporal density in R.B., the patient with reduplicative paramnesia. Right: CT scan reveals moderate, diffuse ventricular enlargement with a particularly prominent right frontal horn.   [From Alexander, M. P., Stuss, D. T., and Benson, D. F. (1979). Capgras syndrome: a reduplicative phenomenon. *Neurology* (NY) 29:334–339. With permission.]

ularly frontal and temporal. Other abilities, including language, simple attention, visuospatial, verbal memory, and overall IQ were intact. IQ (102) was within the normal range. His Wechsler Memory Scale had improved dramatically from the initial stages after trauma, resting within the superior range (WMS MQ = 124). Behaviorally, he was euphoric, apathetic, tangential, and somewhat unkempt in appearance. At no time after the injury did he reveal suspiciousness or psychiatric disturbance other than the focal reduplication.

Characteristics of the change that are relevant to a disorder of awareness may be gleaned from the following interview (E = examiner; S = subject).

E: So you are married now?

S: So I am married now.

E: How many children do you have?

S: This can be confusing, but in any event I am responsible for eight sons and two daughters.

E: That is confusing.

S: Well, between the two girls they, oh I suspect, had five each.

E: You have to slow down now. Two girls? You are married twice? Let's go through this again. You are married once.

S: Married once.

E: How many children did you have from that first marriage?

S: Four boys and one girl, but the second girl who I am married to now, she picked me up on December 5th a year ago.

E: She picked you up?

S: Yes, at the hospital to drive me home for the weekend.

E: She just picked you up like that?

S: Yes.

S: They don't look alike, but they are similar, both brunettes and they are similar in appearance.

E: What do the new children look like?

S: Similar.

E: Similar to the other ones?

S: Yeah.

E: Are they your children?

S: I would suspect so. The eight boys that are in question, six of them are over 6 feet. So they are tall.

E: Both families look like you?

S: Yes, they are similar.

E: Do you think that these two girls knew each other, or the two families know each other?

S: Well the connection that they have is that the second wife I am married to now has a sister and the first wife has a brother who is married to her.

E: You also lived with the first wife.

S: I did, yes.

E: In the same house?

S: The same house.

E: Isn't that unusual?

S: It was unbelievable!

E: So all of a sudden you came out of the hospital and you went back in the same house with a whole different family.

S: Well, that is about the size of it, yes.

E: How can you account for that?

S: I don't know. I tried to understand it myself, and it was virtually impossible to understand it.

. . . .

E: It is almost like the same family but it is not the same.

S: It is not.

E: I think you are pulling my leg.

S: I am not. I am trying to be truthful.

E: You are not trying to pull the wool over my eyes.

S: No, I am not trying to. . . .

E: If somebody would tell you that story, what would you say to them?

S: I would find it hard to believe.

E: Right, that is it exactly.

S: I would find it extremely hard to believe, and I probably should be defending myself more so. I have not to date, I have not tried in any way, shape, or manner or tried to divorce the first wife.

E: Have you ever tried to find her?

S: I have not.

. . . . .

E: So she set up the second wife?

S: She set up the second wife. It was her say so, her doing that the second girl was at the hospital on the Friday.

E: You're kidding, she brought in the whole family the same. That is very thoughtful of her, and she even got a girl who is just like her.

S: Yes. This is the irony of the whole thing is the girl is very similar to her own appearance and she went out and did it herself.

E: Most amazing.

S: Unbelievable—and the only thing I could have done at the time was say, "No, I will not accept it," and I did [accept it].

This individual exhibits many characteristics that could be related to a disturbance of self-awareness. One intangible factor undetectable in the written interview was the quality of his voice, which was full of laughter, joyous, accepting, and overflowing with bonhomie. This tonal unconcern was paralleled behaviorally. He was happy, apathetic, and unmotivated (although his verbalizations at times suggested otherwise); he did absolutely nothing to verify or correct his "bigamous' condition. It is all the more striking considering that the interview indicated that he had full knowledge that the situation was objectively incongruous and "unbelievable."

Despite his correct knowedge of the situation, R.B. was totally convinced that the impossible was true. He adamantly maintained this belief over at least 4 years despite repeated attempts to dissuade him. Seemingly important to this conviction was the nature of the memory. In both the neurology and psychiatric literature, the person or place reduplicated or replaced appears to have a close relation with the patient. For R.B., his "second" wife picked him up for his first visit home after extended hospitalization. With prolonged discontinuity from his previous life at a time of recovering memory, this experience, saturated in warmth (pleasure of visit), intimacy (immediate gratification), and relevance (wife and family), began a new continuity.

These observations can be married to our two theoretical structures. The neuropsychological data relate to the behavioral/anatomical model of Stuss and Benson (1986). In R.B., what were labeled "posterior/basal" functions appear to be intact, e.g., language, overall memory, visuospatial, motor, sensory, general cognitive, and simple attentional abilities. Against this background, those functions frequently labeled "frontal" or "executive" were severely impaired: initiating, monitoring, assessing, evaluating, programming, adapting, and maintaining. In this view, disturbed self-awareness is viewed as intact knowledge disconnected from frontal controlling functions, perhaps due to frontal lobe damage. The ability to initiate the search for the "first" wife, discover pertinent facts, and evaluate their significance was impaired. Frontal system unawareness is not lack of knowledge but impaired judgment of the objective facts in relation to one's own life—a disturbance in self-awareness.

Using James' concepts, there is little doubt that the self is disrupted in R.B. A review of the characteristics of self also indicate that the self is not absolutely destroyed. In this patient there is an "I" who thinks, reports, and feels. Despite the severe injury and protracted disruption in the stream of thought, there is some continuity, some community of self. The warmth, intimacy, and immediacy of the memories result in the strong belief that the family memories before and after the accident belong to him. They are, however, separated in time and perhaps by factors such as the age of the children. It is the emotional salience of each memory that provides the conviction that the two memories are indeed real. What is impaired is his judgment and the reflective condition. The self is disturbed, and awareness is impaired but in a specific way. Disturbances in judgment and control may be reflected in many ways, as demonstrated by the frontal lobe tests. The particular presentation as a reduplication phenomenon is secondary to the disturbance in judgment, in the interaction with the strength and vividness of the two independent memories.

Rehabilitation in a Right Frontal Lobe Damaged Patient

A second example illustrates a more general presentation of disturbed self-awareness after focal frontal lobe damage.

Seizure activity in a highly educated and successful professional businesswoman led to the discovery of a right frontal astrocytoma that was surgically removed. Figure

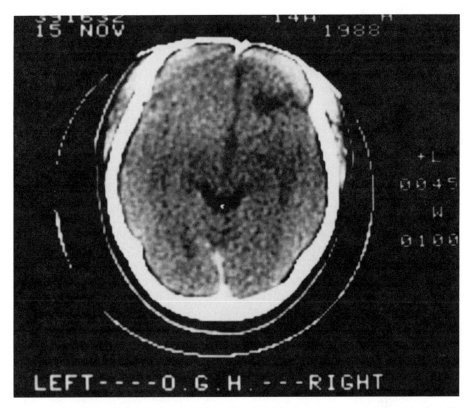

Figure 5–3. CT scan shows the right frontal lesion after tumor removal from patient R.

5–3 depicts the pathology. Subsequently irradiation and chemotherapy eventually eliminated tumor growth. The patient (called R. for confidentiality and brevity's sake) returned to work 1 year after the operation but at a much reduced work load. R. originally denied having any problems. However, at the insistence of her spouse, she eventually was referred for neuropsychological assessment. At that time, she verbally accepted her "deficits."

Neuropsychological examination revealed excellent abilities, even on "frontal lobe" tests (Table 5–1). There were minor exceptions: left-sided motor slowing; perseveration on the California Verbal Learning Test; tangentiality in conversation; mild distractibility; and mild difficulty on certain attentional tasks. Her daily life, however, was characterized by (as the patient herself stated) "all standard frontal lobe signs." She had difficulty getting up, showering, dressing, and getting to work before 11:00 a.m. She would forget to perform even minor daily tasks. In these and other regards, her husband stated that she was a different individual.

Because of her generally excellent results on testing and her high level of prior functioning, rehabilitation was initiated. The following methods were attempted: use of verbal self-regulation to guide behavior; training in the focusing of attention; practice in establishing appropriate goals and monitoring behavior; and increasing the awareness of her problems and the level of functioning of which she was now capable. Rehabilitation over 18 months had limited success. Signs in her office ("stay on task") and verbal self-regulation ("I will finish this one job first") did improve work productivity and punctuality in daily life, but only to a certain limit.

TABLE 5-1   Neuropsychology Results

Test	Result
Simple attention	"Normal"
Mild left side slowing	
Language	Normal
WAIS-R	
VIQ	120
PIQ	104
FSIQ	114
Verbal subscales (percentile)	
Information	95
Digit span	50
Arithmetic	91
Similarities	84
Performance	
Picture arrangement	50
Block design	91
Object assembly	63
Digit symbol	50
Frontal tests	
Porteus maze	Perfect
Wisconsin test	9 Categories
Motor tests	Normal
Memory	
WMS MQ	>143
Consonant trigrams	54/60
CVLT	71/80

At weekly sessions, with therapeutic guidance, appropriate employment goals were established for the following week. Charting the success of achieving these goals attempted to increase R.'s awareness of actual functioning in relation to expected functioning. This objective feedback revealed her lack of success. Even though her stated goals were significantly less than her previous functioning level, her maximum achievement was only 50 percent of the stated goals, reached only once over 18 months. In addition, formal feedback from both her employer and her subordinates was on one occasion so devastating and personal that she was crestfallen. By the next session, however, the implications of this review appeared to have minimal impact on her decisions concerning her work.

Total or partial disability appeared to be a logical conclusion. It would enable her to enjoy her family, obtain a reasonable pension, and possibly find less demanding alternative employment. The patient accepted this decision. During the final therapy meeting, however, the intellectual acceptance of her limitations was abrogated with the verbalization that she could and would return to her previous level of functioning within 1 year.

Role playing was used to evaluate R.'s awareness (knowledge) of her situation and the appropriate steps to take to remedy it. Acting as her own direct supervisor, R. analyzed the facts and made appropriate recommendations concerning her own employment as well as her daily life: continuation of her loss of privilege to drive a car; based on her work performance and medical condition, obtainment of a disability pension; and presentation of practical steps to investigate the best type of pension. When asked, she stated that these conclusions were logical based on the evidence. Once removed from her role-playing position, however, she was no longer able to make the same judgments in relation to her real-life personal situation and was determined to return to work at her presurgery level of functioning.

Several observations may be made concerning this case study. R. was, in many respects, totally "normal" or unimpaired. Not only did she exhibit no disturbance in most abilities tested, her test performance was often superior. Even supposed "frontal lobe" tests were often unimpaired, likely reflecting her superior intelligence.

In contrast, her failure in daily life, at home and work, was dramatic. Although at times she actively denied or minimized problems, most often she acknowledged the deficit. As indicated in the role-playing experiment, her knowledge of her deficits and their effects could be precise. She did not appear to be unaware (in the sense of lacking knowledge) or indeed totally unconcerned, evidenced by her desire to continue therapy to improve. The most significant disturbance occurred in one aspect of self-awareness: the use of the knowledge she possessed in relation to decisions about her future. Behavioral observations also suggested selectivity of attention (that which emphasizes, directs, and unites) was also impaired.

Traumatic Brain Injury

The likely presence of frontal brain disturbance among the multidimensional aspects of traumatic brain injury (TBI) has been suggested (Stuss, 1987), and disturbance of self-awareness after TBI has been proposed (Prigatano, 1988). We have observed a unique phenomenon after TBI. Three of our TBI patients with moderate head injuries described alterations in their recall of remote memories from various periods of their lives. Memories were not lost, but the recalled facts had lost their personal reference, i.e., although the patients could remember the facts, the memories did not belong to them. There was a loss of warmth and immediacy to these memories. This recalled information, previously personal and "episodic" (Tulving, 1983), appeared to have become more like detached, generic "semantic" facts. Although biographical, the memories were no longer truly self- or autobiographical. As the patients recovered over time, there appeared to be at least partial reintegration.

These examples of TBI suggest the possibility of a different and focal disturbance of self, limited to the loss of intimacy and immediacy of memory. This detached, impersonal memory disrupts at least in part the feeling of continuity, the community of self. In this sense, the relation of the patient's past to future decisions is impaired.

It is somewhat premature to conclude that this problem is solely a frontal disturbance of awareness. However, none of the three patients had documented lesions in other brain regions. Evidence accumulated by Tulving (1989) using blood flow measurements suggests that episodic memory is frontal in localization, as he had earlier proposed (Tulving, 1985; see also Chapter 8). Because frontotemporal disturbances are most common in TBI, a frontotemporal (limbic) disconnection is a reasonable postulate to explain this focal disturbance in self-awareness.

CHARACTERISTICS OF FRONTAL LOBE DISORDERS OF AWARENESS

From the history and the presented examples, seven prominent characteristics of disorders of awareness after frontal lobe disturbance may be extracted. Earlier warnings are again repeated: Although many of these observations are related to focal frontal lobe disturbance, a unique relation to frontal pathology cannot yet be concluded. Second, experimental research in groups of patients with focal lesions has not been completed to validate these observations.

1. *"Frontal" disorders of awareness are related to the self.* For this reason, the term "self-awareness" was postulated (Stuss and Benson, 1986). Disturbances of "self-awareness" appear to be essentially different from impaired awareness of deficits in behavioral disorders such as neglect and aphasia. The latter appear more related to specific functional systems such as language. For these systems, impaired awareness of deficit is more directly related to knowledge associated with that particular system. Self-awareness, on the other hand, is related to characteristics of the self (certainly as presented by James) and is more generically related to all behavioral functions.

2. *Disorders of self-awareness can be present with normal sensorium and normal or even superior IQ, memory, and so on.* Whereas self-awareness is disturbed after disorders of arousal, acute confusional states, or diffuse brain dysfunction such as progressive dementias, the presented examples clearly indicate that self-awareness may be disturbed even after limited brain damage or dysfunction. Our examples suggest that the frontal lobes, or more appropriately the frontal systems, play a relevant role in self-awareness. A corollary conclusion is that posterior/basal functions such as sensation and IQ may be normal, whereas self-awareness is severely disturbed.

3. *Fractionation of disturbed self-awareness appears possible.* Different characteristics of the self appear to have been disturbed in the various examples given. One postulate is that this fractionation is related to the specific connections between frontal and other brain regions, as suggested in the TBI example.

4. *Judgment and selectivity are important.* In many of these patients, the primary functional deficit involves frontal abilities, such as initiation, decision-making, judgment of appropriateness, selection of appropriate behaviors, and monitoring of the outcome.

5. *Knowledge is a phenomenon distinct from awareness.* This corollary of the fourth point deserves an independent statement. There often is a striking dissociation between correct knowledge, use of knowledge, or awareness of the implications of such knowledge. At least one aspect of disturbance of self-awareness is a disruption in the judgment of the implications of acquired knowledge, a deficit in self-reflectiveness. Self-awareness is an inherent factor intermingled with the executive control functions of planning, coordinating, and monitoring, although it appears as well to be independent of them.

6. *Immediacy and warmth are essential.* Immediacy and warmth appear to be key characteristics in normal awareness. Examples suggest two possible disturbances based on the characteristics of the immediacy and warmth of memory. In patient R.B., with reduplicative paramnesia, immediacy and warmth left the patient with

a subjective certainty of that memory. In conjunction with the damage to temporal and limbic regions, R.B. was left with a distorted yet irresistible sense of familiarity, but not identity, about the second family. Whereas the ability to assemble the truth about the situation was retained, the ability to reconcile the independent and competing information was lacking because of the frontal disturbance. In the TBI patients, on the other hand, there appeared to be a dissociation between frontotemporal (limbic) regions, perhaps due to focal frontal pathology. There was a loss of the warmth and immediacy, leading to a sensation of dissociation of memories from the personal self. As the patients recovered and judgment returned, there was gradual resolution and reintegration.

7. *Certain aspects of awareness also appear to imply the future.* Many of the patients described appear to live entirely in the present. Implications of the past and the relation to decisions in the future appear to be significantly hindered. Implications are therefore limited in scope. This characteristic has significance, particularly in light of increasing emphasis on the role of the frontal cortex in the temporal integration of behavior (e.g., Fuster, 1985, 1988; Ingvar, 1985).

DISORDERS OF AWARENESS: A PROPOSAL

This chapter has presented concepts of disordered awareness after frontal lobe disturbances. The evidence has suggested several conclusions and concepts for future research: First, damage to the frontal lobe or at least to frontal functions results in a general deficit in self-awareness and not a focal disturbance of awareness such as neglect. Second, within this general concept there are specific characteristics that may be used to define the term. Third, because of the differing characteristics of the self, the examples suggested the possiblity of fractionation of disordered self-awareness. The presentation may be different in different patients, perhaps because of variation in lesion location.

Disorders of awareness after frontal lobe damage are different, at least in part, from disorders secondary to lesions in posterior or basal brain regions. The common theme of dissociation of knowledge or fact from a self-reflectiveness provides us with a broad canvas for speculation. Following Stuss and Benson (1986), knowledge is related to posterior/basal systems, these regions being pertinent to providing the information concerning the internal and external milieu (Nauta, 1971). Damage to one of these specific posterior systems interrupts the feedback loop related to the knowledge of the specific external or internal (e.g., visceral feelings) reality (see Chapter 4). The consequence is specific to the functional system disturbed, e.g., hemiinattention or unawareness of a comprehension deficit.

If, on the other hand, the posterior/basal brain regions are undamaged, knowledge is intact. Denial or even unawareness defined as absence of knowledge would be rare. Error evaluation, if the question is properly structured, is appropriate. If it is accepted that the prefrontal cortex is concerned with the self, damage in this region would result not in loss of knowledge but in a disorder of self-awareness or self-reflectiveness as described above.

Earlier concepts of reciprocal inhibition between frontoparietal regions help us understand this proposal. Magnetic apraxia, observed after focal frontal lobe lesions, was proposed as being secondary to the loss of frontal inhibition over the parietal searching and grasping tendencies (Denny-Brown and Chambers, 1958). Lhermitte's (1986) concept of the "environmental dependency syndrome" similarly proposed a lack of environmental automacy because the parietal lobe was now unapposed without frontal inhibition. Mesulam (1986) related these concepts to disorders of awareness.

> Perhaps the proper psychological distance from the environment reflects the balance of reciprocal inhibition between prefrontal cortex and the posterior parietal network. According to this hypothesis, prefrontal lesions could promote not only an excessive approach to the environment, leading to distractibility and concreteness, but perhaps also an excessive distance from the intrapsychic processes necessary for insight, foresight, and abstraction. In contrast, lesions in the parietal network could promote an avoidance of the extrapersonal world and perhaps an excessive reliance on intrapsychic data, even when these are in conflict with external reality. This state could lead to the anosognosia and psychotic hallucinations that emerge in conjunction with parietal lesions. . . . This janusian view of frontoparietal interactions with one face, under frontal control, directed inward, and the other, under parietal influence, directed outward, may have considerable value for investigating the physiological foundation of complex psychological states, especially those related to self-awareness. [p. 322]

CONCLUSION

The early literature has paved the way for our present understanding and stressed the primary conclusion. The frontal lobes are important for awareness. Although it may be debated whether it is the highest brain function and intimately associated with consciousness, there is little doubt that damage to the frontal lobes results in serious problems in awareness of deficit, with subsequent difficulties in rehabilitation. Indeed, patients with frontal lobe disturbance may be the most difficult to rehabilitate. The implications for treating patients with various disorders that involve frontal systems, such as dementia and head injury, are obvious. Knowledge of disorders of awareness is essential from both clinical and theoretical viewpoints.

ACKNOWLEDGMENTS

M. Lecompte typed the manuscript. Research funding for the new studies reported were funded in part by the Ontario Mental Health Foundation and the Medical Research Council of Canada.

REFERENCES

Ackerly, S. S., and Benton, A. L. (1947). Report of a case with bilateral frontal lobe defect. *Res. Publ. Assoc. Res. Nerv. Ment. Dis.* 27:479–504.

Alexander, M. P., Stuss, D. T., and Benson, D. F. (1979). Capgras syndrome: reduplicative phenomenon. *Neurology* 29:334–339.

Bekhterev, V. M. (1907). *Foundation of the Science of Brain Functions.* Vol. 7. St. Petersburg [in Russian]. Referenced in Luria and Homskaya (1964).

Bianchi, L. (1895). The function of the frontal lobes. *Brain* 18:497–522.

Bianchi, L. (1922). *The Mechanism of the Brain and the Functions of the Frontal Lobes.* New York: William Wood.

Blumer, D., and Benson, D. F. (1975). Personality changes with frontal and temporal lobe lesions. In D. F. Benson and D. Blumer (eds.), *Psychiatric Aspects of Neurologic Disease.* Vol. 1. New York: Grune & Stratton, pp. 151–170.

Brickner, R. M. (1936). *The Intellectual Functions of the Frontal Lobes.* New York: Macmillan.

Capgras, J., and Reboul-Lachaux, J. (1923). L'illusion des "soises" dans un delire systematisé chronique. *Bull. Soc. Clin. Med. Ment.* 2:6–16.

Cummings, J. L. (1985). Organic delusions: phenomenology, anatomical correlation and review. *Br. J. Psychiatry* 146:184–197.

Damasio, A. R. (1979). The frontal lobes. In K. M. Heilman and E. Valenstein (eds.), *Clinical Neuropsychology.* New York: Oxford University Press, pp. 360–412.

Denny-Brown, D. (1951). The frontal lobes and their functions. In A. Feiling (ed.), *Modern Trends in Neurology.* London: Butterworth, pp. 13–89.

Denny-Brown, D., and Chambers, R. A. (1958). The parietal lobe and behaviour. *Res. Publ. Assoc. Res. Nerv. Ment. Dis.* 36:35–117.

De Nobele, E. (1835). *Annales de Medecine Belge.* Referenced in Blumer and Benson (1975).

Feuchtwanger, E. (1923). Die funktionen des stirnhirns ihre pathologie und psychologie. *Monogr. Ges. Neurol. Psychiatr.* 38:4–194. Referenced in Luria and Homskaya (1964).

Flechsig, P. E. (1908). Bemerkungen über die Hörsphaeres des menschlichen Gehirns. *Neurol. Zentralbl.* 27:2–7, 50–57. Referenced in Meyer (1974).

Freeman, W., and Watts, J. W. (1942). *Psychosurgery, Intelligence, Emotions and Social Behavior Following Prefrontal Lobotomy for Mental Disorders.* Springfield, IL: Charles C Thomas.

Freeman, W., and Watts, J. W. (1948). Frontal lobe functions as revealed by psychosurgery. *Dig. Neurol. Psychiatry Inst. Living* 16:62.

Freeman, W., and Watts, J. W. (1950). *Psychosurgery in the Treatment of Mental Disorders and Intractable Pain.* 2nd Ed. Springfield, IL: Charles C Thomas.

Fulton, J. F. (1948). *Functional Localization in the Frontal Lobes and Cerebellum.* Oxford: Clarendon Press.

Fuster, J. M. (1985). The prefrontal cortex, mediator of cross-temporal contingencies. *Hum. Neurobiol.* 4:169–179.

Fuster, J. M. (1988). *The Prefrontal Cortex, Anatomy, Physiology, and Neuropsychology of the Frontal Lobe.* New York: Raven Press.

German, W. J., and Fox, J. C. (1932). Observations following unilateral lobectomies. *Res. Publ. Assoc. Res. Nerv. Ment. Dis.* 13:378–434.

Goldstein, K. (1936). The significance of the frontal lobes for mental performance. *J. Neurol. Psychopathol.* 17:27–40.

Goldstein, K. (1944). Mental changes due to frontal lobe damage. *J. Psychol.* 17:187–208.

Greenblatt, M., and Solomon, H. C. (1966). Studies of lobotomy. In: *The Brain and Human Behavior. Proceedings of the Association for Research in Nervous and Mental Disease.* New York: Hafner, pp. 19–34.

Harlow, J. M. (1868). Recovery after severe injury to the brain. *Publ. Mass. Med. Soc.* 2:327–346.

Heath, R. G., and Pool, J. L. (1948). Bilateral frontal resection of frontal cortex for the treatment of psychoses. *J. Nerv. Ment. Dis.* 107:411–429.

Hoffman, C. K. (1869). *Z. Rat. Med. Leipz.* 34:179. Referenced in Denny-Brown (1951).

Hutton, E. J. (1947). Personality change after leucotomy. *J. Ment. Sci.* 93:31–42.

Ingvar, D. H. (1985). "Memory of the future": an essay on the temporal organization of conscious awareness. *Hum. Neurobiol.* 4:127–136.

James, W. (1890). *The Principles of Psychology.* Vols. 1 and 2. New York: Dover. Republished (1952). Chicago: *Encyclopaedia Britannica.*

Jarvie, H. F. (1954). Frontal lobe wounds causing disinhibition: a study of six cases. *J. Neurol. Neurosurg. Psychiatry* 17:14–32.

Kleist, K. (1934). *Gehirnpathologie.* Leipzig: Barth.

Konow, A., and Pribram, K. H. (1970). Error recognition and utilization produced by injury to the frontal cortex in man. *Neuropsychologia* 8:489–491.

Lewis, S. W. (1987). Brain imaging in a case of Capgras' syndrome. *Br. J. Psychiatry* 150:117–121.

Lhermitte, F. (1986). Human anatomy and the frontal lobes. II. Patient behavior in complex and social situations: the "environmental dependency syndrome." *Ann. Neurol.* 19:335–343.

Lipkin, B. (1988). Capgras syndrome heralding the development of dementia. *Br. J. Psychiatry* 153:117–118.

Luria, A. R. (1969). Frontal lobe syndromes. In P. J. Vinken and G. W. Bruyn (eds.), *Handbook of Clinical Neurology.* Vol. 2. Amsterdam: North Holland, pp. 725–757.

Luria, A. R., and Homskaya, E. D. (1964). Disturbance in the regulative role of speech with frontal lobe lesions. In J. M. Warren and K. Akert (eds.), *The Frontal Granular Cortex and Behavior.* New York: McGraw-Hill, pp. 353–371.

Mazziotta, J. C., and Phelps, M. E. (1986). Positron emission tomography: Studies of the brain. In M. E. Phelps, J. C. Mazziotta, and H. R. Schebert (eds.), *Positron Emission Tomography and Autoradiography: Principles and Applications for the Brain and Heart.* New York: Raven Press, pp. 493–579.

Mesulam, M-M. (1981). A cortical network for directed attention and unilateral neglect. *Ann. Neurol.* 10:309–325.

Mesulam, M-M. (1986). Frontal cortex and behavior. *Ann. Neurol.* 19:320–325.

Meyer, A. (1974). The frontal lobe syndrome, the aphasias and related conditions: contribution to the history of cortical localization. *Brain* 97:565–600.

Milner, B. (1965). Visually-guided maze learning in man: effects of bilateral hippocampal, bilateral frontal, and unilateral cerebral lesions. *Neuropsychologia* 3:317–338.

Morrison, R. L., and Tarter, R. E. (1984). Neuropsychological findings related to Capgras' syndrome. *Biol. Psychol.* 19:1119–1128.

Nauta, W. J. H. (1971). The problem of the frontal lobe: a reinterpretation. *J. Psychiatr. Res.* 8:167–187.

Pick, A. (1903). On reduplicative paramnesia. *Brain* 26:260–267.

Prigatano, G. P. (1988). Anosognosia, delusions, and altered self-awareness after brain injury: a historical perspective. *BNI Quarterly* 4:40–48.

Robinson, M. F., and Freeman, W. (1954). *Psychosurgery and the Self.* Orlando, Grune & Stratton.

Sachs, E. (1927). Symptomatology of a group of frontal lobe lesions. *Brain* 50:474–479.

Shallice, T. (1982): Specific impairments of planning. In D. E. Broadbent and L. Weiskrantz (eds.), *The Neuropsychology of Cognitive Function.* London: The Royal Society, pp. 199–209.

Stengel, E. (1952). The patients' attitude to leucotomy and its effects. *J. Ment. Sci.* 98:382–388.

Stuss, D. T. (1987). Contribution of frontal lobe injury to cognitive impairment after closed head injury: methods of assessment and recent findings. In H. S. Levin, J. Grafman, and H. M. Eisenberg (eds.), *Neurobehavioral Recovery from Head Injury.* New York: Oxford University Press, pp. 166–177.

Stuss, D. T., and Benson, D. F. (1986). *The Frontal Lobes.* New York: Raven Press.

Stuss, D. T., and Benson, D. F. (1987). The frontal lobes and control of cognition and memory. In E. Perecman (ed.). *The Frontal Lobes Revisited.* New York: IRBN Press, pp. 141–158.

Tulving, E. (1983). *Elements of Episodic Memory.* Oxford: Clarendon Press.

Tulving, E. (1985). Memory and consciousness. *Can. Psychol.* 26:1–12.

Tulving, E. (1989). Memory: Performance, knowledge, and experience. *European Journal of Cognitive Psychology,* 1:3–26.

Weinstein, E. A., and Kahn, R. L. (1955). *Denial of Illness: Symbolic and Physiological Aspects.* Springfield, IL: Charles C Thomas.

Welt, L. (1888). Ueber Charakterveränderungen des Menschen in Folge des Lasionen des Stirnhirns. *Dtsch. Arch. Klin. Med.* 42:334. Referenced in Luria and Homskaya (1964).

6

Unawareness of Deficits in Dementia and Schizophrenia

SUSAN M. McGLYNN
AND ALFRED W. KASZNIAK

Dementia and schizophrenia represent brain dysfunctions associated with generalized cognitive impairments. Consequently, one might expect that demented and schizophrenic patients would exhibit disturbed cognition in the domain of awareness. Yet there has been relatively little systematic study of awareness in these populations, in contrast to the substantial amount of research on awareness disturbances in other cognitively impaired populations (McGlynn and Schacter, 1989). The purposes of the present chapter are to: (1) critically review the existing literature concerned with unawareness of deficits in dementia and schizophrenia; (2) describe some techniques used in our own research for quantitatively assessing the degree to which demented patients are aware of their deficits; (3) discuss the methodological problems associated with evaluating awareness in dementing populations; and (4) consider the role of frontal lobe dysfunction in the awareness problems characterizing dementia and schizophrenia.

Unawareness of deficits has been observed in a broad range of neuropsychological syndromes and has significant implications for patient treatment and management. Patients who are unaware of their problems are unlikely to cooperate with treatment plans or accept help from concerned family members. Furthermore, patients may attempt to perform activities that are entirely unrealistic given their disabilities. Both demented and schizophrenic patients who lack awareness of their deficits may pose serious problems for family members and other caretakers. Informing families of the awareness disturbance and possible consequences would help them prepare for and deal with the difficult situations they may confront. In addition to the practical importance of studying awareness, the theoretical insights that may be gained from research in this area could be far-reaching. Examination of disturbed awareness in different neurological disorders such as dementia and schizophrenia, as well as the potential neuro-pathological factors linking the two, may help to elucidate the process by which awareness is compromised.

There is little experimental evidence for unawareness of deficits in the dementing illnesses; however, consideration of clinical descriptions and those few systematic studies that have been done suggest that unawareness phenomena do occur in dementing syndromes. A brief overview of this literature is presented in the next section, followed by some preliminary findings from our own research with Huntington's disease patients. We then turn to unawareness of deficits in schizophrenic patients. The main purpose of this discussion is to raise questions about the processes and mechanisms disrupted in dementing disorders and schizophrenia that may prevent people from being aware of and monitoring their own cognitive functions.

UNAWARENESS OF DEFICITS IN VARIOUS DEMENTING DISORDERS

Patients with certain kinds of dementing illness have been described as lacking awareness or insight into their condition. Frederiks (1985) referred to this phe-nomenon as "anosognosia for dementia." The term *anosognosia* was introduced by Babinski (1914) to describe the lack of knowledge, awareness, or recognition of disease observed in patients with hemiplegia attributable to stroke. The term has since been used more generally to refer to unawareness of any neurological or neuropsychological deficit. In the dementia literature, unawareness of deficits is most frequently reported as a clinical feature of "cortical" dementias, such as Alzheimer's disease and Pick's disease (e.g., Gustafson and Nilsson, 1982; Schneck, Reisberg, and Ferris, 1982; Benson, 1983; Mahendra, 1984; Reisberg, Gordon, McCarthy, and Ferris, 1985; Neary, Snowden, Bowen, et al., 1986). However, lack of insight has also been observed as a striking aspect of Hunting-ton's disease, a hereditary neurological disorder accompanied by what has been classified as a "subcortical" or "frontal-subcortical" dementia syndrome (McHugh and Folstein, 1975; Cummings and Benson, 1984; Joynt and Shoul-son, 1985). In contrast, patients with the predominantly subcortical disorder of Parkinson's disease have been described as exhibiting good comprehension of their illness, even in the most advanced stages of the disease (Danielczyk, 1983).

Awareness of deficits may be a valuable prognostic indicator for ability to function in everyday life. Bergmann, Proctor, and Prudham (1979) examined psychiatric profiles in hospital and community resident elderly persons with dementia and found that lack of insight into their disability was one of the most important features differentiating the two groups. Patients who are unaware of their deficits are unlikely to accept the help and support required to survive in the community and are therefore at risk of being placed in an institutionalized setting.

Alzheimer's disease (AD) is the most prevalent and widely researched dementing illness that occurs during adult life. Clinical descriptions of the more advanced stages of this disease often include loss of insight as a major feature. Schneck et al. (1982) outlined three main phases in the clinical syndrome of AD.

During the initial "forgetfulness" phase patients are described as cognizant of and becoming increasingly anxious about their memory difficulties. As the disease progresses, patients are said to enter the second, "confusional," phase at which time they show definite signs of cognitive impairment, particularly for memory of recent events. According to Schneck et al., patients at this stage reveal a loss of insight into their own deficits, and earlier anxiety is replaced with unawareness of illness. In the most advanced, "dementia," phase patients appear extremely disoriented and may exhibit substantial anxiety despite the continued unawareness of their condition. These phases are thus held to reflect a pattern of decreasing insight and knowledge with increasing severity of the disease process.

Reisberg and colleagues (1985) assessed awareness of deficit in 25 AD patients, five subjects with a primary diagnosis of age-associated cognitive decline consistent with "senescent forgetfulness," and ten control subjects with no memory impairment. Subjects were interviewed and questioned about their own functioning as well as their spouses' functioning. Spouses of subjects were similarly interviewed and questioned about their own functioning and the subject's functioning. Findings revealed that subjects with senescent forgetfulness rated their memory problems as somewhat worse than did the controls, and early "confusional phase" AD patients rated their problems as being considerably worse than did the "forgetfulness phase" AD patients. However, once beyond the early "confusional phase," AD patients tended to rate the degree of their memory impairment as progressively less severe, whereas objective measures of memory function provided evidence of progressive deterioration. Spouses' reports of patients' memory deficit increased consistently as patients' level of impairment increased on objective measures. Patients with moderate to severe memory impairment also tended to minimize their emotional difficulties. They rated their emotional problems as substantially less severe than did their spouses. Patients did exhibit preserved insight into two domains: (1) throughout the illness they showed insight into their ability to communicate with the spouse; and (2) despite marked unawareness of their own deficits during the final phase, patients continued to display awareness of their spouses' cognitive functioning, i.e., patients' ratings of spouses' cognitive abilities closely matched the spouses' ratings of themselves. Based on the latter observation, Reisberg et al. concluded that AD patients were engaging in defensive denial, resulting in an apparent "lack of insight" into their own deficits.

Contrary to the foregoing results, the findings of Neary et al. (1986) suggested that more globally demented patients may have greater insight into their disabilities than those patients at an earlier stage of cognitive deterioration. These investigators found that different subgroups of AD patients demonstrated different degrees of insight. Eighteen patients diagnosed with AD were separated into four groups based on their neuropsychological profiles. A group of 11 patients characterized by a language disorder, amnesia, and a perceptuospatial disorder showed clear signs of anxiety when required to perform difficult tasks, suggesting some awareness of their cognitive problems. A second group ($n = 3$) with amnesia and a perceptuospatial disorder similarly exhibited anxiety with respect to their defects. Two patients with profound apraxia and amnesia tended to minimize their difficulties but possessed some knowledge of their disability. Finally, two patients with amnesia alone admitted to memory impairment but appeared not to understand the severity of the disorder and exhibited no overt anxiety. These findings suggest that there may be substantial variability in awareness among dementia patients.

Other clinical reports of AD have emphasized an early loss of insight in contrast to unawareness during the late stage (Mahendra, 1984; Frederiks, 1985; Joynt and Shoulson, 1985). For example, Frederiks (1985) indicated that the patient is usually unaware of the gradual onset of dementia occurring in both AD and Pick's disease. Similarly, Mahendra (1984) noted the early loss of insight in both AD and Pick's disease. However, Gustafson and Nilsson (1982) found that early loss of insight is a useful dimension for differentiating between AD and Pick's disease. They developed rating scales to identify AD and Pick's disease that evaluated a number of clinical features. Patients with Pick's disease were rated substantially higher than AD patients with respect to early loss of insight on these scales. Thus loss of insight may progress at a different rate in Pick's disease than in AD. Interestingly, both of these dementias are typically associated with signs of frontal lobe pathology (Mahendra, 1984; Kaszniak, 1986), but frontal degeneration is generally more severe in the early stages of Pick's disease than in AD.

Experimental evidence of unawareness of memory dysfunction in AD patients was provided by Schacter, McLachlan, Moscovitch, and Tulving (1986; see also Chapter 8). Alzheimer's patients were given a categorized list and were asked to predict how many items they would be able to recall. Relative to control subjects, AD patients grossly overestimated their ability to remember.

Danielczyk (1983) designed a clinical rating scale consisting of 18 parameters, including "insight into own illness," to assess mental deterioration in four groups of patients: Parkinson's disease (PD), Alzheimer's disease (AD), atypical Parkinson's disease (AP) with signs of vascular disease, and multiple infarction dementia (MID). Although the PD group had suffered from the disease for more than 8 years, there was little disturbance in their memory, reading, writing, orientation, motivation, and initiative, or apraxia. In contrast, the other three groups were impaired to a significantly greater extent on these measures. In addition to the functional differences observed between PD patients and the other groups, electroencephalography (EEG) data revealed significant differences. The "alpha reaction" registered in the EEG of the PD group was near normal, whereas that of all other groups was diminished or absent; moreover, there were significantly fewer "general changes" and "focal signs" in the PD group than in the other three groups. The specific scale for the "insight" parameter ranged from 0 to 3, where 0 indicates no awareness disturbance and 3 reflects a severe disturbance. Patients with PD were found to retain reasonably good insight into their illness, whereas those in the other three groups exhibited disturbed awareness of their deficits. The AD patients showed the least comprehension of their illness, followed by the AP group. The MID patients, though also lacking awareness of their condition, were significantly less impaired on this dimension than the AD group.

The foregoing study suggests that in PD patients with little evidence of cortical dysfunction and dementia there is retention of insight about their illness. In contrast, patients with disorders involving cortical atrophy and cognitive impairment appear to lose insight about their deficits.

Huntington's disease (HD) is generally considered to be a "frontal-subcortical" dementia syndrome; thus one might expect that awareness would be compromised in this group. In fact, there is some evidence suggesting that HD patients lack awareness of their defects. Clinical observations of unawareness of deficits in HD were reported as early as 1923 when Meggendorfer (cited in Bruyn, 1968) conducted a major study on the psychiatric symptoms of HD. He noted that a prominent characteristic of HD is a lack of insight into one's disease. Similarly, Bruyn (1968) included loss of insight as a main feature of the dementia associated with HD. He also noted that, despite marked impairment of intellectual processes, HD patients rarely exhibit confusional states, disorientation, or delirium. Thus the unawareness could not be attributed to confusional disturbances in this population. In a discussion of psychopathology in HD, Wilson and Garron (1979) pointed out that self-report measures would not be a valid method of investigating psychopathology in this syndrome, as insight is often compromised.

More recently, Caine and Shoulson (1983) evaluated 30 patients with HD regarding their insight into the process of their disease. Patients were asked such questions as, "Do you have problems with your memory?" "Has your personality changed since you've had Huntington's?" "What do you see happening to you in the future?" Patients' responses to these questions were judged by the interviewer in terms of degree of awareness. Results revealed that 19 of the 30 patients were judged fully insightful about their condition, 7 exhibited partial insight (i.e., described some deficiency but denied other changes), and 4 completely denied changes in either behavior or intellectual function. Ten of the eleven patients lacking awareness of their deficits had been classified as moderately or severely impaired individuals based on their functional disability in everyday life. Rated functional disability correlated highly with increased caudate atrophy as assessed using computed tomography. Of ten mildly disabled patients, one had partial insight and the other nine were completely realistic in assessing their problems. Consistent with these findings, Mahendra (1984) noted that insight may be preserved until more advanced stages of the disease process. The high frequency of suicide during the initial stages of the disease (Oltman and Friedman, 1961) in contrast to later stages may also be consistent with the notion that insight declines with progression of the disease. Interestingly, Caine and Shoulson (1983) also reported that most of the moderately and severely impaired patients in their study manifested a lack of self-initiated activities, whereas fewer than half of the mildly affected individuals exhibited this apathy. Apathy can be a sign of frontal lobe damage. This finding suggests the possibility that, with progressive frontal degeneration and caudate atrophy, both apathy and lack of insight become apparent.

Bradley (1984) provided a revealing description of an HD patient who appeared to be completely unaware of his movement disturbance.

> He fidgeted, sat about, got up, sat about some more and was euphoric. When I asked about his ability to perform certain movements, he said he was fine and

walked over to the bookcase, picked up a book and threw it into the air and let it crash to the deck. This event did not worry him, he just said it was a mistake. [p. 338]

The possibility that HD patients may be unaware of their choreiform movements has not, to our knowledge, been reported in the literature before. The Bradley (1984) case description suggests that this phenomenon may occur in HD.

Contrary to the above, there also exist several clinical descriptions arguing for a preservation of insight in most HD patients. Caine, Hunt, Weingartner, and Ebert (1978) maintained that the 18 HD patients assessed in their study were acutely aware of their cognitive disabilities. This conclusion was based on the observation that 16 of the 18 patients complained of their inability to perform mental functions at the level they had attained previously. In addition, many patients noted a change of temperament or disposition. These observations were derived from frequent clinical interviews and longitudinal follow-ups. Similar findings were reported by Aminoff, Marshall, Smith, and Wyke (1975). Clinical records suggested that 9 of 11 HD patients seen during assessment of cognitive functions retained insight into their condition. No criteria for assessing awareness were provided. The two patients considered to be lacking awareness were those with the lowest Wechsler Adult Intelligence Scale (WAIS) IQs. Based on his clinical impressions, Lishman (1987) noted that judgment is often severely impaired as part of the widespread intellectual decline in HD, but insight is commonly preserved for a considerable length of time. According to Lishman, the patient may thus be aware of his cognitive deficits, complaining that he feels dulled, slow, and forgetful and that his thinking is confused.

In summary, the paucity of experimental evidence for unawareness of deficits in various dementing illnesses and the conflicting clinical reports of the phenomenon make it impossible to reach any conclusions about the degree to which disturbed awareness occurs in these disorders. Two major methodological shortcomings are evident in studies of anosognosia in dementia. First, clinicians and investigators have often relied solely on their subjective observations of the patient to determine the presence of anosognosia; few investigators have developed quantitative methodologies for objectively evaluating the presence or degree of awareness disturbance. In a number of reports, the criteria for assessing awareness were not even discussed. Second, although the relation of intellectual impairment and generalized confusion to anosognosia is an important issue, the nature and severity of these deficits were rarely assessed in a systematic fashion.

Another problem concerns the justification for inferences drawn from published observations. Reisberg et al. (1985) argued that the discrepancy they observed between AD patients' assessment of their own and others' cognitive functioning indicates that patients are engaging in defensive denial. However, such a discrepancy does not necessarily imply that denial is motivated. It may simply reflect the fact that patients are basing their judgments on past information concerning themselves and their spouse. Because the spouse's level of functioning has presumably not changed substantially, patients' judgments of them are accurate. However, because their own condition has changed, patients' inability to incorporate and monitor new information about themselves results in defective insight. Related to this issue is the possibility that patients' apparent "preserved" insight into spouses' cognitive functioning may be attributable to measurement range problems. That is, because there is little variability in spouses' functioning over time, it is not surprising that patients and spouses ratings appear similar. It is not clear whether patients would exhibit preserved insight in this domain if they had to rate cognitive functioning of others who have, like themselves, changed in their cognitive abilities over time. Finally, most investigators have failed to consider that degree of awareness may vary for different deficits within a given individual. Reports of unawareness in dementia have primarily referred to diminished insight into one's condition or into the process of one's disease, rather than unawareness of a specific deficit. Yet with many neuropsychological syndromes a striking specificity can be observed, whereby patients may be acutely aware of one disability and entirely oblivious of another (McGlynn and Schacter, 1989).

In our own research with dementia patients, we have attempted to develop some systematic techniques for evaluating patients' insight into their conditions. Although this research is in its early stages, there are some suggestive preliminary findings indicating lack of awareness in these populations. Our ongoing study is described in the next section, followed by a discussion of the methodological problems encountered in this investigation.

ASSESSMENT OF AWARENESS IN HUNTINGTON'S DISEASE

No attempts have been made to investigate systematically whether HD patients lack insight into their deficits; yet there are a number of advantages to studying awareness in this dementia group. First, HD patients become progressively demented and could therefore be examined at different stages of their disease to determine the relation between cognitive impairment and development of unawareness. Furthermore, these patients remain relatively verbal and are thus able to answer questions about their condition until the most advanced stages of their disease. Second, HD patients have both memory and motor deficits, permitting assessment of differential awareness of the two impairments. Third, the frontal lobe pathology associated with HD provides a theoretically based reason to suspect that some degree of unawareness may develop in this population.

Consideration of clinical reports of unawareness in HD patients and the literature concerned with anosognosia in other neuropsychological syndromes raises a number of interesting questions with respect to unawareness phenomena in HD. First, given the progressive frontal lobe pathology associated with HD and, to a lesser extent, atrophy in posterior cortical regions, do HD patients lack awareness of their deficits and does degree of awareness correlate with progression of disease and severity of dementia? Second, are there differences in terms of the degree of awareness for different deficits? Third, is it the case that HD patients possess a general awareness of the existence of their deficits but underestimate the degree to which these disabilities affect their performance in everyday life?

Neuropathological investigations of HD reveal atrophy of the basal ganglia, particularly the caudate nucleus and putamen, extending to the frontal, parietal, and occipital cortex as the disease progresses (Bruyn, 1968; Bruyn, Bots and Dom, 1979). Two prominent deficits are evident relatively early in HD: choreiform movements and a severe memory impairment. The chorea consists of irregular, involuntary movements of certain muscles or muscle groups that cause considerable difficulty when performing everyday activities. Patients commonly exhibit dysarthric, incoherent speech, smacking and licking movements of the lips and tongue, facial grimaces, twitching fingers and flexed toes, athetoid twisting movements of the arms, shoulder shrugging, and an unsteady gait (Bradley, 1984; Mahendra, 1984; Joynt and Shoulson, 1985; Lishman, 1987). In the domain of memory function, HD patients have considerable difficulty learning new material on short-term and long-term recall tasks and have significant problems in retrieval of information from long-term memory (Butters, Sax, Montgomery, and Tarlow, 1978; Martone, Butters, Payne, et al., 1984; Butters, Wolfe, Granholm, and Martone, 1986; Wilson, Como, Garron, et al., 1987).

Several investigators have suggested that patients with HD demonstrate impaired "cortical executive functions" closely resembling that observed in classic frontal lobe patients (e.g., Benson and Geschwind, 1975; Blumer and Benson, 1975; Caine et al., 1978). Both HD patients and patients with frontal damage exhibit loss of initiative, slowness, indifference, and apathy. These similarities may be attributable to the close anatomical relation between the frontal region whose destruction likely causes these personality alterations and the basal ganglia affected in HD: Damage affecting either of these regions or their interconnections may lead to similar behavioral manifestations (Blumer and Benson, 1975). The frontal lobe symptomatology observed in HD patients led us to hypothesize that some degree of unawareness occurs in this dementia syndrome.

Our research was designed to assess whether HD patients lack awareness of their deficits and to determine whether patients exhibit differential awareness of their motor disturbance and cognitive impairment. A group of eight HD patients have thus far been examined in this study. Patient information is presented in Table 6–1. Five patients exhibited clear cognitive impairment on the Mini-Mental State Examination (MMSE) (Folstein, Folstein, and McHugh, 1975), as defined by a cutoff score of 25. Patients' scores on the MMSE ranged from 12 to 29. These patients ranged in age from 22 to 68 years and were at various stages of the disease process. According to the Shoulson and Fahn (1979) scale of func-

TABLE 6-1 Huntington's Disease Patient Information

Patient	Age	MMSE	Functional stage
D.A.	40	12	5
H.U.	54	13	5
F.O.	22	14	4
M.O.	34	21	4
H.A.	54	24	3
K.I.	68	26	2
S.C.	54	28	2
S.A.	59	29	2

tional capacity, three patients were at stage 2, one at stage 3, two at stage 4, and two at stage 5. One of the severely demented patients (stage 5) participated only in the initial part of the study. Spouses or other family members of the HD patients served as control subjects. The study included three major components, which are referred to, respectively, as (1) the Daily Difficulties Questionnaire, (2) the Motor Task Performance Predictions, and (3) the Cognitive Task Performance Predictions.

On the *Daily Difficulties Questionnaire* patients were asked to rate, on a 7-point scale, the degree to which they currently experience difficulty performing a variety of activities in everyday life compared to 5 years ago. There are 12 items concerned with motor abilities (e.g., walking up a flight of stairs, signing your name) and 12 items related to cognitive, particularly memory, functions (e.g., remembering a five-item shopping list if you did not have it written down, recalling the order of things you did yesterday). Patients were asked to rate themselves and control subjects on these items. In addition, controls were asked to rate their own functioning and patients' functioning on the questionnaire items. A significant difference between patients' self-ratings and relatives' ratings of patients on this questionnaire would suggest some degree of unawareness on the part of patients. That is, if patients rate themselves as having considerably less difficulty than relatives report them as having, patients may be underestimating their problems. If patients' ratings of relatives closely match relatives' ratings of themselves, it would rule out the possibility that a general impairment of judgment is responsible for patients' underestimation of their difficulties. Finally, analysis of the type of item (motor versus cognitive) contributing most to a patient–relative discrepancy regarding the patient's functioning, may reveal differential awareness of deficits.

The second part of the study, the *Motor Task Performance Predictions,* is specifically concerned with assessing patients' awareness of their choreiform movements. Patients were asked to perform six motor tasks following prediction of their own performance on these tasks (e.g., how many words from a list of ten they can pronounce clearly; how many times they will step off a 10-foot straight line). Control subjects were also asked to estimate patients' motor ability on these tasks. For two of these tasks—the Finger Tapping Test and the Grooved Pegboard—patients and relatives were told how an average person would perform, and they could thus make judgments about patients' performance in comparison to this standard. Predictions of performance on these tasks would be difficult without knowing how people generally perform. Deviations of patients' estimates from objective measures and spouses' predictions provide an index of unawareness of motor deficit. The degree to which patients accurately predict their performance was compared to the accuracy of relatives' predictions.

Finally, on the *Cognitive Task Performance Predictions,* patients' insight into their memory disorder was evaluated using four retrieval tasks: a paired-associate recall test (immediate and delayed), a digit span task, and a verbal fluency task. Patients were asked to predict their performance on each memory task prior to its administration. Relatives were similarly asked to predict patients' performance on these tasks. Patients and relatives were told how the average person performs on the digit span and verbal fluency tasks in order to provide a standard for comparison and ease the task of predicting. Patients' predictions were compared to both their actual performance and to relatives' estimates of patients' retrieval ability in order to determine the degree to which HD patients lack awareness of their memory impairment. The accuracy of patients' estimates of their own performance was compared to the accuracy of relatives' estimates of patients' performance on the memory tests.

Analysis of the Daily Difficulties Questionnaire revealed that patients' ratings of their own difficulties on both the motor and cognitive items are significantly lower than relatives' ratings of patients' problems ($p < 0.01$). These results are presented in Figure 6–1. In contrast, no difference was observed between patients' ratings of relatives and relatives' ratings of themselves (Fig. 6–2). If we assume that relatives are reasonably accurate in their judgments about patients' difficulties, these results suggest that HD patients do not appreciate the severity of their motor and cognitive disabilities. The fact that patients were accurate in their assessment of relatives clearly indicates that patients understood how to use the rating scale, thus eliminating the possibility that their unawareness of their own deficits was simply a consequence of a general impairment of judgment. No main effect of item type was observed, nor was there any interaction between item type and rater. Thus there was no evidence for differential awareness of motor versus cognitive problems. A significant interaction

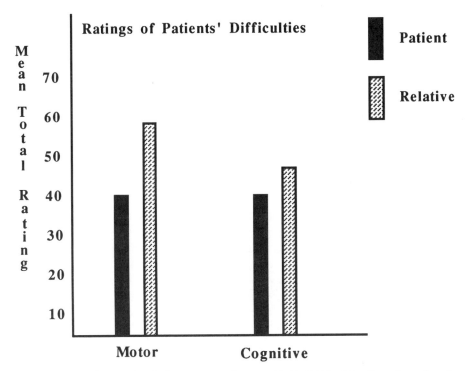

Figure 6–1. Patient and relative mean ratings on Daily Difficulties Questionnaire, for patients' difficulties.

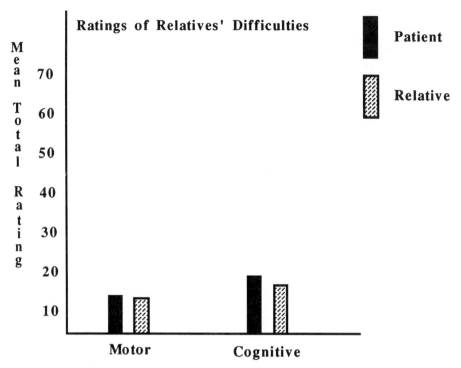

Figure 6–2. Patient and relative mean ratings on Daily Difficulties Questionnaire, for relatives' difficulties.

was found between degree of cognitive impairment and rater (patient versus relative) ($p < 0.05$), indicating that patients who were relatively intact in terms of their cognitive functioning tended to rate themselves as more impaired than their relatives rated them, whereas more demented patients tended to rate themselves as less impaired than relatives reported. This interaction is illustrated in Figures 6–3 and 6–4 for the motor items and cognitive items, respectively.

Contrary to the lack of awareness evident on the questionnaire data, results from the Motor Task Performance Predictions and Cognitive Task Performance Predictions suggest that HD patients are reasonably good at estimating their performance on specific motor tasks and cognitive tasks. Mean accuracy scores for patients' and relatives' predictions are provided in Table 6–2. Accuracy scores were calculated by dividing the predicted performance by the actual performance for each task. Thus an accuracy score of 1.0 indicates a perfect match between predicted performance and actual performance, whereas a score greater or less than 1.0 reflects an overestimation or underestimation of patient performance, respectively. The differences between patients' and relatives' accuracy scores are also provided in Table 6–2.

The accuracy data indicate that patients and relatives are about equally as good at predicting patients' performance on all of the motor tasks and some cognitive tasks. A significant difference between patient and relative accuracy scores is evident on only one of the ten tasks, the paired-associate immediate task, though the observed difference on the paired-associate delayed task

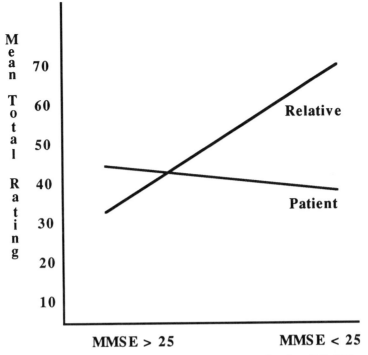

Figure 6–3. Interaction between Mini Mental State Examination (MMSE) scores and rater on Daily Difficulties Questionnaire motor items.

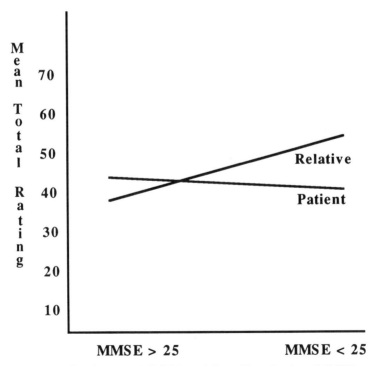

Figure 6–4. Interaction between Mini Mental State Examination (MMSE) scores and rater on Daily Difficulties Questionnaire cognitive items.

TABLE 6–2 Mean Accuracy Scores for Motor and Cognitive Task Performance Predictions

Task	Patient (predicted/actual)	Relative (predicted/actual)	Patient–relative difference
Write word list	1.92	1.13	0.79
Grooved pegboard	1.09	1.15	−0.06
Walk on line	1.03	0.43	0.60
Catch ball	1.59	0.98	0.61
Finger tapping	1.11	1.53	−0.42
Pronounce words	2.24	0.86	1.38
Paired assoc.—immediate	4.38	1.93	2.45*
Paired assoc.—delayed	3.79	1.29	2.50
Digit span	0.98	0.88	0.10
Verbal fluency	1.42	1.54	−0.14

* $p < 0.05$ for paired one-tailed t-test on patient versus relative

approached significance ($p = 0.056$). These results suggest that patients are generally aware of their motor and cognitive disabilities and can make reasonable judgments about how they will perform, given specific tasks in these domains. The seemingly contradictory conclusions of the questionnaire data and the task prediction data may be interpreted in several ways.

First, it is possible that patients were accurately reporting the extent of their problems, whereas relatives were exaggerating the degree to which patients experience difficulty on the everyday activities that appear on the Daily Difficulties Questionnaire. If this situation were the case, one would expect relatives to demonstrate this bias in their predictions of patients' performance on the specific motor and cognitive tasks as well; however, this pattern did not emerge. The finding that patients substantially overpredicted their abilities on two of the prediction tasks also serves to weaken the argument that relatives' inflated ratings of patients' disabilities are responsible for patients' apparent lack of awareness on the questionnaire. Thus it does not appear likely that inaccurate judgment on the part of the relatives can account for the discrepant findings.

Second, patients may be engaging in defensive denial to minimize the psychological impact of their progressive deterioration. The problem with this interpretation is that although patients seem to be underestimating their difficulty on the questionnaire items they are not doing so when predicting their actual performance on most of the specific motor and cognitive tasks. Furthermore, two of the three patients without evidence of cognitive impairment actually rated themselves as more severely disabled on the questionnaire items than did their spouses. This finding suggests that early in the disease process, when patients are beginning to recognize changes in their functioning and would be most likely to use the defense mechanism of denial, they are instead readily admitting and possibly dramatizing their difficulties. Finally, even severely demented patients rated themselves as having considerable difficulty on certain items of the questionnaire but reported having no difficulty on other items that were clearly a severe problem for them. If patients were denying their illness, these kinds of inconsistency in their responses with respect to equally devastating disabilities would not be expected. Thus although defensive denial may play a role in patients' apparent lack of awareness on the questionnaire data, we argue that it is not the major factor accounting for the results.

A third explanation of our findings concerns the different kinds of questions patients are being asked on the questionnaire versus the performance prediction tasks. On the questionnaire, patients are asked to rate the extent to which they currently experience difficulty with various everyday activities compared to 5 years ago. In order to make reasonable judgments on this questionnaire, patients must be aware of how much they have changed over time. The motor and cognitive task performance predictions require patients to judge only their present ability. We propose that the two measures are tapping into different aspects of awareness. McGlynn and Schacter (1989) have pointed out that awareness must not be viewed as a unitary construct whereby patients are either "aware" or "unaware" of their deficits. There may be different components or levels of awareness that can be differentially affected depending on the particular pattern of brain impairment. According to this interpretation, one would not necessarily expect to obtain convergent validity by assessing awareness with a number of measures, as each measure may be sensitive to different dimensions of awareness. The HD patients in this study may be aware of their present level of motor and cognitive functioning, i.e., know that they are below average on these kinds of tasks. However, they may be unaware of the extent to which their performance has deteriorated over the past 5 years. A further study that could test this hypothesis involves asking patients and relatives to predict the patients' current performance on the motor and cognitive tasks as well as their probable performance on these same tasks 5 years ago. If patients' predictions of their earlier performance do not differ from their performance predictions for the present, whereas relatives' predictions are significantly different for the two times, we may conclude that patients lack awareness in the sense that they do not appreciate the progressive deterioration from the "self before" to the "self now."

Another account, not incompatible with the latter, is that patients do lack awareness of their deficits but are able to recruit the limited awareness they still possess to make reasonable performance predictions when presented with specific, concrete motor and cognitive tasks. When asked to engage in a more abstract task of rating how much difficulty they generally have with a variety of motor and cognitive activities in everyday life, such as signing their name or remembering a five-item shopping list, patients are not able to use their preserved self-knowledge to make realistic judgments about their disabilities.

The two interpretations we have proposed to explain the discrepancy between questionnaire and task prediction results do not address the issue of why patients appeared to lack awareness of their deficits when predicting their performance on two of the cognitive tasks. The latter finding suggests that even within a particular measure one may find pockets of unawareness. Even though patients appeared to be aware of their performance abilities on many of the motor and cognitive tasks, they clearly did not appreciate how little they would be able to remember on the paired-associate immediate and delayed tests. Thus not only is it possible to demonstrate dissociations in awareness by asking different questions, as we have on the questionnaire and the prediction tasks, but awareness can also appear fragmented at a far more specific level, as a function of the particular task characteristics patients are asked to consider.

The notion that disruptions in awareness can occur at different levels and in specific domains is further suggested in this study by a number of striking instances of unawareness. Qualitative observations of patients' behavior and their responses to general questions about their situations provide a rich source of information with respect to their awareness.

One of the most demented patients, D.A., was in a wheelchair because of her severe chorea and myoclonic jerks and had extreme difficulty speaking as a consequence of her dysarthria. When asked how many words from a list of ten she would be able to pronounce correctly so others could easily understand her, D.A. reported that she could say all ten. However, her husband accurately predicted that she could not pronounce any of them. When asked how many times she would go off the line while tracing a star-shaped drawing, D.A. predicted five. The husband remarked that if she could hold the pencil at all, which was unlikely, she would probably go off the line about 80 times. It took several attempts for D.A. to grasp the pencil in her fist, and she subsequently made some random marks on the paper wherever the pen happened to make contact. On the paired associate recall test, D.A. predicted that she would be able to recall all ten word pairs on both immediate and delayed tests, whereas her husband predicted 3 and 0, respectively. Her actual performance was zero on both the immediate test and the delayed test. These examples clearly demonstrate that this particular patient was "unaware" in some respects, yet on some of the other motor and cognitive tasks, she was entirely accurate in her predictions.

Another patient, M.O., was generally reasonable when predicting her performance on specific motor and cognitive tasks, yet rated herself as having little or no difficulty on all of the Daily Difficulties Questionnaire items. M.O. is constantly bumping into objects, grimacing, losing her balance, spilling things, dropping her cigarettes while they are burning, and has even accidentally set her bed on fire. When not taking her medication (usually because she has dropped her pills on the floor and cannot pick them up), she exhibits hallucinatory behavior and is unable to look after herself or her house. She commented several times during the testing session that she wants custody of her four children who are currently in foster homes. This patient appears oblivious to her disabilities in everyday life, yet knows that she cannot perform like an average person on specific motor and cognitive tasks.

All patients were asked if they notice their involuntary movements when they look in the mirror. Only three of the eight patients reported noticing any choreiform movements, two of whom reported noticing only finger movements even though they actually exhibited considerable facial grimacing. One patient with little evidence of chorea reported that he did not notice any movements. The other four patients with obvious chorea claimed that they do not see any adventitious movements when they look in the mirror.

The foregoing descriptions certainly suggest that unawareness phenomena do occur in HD, but they also illustrate the variability both within and between individuals in terms of their awareness disturbance. Although the Daily Difficulties Questionnaire was sensitive to a general lack of awareness across patients, there is clearly a need for more sophisticated measures to tap into the complex patterns of unawareness within individuals. The motor and cognitive task performance predictions included in this study represented an attempt to examine patients' awareness in a more concrete and direct fashion, but they were insensitive to the intraindividual awareness disturbances. At this stage, carefully designed single case studies of unawareness in HD patients may prove to be the most appropriate strategy for understanding the awareness disturbances that occur in this population. Until we have a better sense of the manifestations of unawareness phenomena at different stages of HD, it is difficult to develop objective measures for assessing awareness in this group.

NEUROPSYCHOLOGICAL AND NEUROPHYSIOLOGICAL ASPECTS OF SCHIZOPHRENIA

We now turn to a brief review of schizophrenia and unawareness. This subject then leads to a discussion of theoretical issues concerning the possible link between awareness disturbances in dementing disorders and schizophrenia.

Kraepelin's (1919) delineation of "dementia praecox" reflected his belief that schizophrenia is a neurological disease characterized by intellectual and personality deterioration early in adult life. A number of clinical, neuropsychological, and neurophysiological investigations have provided converging evidence for a brain dysfunction in schizophrenia that in many ways resembles certain kinds of dementia, particularly those involving atrophy of the frontal lobes or its connections. Kraepelin's summary of the clinical picture of dementia praecox highlighted the symptomatology often observed in patients with frontal lobe dysfunction.

> [I]n our disease the lower psychic mechanisms as a rule are comparatively little encroached on . . . sensory perception remains . . . well preserved, as also the memory of perceptions, and acquired knowledge and skill. On the other hand judgment is lost, the critical faculty, the creative gift, especially the capacity to make a higher use of knowledge and ability. . . . The patients may also exhibit volition activity of the greatest strength and endurance, but they are wholly incapable of . . . carrying out a well-considered plan." [pp. 221–222]

The resemblance of schizophrenia to frontal lobe dysfunction appears particularly prominent in a subgroup of schizophrenics suffering from "negative" symptoms such as severe social withdrawal, mutism, apathy or loss of goal-directed behavior, attentional dysfunctions, and flat affect (Andreasen and Olsen, 1982; Levin, 1984). Although the early view of schizophrenia as a degenerative brain disease has largely been abandoned, there remain many interesting parallels to the dementing illnesses, particularly Huntington's disease.

A number of neuropsychological studies have provided evidence consistent with clinical descriptions of frontal lobe symptomatology in schizophrenia. For example, schizophrenic patients are severely impaired on tests of word fluency and design fluency—tests particularly sensitive to orbital frontal function (Kolb and Whishaw, 1983). Impaired performance on fluency tests has similarly been reported for dementia patients (Butters et al., 1986). Pronounced deficits of schizophrenics are particularly evident on perceptual and cognitive tasks that involve complex information processing, maintenance of attention, and exercise of rapid psychomotor speed (see Goldstein, 1986, for review). In a discussion of the relation between schizophrenia and prefrontal lobe disease, Goldberg and Costa (1986) emphasized that executive deficits are associated with both disorders. Chapman and Chapman (1973) described the neuropsychological disturbances of schizophrenia as the "general deficit syndrome." This generality of deficit is reminiscent of the broad range of cognitive functions affected in dementia syndromes. In addition to impaired performance on tests sensitive to frontal lobe function, schizophrenics exhibit a memory deficit on tests of verbal and nonverbal memory, suggesting the possibility of some temporal lobe involvement in this disease (Kolb and Whishaw, 1983).

A variety of neurophysiological data suggest a rather complex brain dysfunction in schizophrenic patients, involving areas of the frontal cortex and basal ganglia (Seidman, 1983; Buchsbaum and Haier, 1987). For example, studies have found significantly lower metabolic rates in the basal ganglia of unmedicated schizophrenics than in normal subjects (Sheppard, Gruzelier, Manchanda, et al., 1983). This finding of reduced metabolic activity in the basal ganglia has also been reported for HD (Kuhl, Metter, Riege, and Hawkins, 1985). Other studies have indicated relative metabolic underactivity of the frontal lobes of schizophrenics, similar to that observed in patients with dementia (e.g., Bustany, Henry, Rotrou, et al., 1985; Wolkin, Angrist, Wolf, et al., 1988). Investigators have reported lowered neuronal density in the prefrontal cortex of schizophrenics (Doran et al., 1985, cited in Buchsbaum and Haier, 1987; Benes, Davidson, and Bird, 1986). Several studies employing CT scans and magnetic resonance imaging have found larger lateral and third ventricles, as well as markedly smaller prefrontal "systems" in schizophrenics compared to normal subjects (e.g., Andreasen, Nasrallah, Dunn, et al., 1986; Shelton, Karson, Doran, et al., 1988). Lawson, Waldman, and Weinberger (1988) reported that schizophrenic subjects with enlarged ventricles scored consistently worse on a variety of neuropsychological tests than schizophrenic subjects without evidence of large ventricles. The findings of frontal and basal ganglia changes in schizophrenia are consistent with the psychological deficits associated with the disorder.

Several regional cerebral blood flow studies have employed the Wisconsin Card Sort (WCS) to test for dorsolateral prefrontal cortex (DLPFC) dysfunction in schizophrenics. The WCS is generally considered to be a test of DLPFC cognitive function. Berman, Zec, and Weinberger (1986) found that the increased blood flow to the DLPFC region observed during performance of the WCS in normal subjects was absent in both medication-free and neuroleptically treated chronic schizophrenics. The latter two groups demonstrated marked impairment in their performance on the WCS. Thus it appears that DLPFC physiological impairment in chronic schizophrenics is associated with DLPFC cognitive dysfunction. A similar study of patients with HD also revealed poor performance on the WCS; however, their impairment was attributed to abnormalities in the caudate region rather than DLPFC (Weinberger and Berman, 1985).

Attempts to teach the WCS to chronic schizophrenics have generally failed because patients are unable to use feedback to alter their performance (Goldberg, Weinberger, Berman, et al., 1987). In addition to being unable to monitor their own cognitive behavior, schizophrenics are deficient in the ability to monitor and correct ongoing motor behavior on the basis of internal, self-generated cues (Malenka, Angel, Hampton, and Berger, 1982). Dementia patients with frontal lobe symptomatology also exhibit difficulty recognizing and correcting their errors (Josiassen, Curry, and Mancall, 1983). Impaired self-monitoring characterizes a number of disturbances in self-awareness, self-consciousness, and self-control (Stuss and Benson, 1984) and may be a key factor in understanding why some patients are unaware of their deficits. The literature concerned with unawareness in schizophrenics provides some intriguing parallels to the descriptions of lack of insight in dementia.

UNAWARENESS OF DEFICITS IN SCHIZOPHRENIA

Several studies have indicated that schizophrenics are largely unaware of their abnormal involuntary movements. The motor disturbance in schizophrenia has generally been attributed to the effects of long-term treatment with neuroleptic drugs and is referred to as tardive dyskinesia. However, movement disorders were observed in schizophrenics long before the advent of neuroleptic medication. Crow, Cross, Johnstone, et al. (1982) reported that the incidence of involuntary movements in schizophrenic patients who had never received neuroleptics was not substantially different from that in drug-treated patients. The description of these abnormal movements by Kraepelin (1919) closely resembled clinical descriptions of some of the adventitious movements seen in patients with HD. The symptoms include movements of the tongue and face, athetoid or choreiform movements of the arms, hands, fingers, legs, or toes, and whole body movements. Most studies reporting unawareness of involuntary movements in schizophrenia refer to the motor disturbance of tardive dyskinesia.

Alexopoulos (1979) found that of 18 schizophrenic outpatients diagnosed with tardive dyskinesia, eight were entirely unaware of their movement disorders. Awareness was assessed by a psychiatric interview with each patient. Five of the unaware patients were actively delusional or hallucinating whereas only one of the ten aware patients was delusional. Surprisingly, none of the ten aware patients had complained to their therapists of their symptoms, but they admitted the involuntary movements when questioned directly about them.

Smith, Kucharski, Oswald, and Waterman (1979) employed the Abnormal Involuntary Movement Scale (AIMS) (Guy, 1976) to measure the presence and severity of abnormal movements in 377 psychiatric inpatients. Included on this scale are items assessing patients' reported awareness and distress as a consequence of disturbed movements (range 0 to 4). Each patient was rated by two raters, and test/retest reliabilities were determined by having a different pair of raters assess each patient. The test/retest reliability of the awareness item was low (0.08) primarily because of the variable nature of the patients' responses and the low frequency of reported awareness and distress ($\overline{X} = .15$). Of 113 patients who had an average rating of 3 (moderate) or 4 (severe) for any one item concerning symptoms of abnormal movements, only nine (8%) had mean ratings indicating that they had awareness of their motor disturbance and only four (3.5%) expressed some degree of distress. However, based on clinical observations, the authors believed that many patients were unwilling to report awareness and distress associated with the movements rather than being truly unaware of the symptoms. To address this issue, these patients were asked if they noticed any abnormal movements in other patients. A number of the patients were able to identify accurately the symptoms of tardive dyskinesia in others. Smith and colleagues concluded that although these patients might have been unaware of their own tongue or mouth movements it is unlikely that they did not notice their more obvious hand, feet, or leg movements. As discussed earlier, a similar conclusion was reached by Reisberg et al. (1985) regarding AD patients' apparent lack of insight into their own deficits compared to their preserved ability to assess accurately their spouses' level of functioning. The self–other discrepancy observed in both studies need not imply that patients are engaged in defensive denial. Rather, it may reflect a self-monitoring deficit that prevents patients from recognizing their *own* disturbed behavior while leaving intact the ability to make accurate judgments about others' performance.

Rosen, Mukherjee, Olarte, et al. (1982) found that 23 of 70 patients with tardive dyskinesia, as assessed by the AIMS, indicated an awareness of their abnormal movements, and their awareness increased with the increased severity of their symptoms. Awareness was rated on the AIMS by the authors during a semistructured interview with each patient. Factor analysis on the data revealed that patients seemed aware of their tardive dyskinesia and were distressed by it when they experienced functional impairment, usually when their arms or legs were affected. Myslobodsky, Tomer, Holden, et al. (1985) reported that 15 of the 17 schizophrenic patients they studied with tardive dyskinesia were entirely unaware of or not concerned with their "grotesque orolingual symptomatology," despite the obvious disturbances of speech these symptoms produce. Patients with tardive dyskinesia were also impaired on a picture recall test when compared to schizophrenic patients without the motor disturbance. Myslobodsky et al. conjectured that "a mild memory abnormality, with the lack of concern or anosognosia, is suggestive of an insidious dementia disorder."

In a later study, Myslobodsky, Holden, and Sandler (1986) examined a group of 49 schizophrenic patients with tardive dykinesia, 38 of whom exhibited abnormal movements of the trunk, limbs, or both in addition to dyskinetic movements in the facial region. Only two patients (4%) complained about their motor incapacity when asked directly about the problem. The rest of the sample tended to minimize the motor disturbance or had absolutely no awareness of their motor abnormalities. As Myslobodsky (1986) pointed out, this lack of awareness may account for the fact that even grotesque dyskinesia does not result in social withdrawal but is particularly distressing for the patient's family (Owen, 1979). Myslobodsky (1986) related anosognosia in patients with tardive dyskinesia to some form of cognitive decline associated with dementia disorder. The dementia syndrome was attributed to a neuroleptic-induced deficiency within the dopaminergic circuitry in the right hemisphere.

Many schizophrenic patients exhibit primarily "positive" symptoms consisting in delusions, hallucinations, formal thought disorder, and bizarre behavior. Based on a review of the literature concerned with this subgroup of schizophrenics, Levin (1984) suggested that these patients may suffer from damage of their inferior pareital lobe and the temporoparietal junction and thus exhibit a distinctive pattern of brain impairment. These patients often progress from delusions and hallucinations to a defect state characterized by the negative symptoms, or frontal symptoms, described earlier. Anscombe (1987) provided a description of this process that could easily be mistaken for the gradual loss of insight observed in many dementia patients.

> The loss of self is a gradual process attended by vagueness. As in other processes in which the intellect is affected, the patient goes through an early stage in which it is possible to deny the changes that are taking place, and a later stage in which the failings themselves prevent awareness. In between is a stage of alarm in which the person retains enough insight to be aware of what he is losing. [p. 255]

Greenfeld (1985) indicated that patients who lack awareness of their mental illness are virtually inaccessible to treatment, insisting that they have no illness or symptoms requiring treatment. Two patients were described who had little insight into their psychiatric conditions and who believed that they could perform far beyond their abilities.

Delusions have been considered, by definition, to be outside the realm of patients' awareness. Jaspers (1968) maintained that delusional ideas represent errors in judgment or false beliefs that are "incorrigible." Kihlstrom and Hoyt (1988) viewed delusions as the product of disordered perceptual and attentional processes. According to this view, schizophrenics are entirely unaware of their most fundamental psychological deficit, a perceptual-attentional disorder. Consequently, they search for some explanation for their anomalous experiences, not realizing their own role in constructing the bizarre experiences. Several investigators have been successful in their attempts to modify the abnormal beliefs of schizophrenics (Watts, Powell, and Austin, 1973; Johnson, Ross, and Mastria, 1977; Hole, Rush, and Beck, 1979), suggesting that delusions may not be as intractable as previously believed. Delusions frequently occur in certain dementia syndromes, particularly those associated with subcortical dysfunction (Cummings, 1985). For example, Brothers (1964) regarded schizophrenic behavior as the most common disorder accompanying HD. Myrianthopoulos (1966) reported that HD patients progress to develop severe dementia, suspicious behavior, delusions, and schizophrenic reactions. Dewhurst, Oliver, Trick, and McKnight (1969) found that 50% of HD patients exhibited delusional ideas upon admission. Consequently, patients with HD are often misdiagnosed as schizophrenic (Garron, 1973; McHugh and Folstein, 1975).

Another domain of unawareness in schizophrenia concerns a lack of response to painful stimuli. Earl and Earl (1955) studied a group of chronic schizophrenic patients and employed the cold-pressor test to examine their reaction to painful stimuli. Despite the presence of autonomic changes (e.g., elevated blood pressure) during the test and intact afferent and efferent pathways, patients appeared oblivious to pain during the procedure. The authors concluded that schizophrenic patients lack "appreciation of pain." Talbott and Linn (1978) reported that a substantial proportion of chronic schizophrenic patients who suffer from serious and life-threatening medical and surgical illnesses do not exhibit any pain behavior, discomfort, or distress. The diagnosis of anosognosia was rejected when describing this phenomenon; rather, the absence of pain responses was attributed to patients' rejection of the sick role in their attempts to avoid intimate relationships with treatment staff.

Studies of unawareness in schizophrenia are subject to many of the same criticisms described earlier for unawareness in dementia. First, investigators generally relied on their subjective impressions of patients' awareness, rather than attempting to develop objective measures for assessing awareness. Second, the relation between cognitive impairment and unawareness was not addressed in any systematic way. Third, investigators have tended to focus on unawareness of a particular symptom or experience such as tardive dyskinesia, delusion, or pain. It would be of significant interest to examine whether schizophrenic patients who are unaware of their motor disturbance are similarly unaware of other symptoms associated with their illness. Despite these methodological issues, the literature concerned with unawareness in schizophrenia does suggest that a variety of unawareness phenomena are present in this population. Furthermore, the frontal lobe dysfunction associated with schizophrenia is consistent with evidence suggesting that unawareness of deficits in certain neuropsychological syndromes depends on patterns of brain impairment involving the frontal lobes.

THEORETICAL ISSUES

The literature concerned with unawareness of deficits in dementia and schizophrenia, as well as our own preliminary results from examining unawareness in HD, raise a number of theoretical questions about the processes affected in these diseases that disrupt patients' ability to be aware of and monitor their own state of functioning. This section reviews various theories of anosognosia that may be relevant for understanding unawareness in dementia and schizophrenia.

A number of investigators have proposed that unawareness of deficits reflects primarily motivated use of the psychological defense mechanism of denial (e.g., Goldstein, 1939, 1942; Weinstein and Kahn, 1955; Reisberg et al., 1985). According to this account, anosognosia is considered an expression of the patient's "drive to be well," a means of protection against the recognition of disease or defect. Several problems exist with the motivational account of anosognosia with respect to dementia and schizophrenia. First, most studies assessing unawareness in dementia, including our own study of HD described earlier, indicate that patients are acutely aware of, and openly express anxiety about, changes in their cognitive functioning early in the disease process. It is not until later stages of the disease that patients appear to lose insight into their deficits. The time course for motivated denial would not be expected to follow this pattern of development; rather, if patients are predisposed to deny their defects, they would likely deny or minimize the early signs of disease to avoid facing the potentially devastating or even fatal implications. The gradual loss of insight observed in dementia has also been described with respect to schizophrenia, whereby patients experience a stage of alarm before losing insight into their disturbed cognitive processes.

The gradual development of unawareness in dementia and schizophrenia raises the issue of the role of intellectual deterioration in awareness disturbances. Our preliminary findings from research with HD patients suggest that patients with generalized cognitive impairment are more likely to lack awareness of their disabilities, whereas those with relatively intact cognitive abilities are generally realistic when assessing their difficulties. The study by Reisberg et al. (1985) of unawareness in AD provided additional evidence for a relation between cognitive decline and loss of insight in dementia. This issue has not been investigated in schizophrenia, though clinical descriptions do suggest that as schizophrenic patients become increasingly impaired intellectually they lose awareness of the changes taking place. Thus it appears that cognitive decline may be an important factor contributing to the development of an awareness disturbance in both dementia and schizophrenia.

Several theorists who view anosognosia as a manifestation of intellectual impairment have attributed the disturbance to diffuse cerebral dysfuntion (e.g., Schilder, 1935; Stengel and Steele, 1946; Ullman, 1962). However, in certain dementing disorders such as HD and in schizophrenics with negative symptoms, brain dysfunction is primarily restricted to subcortical structures and the frontal lobes. Stuss and Benson (1986) discussed the possible contribution of frontal lobe damage to the pathogenesis of anosognosia. They maintained that regions of the frontal lobe are involved in self-awareness and monitoring of one's own cognitive function, and that anosognosia could reflect a deficit in self-monitoring. Support for this view has been presented by McGlynn and Schacter (1989). For example, evidence that unawareness of memory deficits is generally observed in cases of amnesia attributable to various etiologies involving the frontal lobes, but not in amnesic patients with restricted lesions in the temporal lobe, strongly suggests that frontal dysfunction contributes to unawareness of deficits. The role of frontal damage in unawareness of deficits is further indicated by the extensive literature on head-injured patients, who often exhibit symptoms of frontal lobe damage in addition to unawareness of deficits.

A striking feature of anosognosia in a variety of neuropsychological syndromes that must be accounted for by any theoretical account is the frequent specificity of the awareness disturbance (e.g., Bisiach, Meregalli, and Berti, 1985; Bisiach, Valler, Perani, et al., 1986; McGlynn and Schacter, 1989). For example, stroke patients are often entirely unaware of their hemiplegia but may complain about other equally serious defects. Observations of the specificity of anosognosia have argued against the view that the unawareness is attributable to a generalized intellectual impairment. However, there are also a number of reports indicating that brain-damaged patients can be unaware of multiple deficits simultaneously. Two theoretical frameworks for anosognosia have attempted to account for the specific disruptions of awareness observed in various neuropsychological disorders as well as awareness disturbances involving multiple deficits (Bisiach et al., 1985; McGlynn and Schacter, 1989).

There have been no systematic studies investigating the issue of specificity in dementia and schizophrenia, with the exception of our own research with HD patients. Results from our study thus far suggest that HD patients generally lack awareness of their motor deficit and their memory impairment. However, individual patients may exhibit variable awareness depending on the particular motor tasks or memory tasks on which they are asked to report. Thus the question of specificity in dementia remains unclear at this time. Based on current views of anosognosia as a disruption of executive functions and the rather extensive frontal pathology associated with certain dementing disorders and schizophrenia, it would not be surprising to find that dementia patients and schizophrenics exhibit a general self-monitoring deficit that renders them unable to maintain awareness of their numerous disabilities. Nor would it be surprising to discover that intellectual impairment correlates highly with unawareness in these disorders, given that frontal dysfunction produces a broad range of cognitive deficits. The finding that PD patients without cognitive impairment and EEG abnormalities exhibit good awareness of their condition, whereas those with AD, MID, and PD with vascular disease demonstrate a loss of insight (Danielczyk, 1983), is suggestive of a relation between cortical involvement, cognitive decline, and unawareness. At this early stage, one can only speculate about the neural substrates of unawareness in dementia and schizophrenia. Although our intention is not to suggest that dementia and schizophrenia involve the same kinds of brain pathology, we do want to point out that both populations exhibit unawareness phenomena as well as many similar symptoms of frontal lobe dysfunction. The awareness disturbances observed in these seemingly disparate groups may be attributable to disruption of similar mechanisms in particular regions of the frontal lobe.

REFERENCES

Alexopoulos, G. S. (1979). Lack of complaints in schizophrenics with tardive dyskinesia. *J. Nerv. Ment. Dis.* 167:125–127.

Aminoff, M. J., Marshall, J., Smith, E. M., and Wyke, M. A. (1975). Pattern of intellectual impairment in Huntington's chorea. *Psychol. Med.* 5:169–172.

Andreasen, N., Nasrallah, H. A., Dunn, V., Olsen, S. C., Grove, W. M., Ehrhardt, J. C., Coffman, J. A., and Crossett, J. H. W. (1986). Structural abnormalities in the frontal system in schizophrenia. *Arch. Gen. Psychiatry* 43:136–144.

Andreasen, N. C., and Olsen, S. (1982). Negative vs. positive schizophrenia. *Arch. Gen. Psychiatry* 39:789–794.

Anscombe, R. (1987). The disorder of consciousness in schizophrenia. *Schizophr. Bull.* 13:241–260.

Babinski, M. J. (1914). Contribution a l'etude des troubles mentaux dans l'hemiplegie organique cerebrale (anosognosie). [Contribution to the study of mental disturbance in organic cerebral hemiplegia (anosognosia)]. *Rev. Neurol. (Paris)* 12:845–848.

Benes, F. M., Davidson, J., and Bird, E. D. (1986). Quantitative cytoarchitectural studies of the cerebral cortex of schizophrenics. *Arch. Gen. Psychiatry* 43:31–35.

Benson, D. F. (1983). Subcortical dementia: a clinical approach. In R. Mayeux and W. G. Rosen (eds.), *The Dementias*. New York: Raven Press, pp. 185–193.

Benson, D. F. and Geschwind, N. (1975). Psychiatric conditions associated with focal lesions of the central nervous system. In S. Arieti and M. F. Reiser (eds.), *American Handbook of Psychiatry.* Vol. 4. New York: Basic Books, pp. 208–243.

Bergmann, K., Proctor, S., and Prudham, D. (1979). Symptom profiles in hospital and community resident elderly persons with dementia. In F. Hofmeister and C. Muller (eds.), *Brain Function in Old Age.* New York: Springer Verlag, pp. 60–67.

Berman, K. F., Zec, R. F., and Weiberger, D. R. (1986). Physiologic dysfunction of dorsolateral prefrontal cortex in schizophrenia. II. Role of neuroleptic treatment, attention, and mental effort. *Arch. Gen. Psychiatry* 43:126–135.

Bisiach, E., Meregalli, S., and Berti, A. (1985). Mechanisms of production-control and belief-fixation in human visuospatial processing: clinical evidence from hemispatial neglect. Presented to the Eighth Symposium on Quantitative Analyses of Behavior, Harvard University, June 1985.

Bisiach, E., Vallar, G., Perani, D., Papagno, C., and Berti, A. (1986). Unawareness of disease following lesions of the right hemisphere: anosognosia for hemiplegia and anosognosia for hemianopia. *Neuropsychologia* 24:471–482.

Blumer, D., and Benson, D. F. (1975). Personality changes with frontal and temporal lobe lesions. In D. F. Benson and D. Blumer (eds.), *Psychiatric Aspects of Neurological Disease,* Orlando: Grune & Stratton, pp. 151–170.

Bradley, K. (1984). Diseases of the basal ganglia. In J. S. McKenzie, R. E. Kemm, and L. N. Wilcock (eds.), *The Basal Ganglia.* New York: Plenum Press, pp. 333–341.

Brothers, C. R. D. (1964). Huntington's chorea in Victoria and Tasmania. *J. Neurol. Sci.* 1:405–420.

Bruyn, G. (1968). A historical, clinical and laboratory synopsis. In P. Vinken and G. W. Bruyn (eds.), *Handbook of Clinical Neurology.* Vol. 6. Amsterdam: North Holland, pp. 298–378.

Bruyn, G. W., Bots, G. Th. A. M., and Dom, R. (1979). Huntington's chorea: current neuropathological status. *Adv. Neurol.* 23:83–93.

Buchsbaum, M. S., and Haier, R. J. (1987). Functional and anatomical brain imaging: impact on schizophrenia research. In D. Shore (ed.), *Special Report: Schizophrenia.* Rockville, MD: National Institute of Mental Health, pp. 129–146.

Bustany, P., Henry, J. F., Rotrou, J., Singnoret, P., Cabanis, E., Zarifian, E., Ziegler, M., Derlon, J. M., Crouzel, C., Soussaline, F., and Comar, D. (1985). Correlations between clinical state and PET measurement of local brain protein synthesis in Alzheimer's dementia, Parkinsons's disease, schizophrenia and gliomas. In T. Greitz, D. H. Ingvar, and L. Widen (eds.), *The Metabolism of the Human Brain Studied with Positron Emission Tomography.* New York: Raven Press, pp. 241–250.

Butters, N., Sax, D., Montgomery, K., and Tarlow, S. (1978). Comparison of the neuropsychological deficits associated with early and advanced Huntington's disease. *Arch. Neurol.* 35:585–589.

Butters, N., Wolfe, J., Granholm, E., and Martone, M. (1986). An assessment of verbal recall, recognition and fluency abilities in patients with Huntington's disease. *Cortex* 22:11–32.

Caine, E. D., and Shoulson, I. (1983). Psychiatric syndromes in Huntington's disease. *Am. J. Psychiatry* 140:728–733.

Caine, E. D., Hunt, R. D., Weingartner, H., and Ebert, M. H. (1978). Huntington's dementia. *Arch. Gen. Psychiatry* 35:377–384.

Chapman, L. J., and Chapman, J. P. (1973). *Disordered Thought in Schizophrenia.* Englewood Cliffs, NJ: Prentice-Hall.

Crow, T. J., Cross, A. J., Johnstone, E. C., Owen, F., Owens, D. G. C., and Waddington,

J. L. (1982). Abnormal involuntary movements in schizophrenia: are they related to the disease process or its treament? Are they associated with changes in dopamine receptors? *J. Clin. Psychopharmacol.* 2:336–340.

Cummings, J. L. (1985). Organic delusions: phenomenology, anatomical correlations, and review. *Br. J. Psychiatry* 146:184–197.

Cummings, J. L., and Benson, D. F. (1984). Subcortical dementia. *Arch. Neurol.* 41:874–879.

Danielczyk, W. (1983). Various mental behavioral disorders in Parkinson's disease, primary degenerative senile dementia, and multiple infarction dementia. *J. Neural Transm.* 56:161–176.

Dewhurst, K., Oliver, J., Trick, K. L. K., and McKnight, A. L. (1969). Neuropsychiatric aspects of Huntington's disease. *Confin. Neurol.* 31:258–268.

Earl, A., and Earl, E. V. (1955). The blood pressure response to pain and emotion in schizophrenia. *J. Nerv. Ment. Dis.* 121:132–139.

Folstein, M. F., Folstein, S. E., and McHugh, P. R. (1975). "Mini-mental state." *J. Psychiatr. Res.* 12:189–198.

Frederiks, J. A. M. (1985). The neurology of aging and dementia. In J. A. M. Frederiks (ed.), *Handbook of Clinical Neurology.* Vol. 2. Amsterdam: Elsevier, pp. 199–219.

Garron, D. C. (1973). Huntington's chorea and schizophrenia. *Adv. Neurol.* 1:1872–1972.

Goldberg, E., and Costa, L. D. (1986). Qualitative indices in neuropsychological assessment: an extension of Luria's approach to executive deficit following prefrontal lesions. In J. Grant and K. M. Adams (eds.), *Neuropsychological Assessment of Neuropsychiatric Disorders.* New York: Oxford University Press, pp. 48–64.

Goldberg, T. E., Weinberger, D. R., Berman, K. F., Pliskin, N. H., and Podd, M. H. (1987). Further evidence for dementia of the prefrontal type in schizophrenia? *Arch. Gen. Psychiatry* 44:1008–1014.

Goldstein, G. (1986). The neuropsychology of schizophrenia. In J. Grant and K. M. Adams (eds.), *Neuropsychological Assessment of Neuropsychiatric Disorders.* New York: Oxford University Press, pp. 147–171.

Goldstein, K. (1939). *The Organism.* New York: American Book Company.

Goldstein, K. (1942). *Aftereffects of Brain Injuries in War.* Orlando: Grune & Stratton.

Greenfeld, D. (1985). *The Psychotic Patient.* New York: The Free Press.

Gustafson, I., and Nilsson, L. (1982). Differential diagnosis of presenile dementia on clinical grounds. *Acta Psychiatr. Scand.* 65:194–207.

Guy, W. (1976). *ECDEU Assessment Manual for Psychopharmacology.* Washington, D.C.: Department of Health, Education, and Welfare, pp. 534–537.

Hole, R. W., Rush, A. J., and Beck, A. T. (1979). A cognitive investigation of schizophrenic delusions. *Psychiatry* 42:312–319.

Jaspers, K. (1968). Delusion and awareness of reality. *Int. J. Psychiatry* 6:25–40.

Johnson, W. G., Ross, J. M., and Mastria, M. A. (1977). Delusional behavior: an attributional analysis of development. *J. Abnorm. Psychol.* 86:421–426.

Josiassen, R. C., Curry, L. M., and Mancall, E. L. (1983). Development of neuropsychological deficits in Huntington's disease. *Arch. Neurol.* 40:791–796.

Joynt, R. J., and Shoulson, I. (1985). Dementia. In K. M. Heilman and E. Valenstein (eds.), *Clinical Neuropsychology.* 2nd Ed. New York: Oxford University Press, pp. 453–479.

Kaszniak, A. (1986). The neuropsychology of dementia. In J. Grant and K. M. Adams (eds.), *Neuropsychological Assessment of Neuropsychiatric Disorders.* New York: Oxford University Press, pp. 172–220.

Kihlstrom, J. F., and Hoyt, I. P. (1988). Hypnosis and the psychology of delusions. In T. F. Oltmanns and B. A. Maher (eds.), *Delusional Beliefs.* New York: Wiley, pp. 66–109.

Kolb, B., and Whishaw, I. Q. (1983). Performance of schizophrenic patients on tests sensitive to left or right frontal, temporal, or parietal function in neurological patients. *J. Nerv. Ment. Dis.* 171:435–443.

Kraepelin, E. (1919). *Dementia Praecox and Paraphrenia.* Edinburgh: Livingstone.

Kuhl, D. E., Metter, E. J., Riege, W. H., and Hawkins, R. A. (1985). Patterns of cerebral glucose utilization in dementia. In T. Greitz, D. H. Ingvar, and L. Widen (eds.), *The Metabolism of the Human Brain Studied with PET.* New York: Raven Press, pp. 419–432.

Lawson, W. B., Waldman, I. N., and Weinberger, D. R. (1988). Schizophrenic dementia: clinical and computed axial tomography correlates. *J. Nerv. Ment. Dis.* 176:207–212.

Levin, S. (1984). Frontal lobe dysfunctions in schizophrenia. II. Impairments of psychological and brain functions. *J. Psychiatr. Res.* 18:57–72.

Lishman, W. A. (1987). *Organic Psychiatry. The psychological consequences of cerebral disorder.* Blackwell Scientific Publications, pp. 393–400.

Mahendra, B. (1984). *Dementia.* Lancaster: MTP Press.

Malenka, R. C., Angel, R. W., Hamptom, B., and Berger, P. A. (1982). Impaired central error-correcting behavior in schizophrenia. *Arch. Gen. Psychiatry.* 39:101–107.

Martone, M., Butters, N., Payne, M., Becker, J. T., and Sax, D. S. (1984). Dissociations between skill learning and verbal recognition in amnesia and dementia. *Arch. Neurol.* 41:965–970.

McGlynn, S. M., and Schacter, D. L. (1989). Unawareness of deficits in neuropsychological syndromes. *J. Clin. Exp. Neuropsychol.* 11:143–205.

McHugh, P. R., and Folstein, M. F. (1975). Psychiatric syndromes of Huntington's chorea: a clinical and phenomenologic study. In D. F. Benson and D. Blumer (eds.), *Psychiatric Aspects of Neurologic Disease.* Orlando: Grune & Stratton, pp. 267–285.

Myrianthopoulos, N. T. (1966). Review article: Huntington's chorea. *J. Med. Genet.* 3:298–313.

Myslobodsky, M. S. (1986). Anosognosia in patients with tardive dyskinesia: a symptom of "tardive dysmentia" or "tardive dementia"? *Schizoph. Bull.* 12:1–6.

Myslobodsky, M. S., Holden, T., and Sandler, R. (1986). Parkinsonian symptoms in tardive dyskinesia. *S. Afr. Med. J.* 69:424–426.

Myslobodsky, M. S., Tomer, R., Holden, T., Kempler, S., and Sigal, M. (1985). Cognitive impairment in patients with tardive dyskinesia. *J. Nerv. Ment. Dis.* 173:156–160.

Neary, D., Snowden, J. S., Bowen, D. M., Sims, N. R., Mann, D. M. A., Benton, J. S., Northen, B., Yates, P. O., and Davison, A. N. (1986). Neuropsychological syndromes in presenile dementia due to cerebral atrophy. *J. Neurol. Neurosurg. Psychiatry* 49:163–174.

Oltman, J. E., Friedman, S. (1961). Combination of general paresis and Huntington's chorea. *Disord. Nerv. Syst.* 22:507–509.

Owen, R. T. (1979). Dyskinesias. *Drugs Today* 15:65–80.

Reisberg, B., Gordon, B., McCarthy, M., and Ferris, S. H. (1985). Clinical symptoms accompanying progressive cognitive decline and Alzheimer's disease. In V. L. Melnick and N. N. Dubler (eds.), *Alzheimer's Dementia.* Clifton, NJ: Humana Press, pp. 19–39.

Rosen, A. M., Mukherjee, S., Olarte, S., Varia, V., and Cardenas, C. (1982). Perception of tardive dyskinesia in outpatients receiving maintenance neuroleptics. *Am. J. Psychiatry* 139:372–373.

Schacter, D. L., McLachlan, D. R., Moscovitch, M., and Tulving, E. (1986). Monitoring of recall performance by memory-disordered patients. *J. Clin. Exp. Neuropsychol.* 8:130. (abstract).

Schilder, P. (1935). *The Image and Appearance of the Human Body.* London: Kegan Paul, Trench, Trubner & Co.

Schneck, M. K., Reisberg, B., and Ferris, S. H. (1982). An overview of current concepts of Alzheimer's disease. *Am. J. Psychiatry* 139:165–173.

Seidman, L. J. (1983). Schizophrenia and brain dysfunction: an integration of recent neurodiagnostic findings. *Psychol. Bull.* 94:195–238.

Shelton, R. C., Karson, C. N., Doran, A. R., Pickar, D., Bigelow, L. B., and Weinberger, D. R. (1988). Cerebral structural pathology in schizophrenia: evidence for a selective prefrontal cortical defect. *Am. J. Psychiatry* 145:154–163.

Sheppard, G., Gruzelier, J., Manchanda, R., Hirsch, S. R., Wise, R., Frackowiak, R., and Jones, T. (1983). 15 O-position emission tomographic scanning in predominantly never-treated acute schizophrenic patients. *Lancet* 2:1448–1452.

Shoulson, I., and Fahn, S. (1979). Huntington's disease: clinical care and evaluation. *Neurology* 29:1–3.

Smith, J. M., Kucharski, L. T., Oswald, W. T., and Waterman, L. J. (1979). A systematic investigation of tardive dyskinesia in inpatients. *Am. J. Psychiatry* 136:918–922.

Stengel, E., Steele, G. D. F. (1946). Unawareness of physical disability (anosognosia). *Br. J. Psychiatry* 92:379–388.

Stuss, D. T., Benson, D. F. (1984). Neuropsychological studies of the frontal lobes. *Psychol. Bull* 95:3–78.

Stuss, D. T., Benson, D. F. (1986). *The Frontal Lobes.* New York: Raven Press.

Talbott, J. A., and Linn, L. (1978). Reactions of schizophrenics to life-threatening disease. *Psychiatr. Q.* 50:218–227.

Ullman, M. (1962). *Behavioral Changes in Patients Following Strokes.* Springfield, IL: Charles C Thomas.

Watts, F. N., Powell, G. E., and Austin, S. V. (1973). The modification of abnormal beliefs. *Br. J. Med. Psychol.* 46:359–363.

Weinberger, D. R., and Berman, K. F. (1985). Huntington's disease and subcortical dementia: rCBF evidence. *Neurology* (suppl. 1):109.

Weinstein, E. A., and Kahn, R. L. (1955). *Denial of Illness: Symbolic and Physiological Aspects.* Springfield, IL: Charles C Thomas.

Wilson, R. S., and Garron, D. C. (1979). Cognitive and affective aspects of Huntington's disease. *Adv. Neurol.* 23:193–201.

Wilson, R. S. Como, P. G., Garron, D. C., Klawans, H. L., Barr, A., and Klawans, D. (1987). Memory failure in Huntington's disease. *J. Clin. Exp. Neuropsychol.* 9:147–154.

Wolkin, A., Angrist, B., Wolf, A., Brodie, J. D., Wolkin, B., Jaeger, J., Cancrow, R., and Rotrosen, J. (1988). Low frontal glucose utilization in chronic schizophrenia: a replication study. *Am. J. Psychiatry* 145:251–253.

7

Disturbances of Self-Awareness of Deficit After Traumatic Brain Injury

GEORGE P. PRIGATANO

Outcome statistics on psychosocial adjustment after severe traumatic brain injury (TBI) make it clear that an adequate understanding of the higher cerebral deficit associated with this condition and adequate rehabilitation programs have not yet been developed. When the period of observation lasts 2 to 4 years after injury, approximately one-third of severe TBI patients are able to resume reasonably productive life styles. However, when the period of follow-up is much longer (10 to 15 years after injury), the percentage may be less than 10% (Thomsen, 1984; Prigatano, Klonoff, and Bailey, 1987).

Although many factors potentially contribute to this phenomenon, clinically it often appears that severely brain-injured patients do not adequately perceive significant changes in their higher cerebral functioning. Consequently, they may choose a level of work that is not appropriate for their abilities, with catastrophic social consequences. The same problem is seen in their interpersonal relationships. They often do not recognize how impulsive, irritable, childish, or demanding they are in certain circumstances. Thus they frequently alienate family and friends, and they appear confused and bewildered in the face of these interpersonal failures. The result is often social isolation (Prigatano and Others, 1986a). In some instances frank delusional ideation emerges (Prigatano, O'Brien, and Klonoff, 1988).

This chapter reviews the sparse literature on the complex disturbances of impaired self-awareness after TBI. Clinical descriptions are presented, and a model for understanding this important neuropsychological impairment is suggested. Implications for rehabilitation also are briefly considered.

A drawing by a young woman who suffered traumatic brain injury highlights this problem and places it into a personal context (Fig. 7–1). The patient stated that she is a normal person with part of her head off in "never, never land"

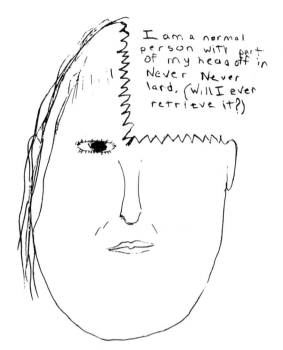

Figure 7–1. TBI patient drawing. See text.

and asked the question of whether she will ever "retrieve it." This experience of normality despite brain damage, coupled with the *simultaneous perception* of an altered sense of self, is the clinical definition and manifestation of what is referred to as a disturbance in self-awareness of deficit after traumatic brain injury.

CLINICAL EXAMPLES

The general problem of altered self-awareness and its specific manifestations after TBI was first made obvious to me when attempting to rehabilitate a young adult brain-injured patient 9 months after injury. Bifrontal lobe contusions had been documented, yet he performed nearly normally on many of the psychometric tests given to him. He showed a surprising lack of insight into his poor social judgment and its behavioral impact on others. On one occasion, the patient was observed ordering food in a hospital cafeteria. He stood next to an attractive physical therapist and began to engage her in conversation. As the woman walked up in line, he stood next to her staring at her in a rather socially inappropriate manner. He began to walk almost parallel to her as she moved up in line. He then began to comment about her attractiveness. She was obviously uncomfortable but acknowledged his comments briefly. The patient continued to make comments and specifically mentioned that her hair was pretty. Again, she briefly acknowledged him but said little. It was obvious to all around her that she was uncomfortable and uninterested in further dialogue. Yet the patient persisted in making more and more comments until he finally asked her where she had gotten her beautiful hair. By now indignant, she angrily answered: "I grow it out of my head!" The patient smiled and said in a boyish manner, "Oh!" He then appeared to recognize his negative impact on her but was perplexed as to what had displeased her.

About an hour later, I had the opportunity to ask this patient what had occurred during lunch. He remembered the young woman and the dialogue but did not recognize any aberrant behavior on his part. When told that the woman in question was upset with him, he thought that I was exaggerating the situation. When asked what it would take to convince him that in fact his behavior was socially inappropriate, he said that he would have to hear it directly from the woman. Because this potentially would make her uncomfortable, it was agreed that this woman would talk to a female therapist and convey her personal reactions via the therapist. When the female therapist reported back that, in fact, the woman was insulted by the patient's comments, the patient seemed honestly surprised. His reaction was one of disbelief over his inappropriate behavior. He eventually accepted feedback that he had acted inappropriately but was not convinced that he had done anything "that wrong." This patient, it must be added, had no major premorbid personality difficulties prior to his injury. His lack of awareness seemed to be secondary to underlying neuropsychological impairment.

A second clinical example emerged when analyzing initial outcome data of a neuropsychologically oriented rehabilitation program (Prigatano and others, 1986a). The first group of patients seen in that program were classified as either "treatment successes" or "treatment failures." The criteria for determining whether patients belonged in one category or the other centered on their ability to be productive in their lives, maintain adequate interpersonal relationships with others particularly family members, and show some degree of involvement or active participation in rehabilitation activities. Patients and rehabilitation staff independently made ratings on a simple question that was posed to the patient: "How aware are you today of the impact of your brain injury on your daily behavior?" All those deemed treatment successes stated (after 6 months of treatment) that they were not totally aware (Table 7–1). In contrast, every one of the treatment failures insisted that they were totally aware, some even after 12 months of daily rehabilitative work. The staff independently made their ratings of the degree of awareness for each patient. The "successful" patients showed ratings similar to those prepared by the staff. The opposite was true for each patient who was classified as a "failure."

These clinical observations made it clear that the phenomenon of altered self-awareness after TBI was worthy of further investigation. Yet the literature is rather sparse as it relates to this phenomenon in post-acute TBI patients. A review by McGlynn and Schacter (1989), however, considered the problem of altered self-awareness in various patient groups.

SELECTED LITERATURE REVIEW OF IMPAIRED AWARENESS AFTER TBI

The work of Oddy, Coughlan, Tyerman, and Jenkins (1985) demonstrated the importance of impaired awareness of behavioral limitations after traumatic

TABLE 7–1 Comparison of Staff and Patient Ratings on
Awareness of Implication after Brain Injury

Patient	Time after rehabilitation (months)	Patient rating	Staff rating
"Success"			
D.B.	6	9	9
B.W.	6	9	9
M.L.	12	9	9
A.M.	6	8	6
"Failure"			
S.D.	6	10	2
	12	10	6
T.W.	6	10	4
	12	10	8
C.P.	6	10	6
	12	9	4

brain injury. Oddy and his colleagues asked patients and their families to describe the behavioral problems they encountered 7 years after traumatic brain injury. Table 7–2 lists the observations made. The first point to note is that the patients tended to underestimate the frequency of problems compared to relatives' reports. For example, at 7 years after injury 53% of the patients mentioned residual memory problems as a common long-term neuropsychological difficulty. In contrast, 79% of the families mentioned memory problems as significant sequelae. Next, the families noted two problems that patients never reported. Seven years after traumatic brain injury, 40% of the families reported that the patient behaved in a much more childish manner. They also reported that 40% of the patients refused to admit to difficulties. Such refusal may be more than psychological denial. In fact, it may reflect what might broadly be called "organic" unawareness.

Parenthetically, it has been noted elsewhere that when TBI patients are asked during neuropsychological interviews to rate the severity of their behavioral problems, they often underestimate the severity of the problem compared to relatives' report (Prigatano, Pepping, and Klonoff, 1986b). These data suggest that impaired self-awareness after brain injury has important diagnostic and rehabilitation implications.

Fordyce and Roueche (1986), using the Patient Competency Rating Scale developed at Presbyterian Hospital's Neuropsychological Rehabilitation program (Prigatano and Others, 1986a), compared behavioral ratings made by patients, relatives, and rehabilitation staff. They noted that patients typically rated themselves "higher" (more competent) than did their relatives, and that relatives typically rated the patient "higher" than did the rehabilitative staff. That is, the patients saw themselves as having fewer behavioral problems than did the relatives; and the relatives reported fewer behavioral problems than did the staff. For the purpose of this chapter, however, the more interesting finding is that the patients' ratings were unrelated to whether they were "vocationally active" or "inactive." In contrast, the ratings of family and rehabilitation staff were related to this important outcome measure. This finding provided indirect evidence that patients were not only showing poor insight into their behavioral limitations, but their judgments did not correlate with their actual vocational behaviors.

Other research that touched on the problem of altered self-awareness after TBI was reported by Sunderland, Harris, and Baddeley (1983). Their TBI patients, who showed a period of posttraumatic amnesia (PTA) of 24 hours or more, were asked to rate themselves in terms of their memory skills. Patients were then tested on various psychometric measures of memory. Relatives made their own independent ratings of patients' memory capacity, and their scores were correlated with the patients' memory test performances. An orthopedic control group was studied in a similar fashion. For postacute TBI patients, the relatives' ratings of patients' memory skills tended to correlate with patients' actual memory performance (five of nine memory measures had significant correlations). In contrast, only three of the nine correlations were significant for the patients' report compared to their actual performance. The magnitude of the correlations were also generally lower. During the acute phase, neither TBI patients' nor relatives' judgment about memory function was actually correlated with performance on memory tests. For these groups, all correlations were nonsignificant. This finding is interesting, as one frequently sees in the acute setting both the patient and family greatly underestimating the severity of the neurobehavioral deficits.

TABLE 7–2 Symptoms Reported by Patients and Relatives 7 Years after Head Injury

Symptom	%
Patients	
Trouble remembering things	53
Difficulty concentrating	46
Easily affected by alcohol	38
Often knocks things over	31
Often loses temper	31
Difficulty becoming interested	28
Likes to keep things tidy	28
Sometimes loses way	28
Eyesight problems	28
Difficulty following conversation	28
Relatives	
Trouble remembering things	79
Difficulty concentrating	50
Difficulty speaking	50
Easily affected by alcohol	43
Difficulty becoming interested	43
Becomes tired easily	43
Often impatient	43
Sometimes behaves childishly	40
Likes to keep things tidy	40
Refuses to admit difficulties	40

A later report by Sunderland, Harris, and Gleave (1984) reported on TBI patients who had severe injuries (PTA of at least 24 hours) versus mild injuries (PTA no longer than 10 minutes). Again, subjects rated their memory skills on a questionnaire, and independent relatives ratings were obtained. No objective measures of memory function were made in this study. However, when asked to rate how much of a "nuisance" their memory and concentration difficulties were, 33% of the severe head injury patients said that these problems *were not a nuisance at all.* Thirty-three percent of the mild head injury patients reported the same rating. Despite several studies demonstrating that more severe injuries carry with them greater memory deficits (Levin, Benton, and Grossman, 1982), the severe head injury group did not differ in their report about the impact of the problem on their daily lives compared to mild head injury patients. This report may be considered indirect evidence of impaired awareness of deficit after TBI, particularly in severely injured patients. Interestingly, in the latter study, 34% of the relatives of the severely head-injured patients reported memory problems being severe or moderate. In the mildly head-injured group, only 18% of the relatives reported such a magnitude of difficulty.

Clinicians may be further surprised, however, that 41% of the relatives of severely head-injured patients considered that memory was not a major "nuisance" at all for the patients. This finding is contrary to what is expected and raises the question of whether relatives tend to underestimate patients' problems, at least at certain points during the recovery phase (Romano, 1974; Bond, 1988). To help explain these behavioral observations and to set the stage for the research we conducted on impaired awareness of behavioral limitations after brain injury, a brief review of the neuropathology associated with severe head injuries and some observations on animals who suffered comparable lesions are considered.

RELATED STUDIES

Traditional studies of the neuropathology associated with severe acceleration/deceleration injuries emphasize the importance of injury to the anterior tips of the frontal and temporal regions of the brain. Not infrequently, these lesions are bilateral (Russell, 1971; Levin et al., 1982; Adams, Graham, and Gennarelli, 1985). In one study with rhesus monkeys who underwent bilateral prefrontal and anterior temporal cortex surgical ablations (Franzen and Myers, 1973), there was a notable change in the monkeys' social behavior. It was reported that the lesioned monkeys approached without hesitation any animal irrespective of that animal's dominant status. There was no evidence that the monkeys could not adequately perceive other animals' size, physical characteristics, or other relevant features that would warn about one monkey being physically dominant over another. Rather, what seemed to be altered was the ability of the monkey to perceive his relationship with another monkey, which could well relate to impaired perception of the self. Knowing who one is often depends on knowing who one is in relation to someone else.

This type of behavioral disturbance is reminiscent of what is seen in many severely TBI patients. Frequently, they approach any individual without the normal social hesitation and do not take into consideration the impact of their actions on someone they have met for the first time. Also, within the work environment, they frequently speak to individuals about personal matters without any apparent recognition of the impact it might have on their relationship. The end result for the lesioned monkeys was that their inappropriate social behavior often resulted in retaliation from dominant males. Versions of the same situation occur for TBI patients suffering anterior frontal and temporal lesions as society recoils from their inappropriate behavior.

In the study of Franzen and Myers (1973), it was also reported that lesioned animals lose the use of common facial expressions, postures, and gestures necessary for social interaction. Moreover, it was observed that other group members could no longer predict the behavior of these lesioned animals. Consequently, they were isolated from many forms of group interaction. This problem of social isolation as noted above is often seen after severe TBI in humans.

It therefore appears that lesions commonly suffered with severe closed head injury may well put the individual at high risk for impaired self and, consequently, social awareness. To begin to investigate this problem, a retrospective study of 64 TBI individuals seen at the Barrow Neurological Institute was conducted. Data obtained from this study are briefly reviewed.

OBSERVATIONS ON IMPAIRED AWARENESS OF BEHAVIORAL LIMITATIONS AFTER BRAIN INJURY

A cross section of TBI patients were studied using the Patient Competency Rating Scale (PCRS). This scale consists of 30 items. The patient is asked to rate, on a 5-point scale, how easy or difficult it is to carry out a given behavioral activity. Some activities were simple and easy to judge (e.g., How much of a problem do I have when dressing myself?). Other items appear to require more insight (e.g., How much of a problem do I have when remembering what I had for dinner last night?). Still other items require a fairly high degree of self and social awareness (e.g., How much of a problem do I have in controlling my temper? How much of a problem do I have in recognizing when something I have said is upsetting to someone else?).

In addition to having the patient fill out this questionnaire, a close relative or friend rated the patient on each of the same items. This practice allows some comparison of the patients' perception of his or her abilities versus an informed other's perception of the patient's abilities.

The TBI patients studied ranged in age from 16 to 64 years, with a mean age of 29.7 years. The average educational level was 13.3 years. The mean chronicity (i.e., the difference between date of injury and date examined) was 16 months, but there was great variability (ranging from 1 to 153 months). The average Glasgow Coma Scale (GCS) score for the patients was 9.68 [a GCS of 3 to 8 is considered to reflect a severe injury, 9 to 12 a moderate injury, and 13 to 15 a mild injury (Jennett and Teasdale, 1981), but again there was great variability. Details concerning the experimental design and subject characteristics can be found in Prigatano and Altman (in press) and Prigatano, Altman, and O'Brien (1990).

As a group, TBI patients tended to underestimate their social and emotional problems (Prigatano, Altman, and O'Brien, 1990). Their relatives reported that these patients typically overestimated their ability to handle arguments, recognize when something they have said has upset others, and control their temper when angered. In contrast, patients and relatives often agreed about the patient's ability to carry out basic self-care activities. It is in the area of judging their most complex interpersonal skills that impaired perception is clearly demonstrated in TBI patients. Interestingly, it appears that standard neuropsychological test findings fail to predict these complex interpersonal behaviors but do correlate with basic activities of daily living.

This finding can be interpreted in at least in two ways. First, neuropsychological deficits may have no bearing on impaired self-awareness as it emerges in social interventions. Thus impaired self-awareness may be primarily related to nonneurological variables (e.g., long-term personality characteristics of the patient or their social situation). Second, what is measured by standard neuropsychological tests may fail to capture more complex neuropsychological impairments underlying this disturbance. The latter of the two possibilities is more likely, given clinical experience with this patient population.

A second report on this group of 64 patients explored in more detail the neuroradiographic and neuropsychological correlates of impaired awareness of behavioral limitations after TBI (Prigatano and Altman, in press). The 64 patients were subclassified into three groups depending on their ratings and their relative's ratings on the PCRS. As indicated above, this scale required the patient and family to rate behavioral competence on a wide variety of behavioral tasks.

Collapsing across all items on the PCRS, group I patients were those who tended to overestimate their behavioral competence relative to their family member's ratings. Group II patients had behavioral ratings similar to those in their relative's reports concerning behavioral competence. Group III underestimated their behavioral competence compared to that in the relatives' reports.

Somewhat surprisingly, the severity of TBI, as measured by the GCS score, was not strongly related to group membership. Also, neuropsychological impairment, as measured by subtests from the Wechsler Adult Intelligence Scale (WAIS)—Revised form, the Wechsler Memory Scale—Revised form, and the Wisconsin Card Sorting test did not relate to group membership. As predicted, however, group I patients had more evidence of decreased speed of finger-tapping in the left hand. Although this finding was in accordance with the hypothesis that patients who showed impaired awareness of behavioral deficits often demonstrate right hemisphere disease, it was also noted that the right hand speed of finger-tapping in this group was below what would be clinically expected. This finding raised the possibility of greater bilateral cerebral impairment in those patients who show less insight into their behavioral limitations.

Neuroradiographic studies of these patients provided evidence that this situation may in fact be the case. Group I patients had suffered a greater number of lesions as visualized on magnetic resonance imaging (MRI) or computed tomography (CT) findings. This finding implied a higher incidence of potentially

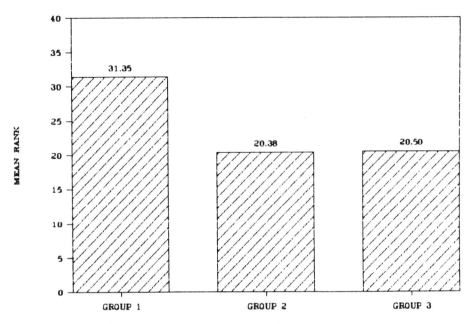

Figure 7-2. Neuroradiographic lesions reported.

bilateral cerebral lesions. Figure 7-2 illustrates the mean ranking (of frequency) of reported lesions by neuroradiologists for each of the three groups. On the average, group I had 3.07 lesions that could be visualized on neuroradiographic examination; group II had 2.6 lesions; and group III had 2.11 lesions. These differences were statistically significant (Prigatano and Altman, in press).

The group sizes were too small to test reliably for differences in lesion location; however, Figure 7-3 demonstrates that group I patients had a relatively high incidence of both frontal and parietal lesions. These findings are compatible with some theoretical ideas suggested by Mesulam (1985).

THEORETICAL IMPLICATIONS

Mesulam (1985) suggested that the cerebral cortex be described in terms of the type of stimuli it responds to rather than the classic subdivisions of this region of the brain. He pointed out that the traditional view was that the cerebral mantle could be subdivided into two types of cortex. One was primary motor and sensory cortex, and the other was called "association" cortex. Figure 7-4, taken from Mesulam's book, reanalyzes different areas of brain tissue and places them in perspective to Brodmann's architectonic map. The most readily identified cortical tissue is, of course, the primary motor and sensory cortex as defined by early neurologists. This area (depicted in blue in Figure 7-4) responds primarily to one type of stimuli. The rest of the cortex was deemed "association" cortex by traditional neurologists. Mesulam (1985) suggested that the association cortex

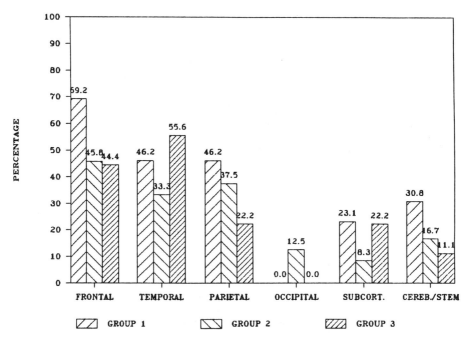

Figure 7–3. Percentage of group by site of lesion.

could theoretically be subdivided into what he termed "unimodal" and "heter-omodal" cortex. Unimodal cortex responds primarily to one type of stimulus, although the stimuli it typically responds to are more complex in nature. The unimodal cortex is depicted in yellow in Figure 7–4. For example, the inferior portion of the temporal lobe frequently responds to complex visual discrimination stimuli.

The rest of the cerebral cortex is considered to be "heteromodal" cortex according to Mesulam's (1985) analysis. It is depicted in pink in Figure 7–4. Inspection of this figure indicates that these regions include not only large por-

Figure 7–4. Distribution of functional zones in relation to Brodmann's map of the human brain. The boundaries are not intended to be precise. Much of this information is based on experimental evidence obtained from laboratory animals and needs to be confirmed in the human brain. AA = auditory association cortex; AG = angular gyrus; A1 = primary auditory cortex; CG = cingulate cortex; INS = insula; IPL = inferior parietal lobule; IT = inferior temporal gyrus; MA = motor association cortex; MPO = medial parietooccipital area; MT = middle temporal gyrus; M1 = primary motor area; OF = orbitofrontal region; PC = prefrontal cortex; PH = parahippocampal region; PO = parolfactory area; PS = peristraite cortex; RS = retrosplenial area; SA = somatosensory association cortex; SG = supramarginal gyrus; SPL = superior parietal lobule; ST = superior temporal gyrus; S1 = primary somatosensory area; TP = temporopolar cortex; VA = visual association cortex; V1 = primary visual cortex. (From Mesulam, M. M. *Principles of Behavioral Neurology.* Philadelphia: Davis, 1985. With permission.)

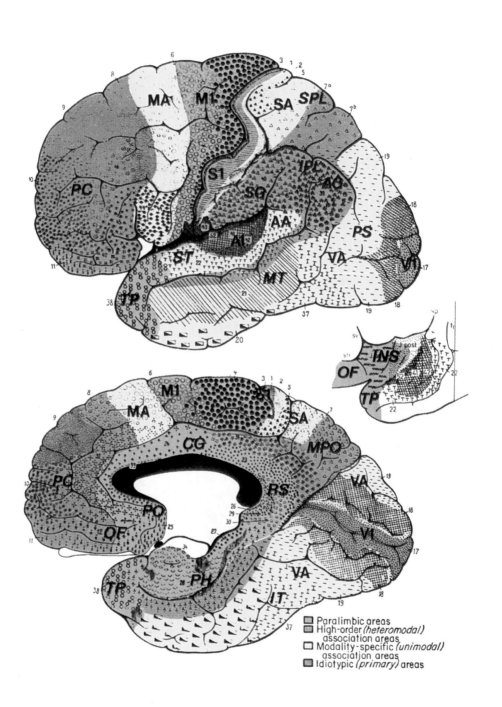

Paralimbic areas
High-order (heteromodal)
   association areas
Modality-specific (unimodal)
   association areas
Idiotypic (primary) areas

tions of the frontal lobe and the prefrontal cortex but also areas in the inferior parietal lobule, the superior marginal gyrus, and the angular gyrus. These areas seem to develop last, from a phylogentic and ontogenetic point of view. Moreover, these regions are important for interfacing information from the external world (which is primarily obtained through the sensorimotor cortex) with information that is received "internally" (primarily from what might be called the paralimbic regions).

Using Mesulam's (1985) analysis, the regions depicted in green in Figure 7–4 are defined as paralimbic cortex. These regions are responsive primarily in internal bodily states. The anterior tip of the temporal lobe (which is at high risk in severe acceleration/deceleration injuries) is made up primarily of this type of neural tissue. It is to be expected therefore that injuries affecting primarily the prefrontal cortex and the anterior temporal lobe would produce significant impairment in the integration of information concerning extrapersonal and intrapersonal space, to use Mesulam's (1985) terms. Disturbances in self-awareness may reflect damage to this type of integration. The capacity for self-perception may rest in those cortical regions that Mesulam (1985) considered heteromodal.

In this model, capacity for self-awareness is not a pure function of frontal lobe activity. Depending on the nature of the cerebral activity involved, different "types" of awareness or impaired awareness might be measured. If one is exploring self-awareness about social judgment, the ability to anticipate change, and so on, the prefrontal regions may be important. In contrast, self-awareness of body and body image may be more influenced by the inferior parietal lobe. Self-perception of linguistic output may be highly dependent on the integrity of the superior marginal and angular gyrus as well as the superior portion of the temporal lobe (see Chapter 3). This model would bring together many of the observations made in this book. As several writers have indicated, one can frequently observe altered self-awareness as a result of injury to frontal, parietal, and temporal regions (McGlynn and Schacter, 1989; see also Chapters 2, 3, 5, and 8).

Mesulam's model may provide the most heuristic approach for understanding these complex and interrelated problems. In this light, one would anticipate different types of awareness disturbances associated with different injuries to various brain regions. This observation has led us to study in more detail two patients who have suffered similar neuropathological lesions but in different brain locations.

RIGHT FRONTAL OLIGODENDROGLIOMA VERSUS RIGHT PARIETAL OCCIPITAL OLIGODENDROGLIOMA

One study compared the behavioral insights of a patient with a right frontal tumor to a patient who had a right parietal occipital mass lesion (Prigatano and O'Brien, in press). The neoplasm in both cases was an oligodendroglioma that was surgically resected. The patient with the frontal tumor was similar to the TBI patients insofar as he demonstrated primary lack of insight into his social awareness. The "parietal" patient, however, had no such difficulties in his self-perceptions in these areas. He showed more difficulty in perceiving his ability to carry out complex perceptual motor tasks (such as his ability to dress himself). We are continuing to study these two patients, but their initial data suggest that there may be different awareness problems associated wtih different brain regions. These observations are certainly compatible with those made by Pribram (1987) and Bisiach, Vallar, Perani, et al. (1986). The latter authors have concluded that "awareness of the failure of a particular function betrays a disorder of the highest level of organization of that function."

It appears that this situation is in fact the case. Lesions of the prefrontal region may produce disturbances in the highest perception of one's social and interpersonal behavior. Lesions of the parietal area may produce lack of insight into problems dealing with the highest perceptual, sensory, and motor functions. In light of the observtions made by other authors in this volume, it also appears that lesions in the superior marginal gyrus and superior temporal lobe may affect the ability of the patient to perceive errors of linguistic output (see Chapter 3).

Studies of anosognosia after various types of brain injury have reported the high incidence of bilateral versus unilateral lesions (see Weinstein and Kahn, 1955; see also several chapters in this book). It may well be therefore that multiple brain regions are correlated with impaired awareness of behavioral limitations. If a single lesion is present, the degree of impaired awareness may be substantially reduced. This point is worthy of further investigation.

ANTON'S SYNDROME IN LIGHT OF THE PRESENT MODEL OF IMPAIRED SELF-AWARENESS AFTER BRAIN INJURY

A possible exception to the model being proposed to account for impaired self-awareness of behavioral limitations is Anton's syndrome, which is defined as denial of blindness when there is evidence that cortical blindness is indeed present (Weinstein and Kahn, 1955). Anton's syndrome is most frequently associated with bilateral vascular lesions in the occipital cortex, particularly involving the calcarine fissure. Primary sensory cortex therefore is destroyed in this type of anosognostic phenomenon. Although this syndrome has rarely been reported following traumatic brain injury, it raises questions concerning the model that heteromodal cortex versus primary sensory cortex is important for permanent alterations of awareness of disability.

As in the case of anosognosia for hemiplegia, recovery from Anton's syndrome (e.g., the anosognostic component) can occur once the acute phase of the illness has disappeared. That is, with the passage of time, awareness of blindness and awareness of hemiplegia may dramatically improve in patients suffering acute vascular insults. In such cases, the neuropathological lesions undoubtedly affect not only basic sensory inputs but most likely produce broad areas of brain dysfunction. This problem may be temporary, secondary to problems of cerebral edema, or it may be permanent depending on whether other cortical tissue is directly damaged.

The fact that frequently there is recovery of the frank anosognosia is important for the present model. Improvement may occur precisely because heteromodal areas are preserved and ultimately respond to a variety of sensory inputs, which correct the initial faulty misperception caused by primary sensory lesions. If only a primary sensorimotor lesion is present, it would be predicted that lack of insight into disturbed neurological function will eventually return because it is primarily the heteromodal regions that are of ultimate importance in the phenomenon of self-awareness. A review of impaired awareness of neuropsychological syndromes discussed Anton's syndrome (McGlynn and Schacter, 1989). It highlighted the finding that, when permanent anosognosia for blindness persists, autopsy studies suggest bilateral lesions in such heteromodal areas as the angular gyrus and the superior and temporal gyri.

IMPLICATIONS FOR REHABILITATION

Disorders of self-awareness have two major implications for rehabilitation. The first is that if patients do not recognize their own altered higher cerebral functioning, they may continue in a number of socially maladapted responses. These responses, particularly after severe TBI, often result in choosing work activities that are not within their realm of behavioral competence and continuing in socially inappropriate behaviors with the consequence of social isolation (Prigatano, 1987; Prigatano et al., 1987). Such patients can become a tremendous financial drain on society as well as a major personal drain on family members (Klonoff and Prigatano, 1987). Rehabilitation efforts that have employed a "holistic approach" (Ben-Yishay, Rattock, Lakin, et al., 1985; Prigatano and Others, 1986a; Ben-Yishay and Prigatano, 1990) have attempted to use a variety of individual and small group activities to help patients achieve a realistic perception of their impact on others and the need to compensate for permanent residual neurobehavioral disorders. The data presented in Table 7–1 highlight the importance of realistic *self-appraisal* of behavioral strengths and weaknesses for ultimate psychosocial outcome after severe TBI.

In addition, there is a second important role of *self-awareness* in neurorehabilitation that is especially true during the acute and intermediate phases of recovery (i.e., particularly during the first year after injury). Given the model adapted from Mesulam (1985) described above, self-awareness emerges primarily in areas of the brain deemed heteromodal cortex. This region is important for integrating what might broadly be called "cognitive" and "affective" components of experience. Learning any new behavior, as well as attempts at relearning "old" behaviors, might well require involvement from these structures. That is, awareness of various components of the self (or higher cerebral mediated activities) is by definition important for the relearning necessary in neurorehabilitation.

There are clinical vignettes that highlight this point. As described elsewhere (Prigatano, 1988), one young adult female patient who suffered severe TBI was working on vocal quality and control 3 months after injury. Her speech and language therapist viewed the patient's voice quality as being "abnormally high-pitched and breathy." The patient did not perceive any change in her voice quality, but family members did. During one therapy session the patient was repeatedly reading the phrase: "The scum is on the pond." The alert therapist noted that the patient at one point suddenly stopped and looked surprised. The patient spontaneously noted, "That's my voice. I can't believe I found my voice on 'the scum is on the pond.'"

The patient's sudden self-awareness of her changed neurobehavioral function helped her to begin to modify her behavior, and so it was a crucial component to her neuro-reeducation.

A second notable example, which highlights that the perception of what is normal for an individual can be affected after brain injury, comes from the insightful writings of Brodal (1973). As a noted neuroanatomist, Professor Brodal was in the unique position of being able to describe his own recovery from a right hemisphere basal ganglia stroke that had produced a left-sided hemiparesis. In his report (Brodal, 1973) he emphasized the tremendous amount of energy required for moving muscles after brain injury and pointed out that one of the values of passive range of movements, a common training procedure used in physical therapy, was that it provided him with a sense of the correct movement. The perception of what is a correct movement was somehow lost following his stroke. This subjective sense of what is normal versus not normal may thus be altered after various types of brain injury. It may well reflect the underlying problem of altered awareness of self during disturbed brain function.

As noted earlier in the chapter, the drawing of one patient reflected a feeling of being both normal and yet different at the same time, which is a common phenomenological experience of many severe TBI patients. Better understanding of this phenomenon may shed needed insight on which retraining procedures are most appropriate for brain dysfunctional patients. In addition, a better understanding of this complex problem of altered self-awareness after brain injury may well provide major insights into the basic mind/body question, which is at the core of behavioral neurology and clinical neuropsychology.

REFERENCES

Adams, J. H., Graham, D. I., and Gennarelli, T. A. (1985). Contemporary neuropathological considerations regarding brain damage in head injury. In D. P. Becker and J. T. Povlishock (eds.), *Central Nervous System Trauma Status Report*. Bethesda: Institute of Neurological and Communicative Disorders and Stroke, National Institutes of Health, pp. 65–77.

Ben-Yishay, Y., and Prigatano, G. P. (1990). Cognitive remediation. In E. Griffith and M. Rosenthal (eds.), *Rehabilitation of the Adult and Child with Traumatic Brain Injury*. Philadelphia: Davis, pp. 393–409.

Ben-Yishay, Y., Rattok, J. Lakin, P., Piasetsky, E. D., Ross, B., Silver, S., Zide, E., and Ezrachi, O., (1985). Neuropsychological rehabilitation: quest for a holistic approach. *Semin. Neurol.* 5:252–258.

Bisiach, E., Vallar, G., Perani, D., Papagno, C. and Berti, A. (1986). Unawareness of disease following lesions of the right hemisphere: anosognosia for hemiplegia and anosognosia for hemianopia. *Neuropsychologia* 24:471–482.

Bond, M. R. (1988). Preface. *J. Head Trauma Rehabil.* 3(4):vii–ix.

Brodal, A. (1973). Self-observations and neuro-anatomical considerations after a stroke. *Brain* 96:675–694.

Fordyce, D. J., and Roueche, J. R. (1986). Changes in perspectives of disability among patients, staff, and relatives during rehabilitation of brain injury. *Rehabil. Psychol.* 31:217–229.

Franzen, E. A., and Myers, R. E. (1973). Neural control of social behavior: prefrontal and anterior temporal cortex. *Neuropsychologia* 11:141–157.

Jennett, B., and Teasdale, G. (1981). *Management of Head Injuries.* Philadelphia: Davis.

Klonoff, P. S., and Prigatano, G. P. (1987). Reactions of family members and clinical intervention after traumatic brain injury. In M. Ylvisaker and E. R. Gobble (eds.), *Community Re-entry for Head Injured Adults.* Boston: College Hill Press, pp. 381–402.

Levin, H. S., Benton, A. L., and Grossman, R. C. (1982). *Neurobehavioral Consequences of Closed Head Injury.* New York: Oxford University Press.

McGlynn, S. M., and Schacter, D. L. (1989). Unawareness of deficits in neuropsychological syndromes. *J. Clin. Exp. Neuropsychol.* 11:143–205.

Mesulam, M. M. (1985). *Principles of Behavioral Neurology.* Philadelphia: Davis.

Oddy, M., Coughlan, T., Tyerman, A., and Jenkins, D. (1985). Social adjustment after closed head injury: a further follow-up seven years after injury. *J. Neurol. Neurosurg. Psychiatry* 48:564–568.

Pribram, K. H. (1987). The subdivisions of the frontal cortex revisited. In E. Perecman (ed.), *The Frontal Lobes Revisited.* New York: IRBN Press, pp. 11–39.

Prigatano, G. P. (1987). Neuropsychological deficits, personality variables and outcome. In M. Ylvisaker and E. M. R. Gobble (eds.), *Community Re-entry for Head Injured Adults.* Boston: College Hill Press, pp. 1–23.

Prigatano, G. P. (1988). Emotion and motivation in recovery and adaptation to brain damage. In S. Finger, T. LeVere, C. Almli, and D. Stein (eds.), *Brain Injury and Recovery: Theoretical and Controversial Issues.* New York: Plenum Press, pp. 335–350.

Prigatano, G. P., and Altman, I. M. (in press). Impaired awareness of behavioral limitation after brain injury. *Archives Physical Medicine and Rehabilitation.*

Prigatano, G. P., and O'Brien, K. P. (in press). Awareness of deficit in patients with frontal vs. parietal lesions: 2 case reports. *BNI Q.,* in press.

Prigatano, G. P., and Others. (1986a). *Neuropsychological Rehabilitation After Brain Injury.* Baltimore: Johns Hopkins University Press.

Prigatano, G. P., Pepping, M., and Klonoff, P. (1986b). Cognitive, personality and psychosocial factors in the neuropsychological assessment of brain-injured patient. In B. Uzzell and Y. Gross (eds.), *Clinical Neuropsychology of Intervention.* Boston: Martinus Nijhoff, pp. 135–166.

Prigatano, G. P., Klonoff, P. S., and Bailey, I. (1987). Psychosocial adjustment associated with traumatic brain injury: statistics BNI neurorehabilitation must best. *BNI Q.* 3:18–21.

Prigatano, G. P., O'Brien, K. P., and Klonoff, P. S. (1988). The clinical management of delusions in post acute traumatic brain injured patients. *J. Head Trauma Rehabil.* 3(3):23–32.

Prigatano, G. P., Altman, I. M., and O'Brien, K. P. (1990). Behavioral limitations that brain injured patients tend to underestimate, *Clinical Neuropsychologist,* pp. 163–176.

Romano, M. D. (1974). Family response to traumatic head injury. *Scand. J. Rehabil. Med.* 6:1–6.

Russell, W. R. (1971). *The Traumatic Amnesias.* London: Oxford University Press.

Sunderland, A., Harris, J. E., and Baddeley, A. D. (1983). Do laboratory tests predict everyday memory? A neuropsychological study. *J. Verbal Learn. Verbal Behav.* 22:341–357.

Sunderland, A., Harris, J. E., and Gleave, J. (1984). Memory failures in everyday life following severe head injury. *J. Clin. Neuropsychol.* 6:127–142.

Thomsen, I. V. (1984). Late outcome of very severe blunt head trauma: 10–15 year second follow-up. *J. Neurol. Neursurg. Psychiatry* 47:260–268.

Weinstein, E. A., and Kahn, R. I. (1955). *Denial of Illness.* Springfield, IL: Charles C Thomas.

8

Unawareness of Deficit and Unawareness of Knowledge in Patients with Memory Disorders

DANIEL L. SCHACTER

Unawareness of deficit represents a counterintuitive and sometimes bizarre feature of various neuropsychological syndromes. The notion that a person could be unaware of such visibly disabling disorders as hemiplegia, hemianopia, aphasia, or even complete blindness seems so contrary to everyday experience that one is tempted to think of the phenomenon as an infrequent curiosity that need not command much theoretical attention, even though the literature shows clearly that unawareness of deficit is observed in large numbers of patients (see McGlynn and Schacter, 1989, for comprehensive review).

The fact that unawareness of deficit is often observed in patients with memory disorders does not seem nearly as surprising as does the occurrence of unawareness in the syndromes noted above. After all, if patients have difficulty remembering recent experiences and acquiring new information, it seems to follow that they would have similar difficulty remembering that they have a memory problem. It is perhaps more surprising to learn that many memory-disordered patients—including some who are severely amnesic—are acutely aware of their deficits. This observation indicates that unawareness of deficit in amnesic patients cannot be accounted for simply by claiming that patients fail to remember that they have a deficit (e.g., Whitlock, 1981) and thus raises questions concerning the mechanisms underlying awareness and unawareness of memory disorder.

The purposes of this chapter are twofold. The first is to consider empirical observations on awareness and unawareness of memory deficit in various patient groups and discuss pertinent methodological and conceptual issues. The second is to consider the relation between unawareness of deficit and a phenomenon that is referred to generically as "unawareness of knowledge." Research has established firmly that information presented during a specific episode can facilitate amnesic patients' performance on various implicit memory tests (Graf and Schacter, 1985; Schacter, 1987b), even though patients have no conscious recollection of the episode: The patients are unaware that they have acquired any knowledge (e.g., Warrington and Weiskrantz, 1974; Moscovitch, 1982; Graf, Squire, and Mandler, 1984; Schacter, 1985). Similar dissociations have been observed in a variety of neuropsychological syndromes in which patients' performance reveals that they possess knowledge of which they are unaware (Schacter, McAndrews, and Moscovitch, 1988). The latter part of this chapter examines the relation between unawareness of deficit and unawareness of knowledge within the context of some theoretical ideas (cf., Schacter, 1990).

AWARENESS AND UNAWARENESS OF MEMORY DEFICIT: EMPIRICAL OBSERVATIONS

This section considers evidence on awareness of deficit that is derived from three sources: clinical observations, questionnaire studies, and experimental paradigms.

Clinical Observations

In a pioneering article describing the syndrome that now bears his name, Korsakoff (1889) noted that most of his patients showed little awareness of or concern about their memory disorders; only two of his patients showed clear evidence of awareness, by taking active steps to cover up their memory problem. Talland (1965), in his classic monograph on Korsakoff syndrome, claimed that none of his patients were aware of the "full extent" of their disorder and reported that some "denied any memory disturbance even in the face of the most striking evidence" (p. 29). Talland believed that patients' frequently evasive responses about their memory deficit "does not prove awareness of that difficulty" (p. 29) but instead reflects difficulty retrieving appropriate information. Talland noted further that patients typically attributed their presence in the hospital to physical defects, rather than to memory or cognitive problems. Other clinical observers have also noted that Korsakoff patients typically exhibit little or no awareness of their memory problem (e.g., Zangwill, 1966; Victor, Adams, and Collins, 1971).

A prominent feature of Korsakoff's syndrome is the presence of neuropsychological signs of frontal lobe impairment (e.g., Butters and Cermak, 1980; Schacter, 1987c; Squire, 1987). As McGlynn and Schacter (1989) pointed out, impaired awareness of memory disorder has been described in other patients with signs of frontal pathology. Jahro (1973) reported that patients with penetrating brain injuries were more likely to exhibit unawareness of memory deficit when frontal regions were damaged than when they were not. In a study of patients with ruptured aneurysms of the anterior communicating artery (ACAA), Vilkki (1985) noted that three patients with frontal lesions were unaware of their memory problems, whereas two patients with no frontal signs showed intact awareness. Luria (1976) provided striking descriptions of unawareness in ACAA patients, exemplified by the following exchange.

> *How is your memory?* "My memory is not bad . . . I don't complain of any loss of memory . . . I consider that my memory is normal. . . ." *Why then do you tell me now sometimes that it is August, sometimes that it is May?* "I don't know." [p. 276]

Luria described similar examples of unawareness in patients with massive frontal lobe tumors. In contrast, he noted that patients with amnesia attributable to third ventricle lesions or pituitary tumors expressed acute awareness of their memory problems, complaining that their memories were no longer any good (p. 342).

Excellent awareness of memory disorder has also been observed in other patients who are free of frontal signs. The extensively studied patient N.A., who developed a severe verbal memory deficit following a stab wound in the left dorsomedial nucleus of the thalamus, can provide lucid descriptions of his memory problems (Kaushall, Zetin, and Squire, 1981). Another well-studied patient, H.M., who became globally amnesic after medial temporal lobe resection, was reported to be aware of his deficit (Milner, Corkin, and Teuber, 1968). Consistent with this observation, encephalitic patients with amnesia attributable to temporal lobe lesions also appear to be well aware of their deficits on clinical observation (Rose and Symonds, 1960). Some of these patients have provided succinct, penetrating accounts of their condition: "There's nothing wrong with me physically but mentally things as they happen don't seem to impress themselves on my mind" (p. 195). Similar observations have been made in cases of transient global amnesia—a temporary though severe form of anterograde amnesia that can be produced by ischemia of the medial temporal lobes (Pansford and Donnan, 1980; Jenson and Olivarius, 1981). For instance, a patient described by Evans (1966) suddenly became amnesic after taking a bath: "His first words were 'Am I going mad? I can't remember anything'" (p. 543). An instructive feature of this case and other instances of transient global amnesia like it (e.g., Byer and Crowley, 1980; Roman-Campor, Poser, and Wood, 1980; Fisher, 1982) is that patients exhibit awareness of their memory disorder immediately after its onset. Thus when intact awareness is observed in amnesic patients, it need not be something that is "learned" slowly over time as patients experience more and more episodes of forgetting.

Clinical observation, though useful descriptively, entails well known methodological limitations that restrict the force of the conclusions that can be drawn from it. Nevertheless, the observation that unawareness of memory deficit is linked to frontal lobe pathology receives support from several more rigorous studies, as discussed in the next two sections.

Questionnaire Studies

Most empirical studies of memory and amnesia have relied on either experimental paradigms or clinical test batteries. In recent years, however, a significant number of studies have used questionnaire techniques in which people are required to provide self-reports about various aspects of their own memory function (Herrmann, 1982). As Schacter, Glisky, and McGlynn (1990) pointed out, the initial goal of questionnaire studies of memory-impaired patients is to provide ecologically valid information about the impact of memory disorders on everyday life.

Thus, for example, Sunderland, Harris, and Baddeley (1983) administered a questionnaire that included 35 items, each concerned with different aspects of everyday memory function, to a group of severely head-injured patients and their relatives. Patients were required to rate how much difficulty they believed they had with each item in their everyday lives (i.e., remembering to do things, remembering people's names, and so forth); relatives were required to rate patients' everyday memory function on the same items. Sunderland et al. were particularly interested in the relation between patients' questionnaire responses and their performance on standard laboratory tests of memory. They found no correlation between the two and suggested that laboratory tests do not tap the same processes that underlie everyday memory function. An alternative interpretation, however, is that the absence of correlation between test performance and questionnaire responses can be attributed in part or entirely to patients' lack of awareness of their memory difficulties. If patients were not fully aware of their memory deficits, they could hardly be expected to provide accurate information about what kinds of problem they experienced in everyday life.

Two types of data from the Sunderland et al. study are consistent with the latter interpretation: First, relatives' questionnaire ratings were positively correlated with patients' test performance and uncorrelated with patients' self-report on the questionnaire; and second, patients rated their memory function no differently than did control subjects, even though patients performed significantly worse than controls on laboratory memory tests. Further questionnaire studies of head-injured patients have confirmed that patients' subjective rating of their own memory function typically shows little if any correlation with either relatives' ratings or objective test performance (Rimel, Giordani, Barth, et al., 1981; Sunderland, Harris and Baddeley, 1984; Cockburn, Wilson, and Baddeley, 1986; Boake, Freedland, Ringholz, et al., 1987).

A plausible alternative to the "unawareness" interpretation of the foregoing results relates to what Hermann (1982) termed the "memory introspection paradox": Completing a questionnaire is itself a memory task, so people with poor memories are less likely to remember instances of memory failure than are people with good memories. Thus it would not be surprising if memory-impaired patients provided inaccurate questionnaire responses because they would likely be unable to retrieve the appropriate information (Sunderland et al., 1983; Brooks and Lincoln, 1984; Hart and Hayden, 1986). One implication of this view is that inaccurate responding on a self-report memory questionnaire must be observed in virtually all patients with memory disorders. However, data contrary to such an expectation have been provided by Bennett-Levy, Polkey, and Powell (1980), who found that patients with memory disorders attributable to temporal lobectomy provided generally accurate assessments of their memory problems on a questionnaire. This finding, when considered in relation to the studies showing that head-injured patients generally provide inaccurate subjective assessments of their memory functions, may relate to the frontal lobe issue discussed earlier: Head-injured patients typically have extensive frontal lobe damage, whereas the temporal lobectomy patients did not have significant frontal lobe impairment. Moreover, head-injured patients exhibit impaired awareness in various other cognitive, social, and behavioral domains (e.g., Hackler and Tobis, 1983; Prigatano and others, 1986). These considerations suggest that amnesic patients without frontal signs may be able to provide reasonably accurate self-assessments on a memory questionnaire, whereas patients with frontal signs cannot. Consistent with this expectation, Parkin, Bell, and Leng (in press) found that a group of four temporal lobe amnesics showed awareness of their memory problem in response to a questionnaire probe, whereas a group of five Korsakoff patients did not.

Further pertinent data were provided in a study by McGlynn, Schacter, and Glisky (1989) that developed new questionnaire techniques to study subjective assessment of memory disorders in two amnesic patients; that study is described here in some detail. The first patient (B.Z.) was a 40-year-old, college-educated man who suffered a ruptured ACAA in June 1985. Neuropsychological evaluation revealed above-average intelligence: B.Z.'s Full-scale IQ on the Wechsler Adult Intelligence Scale-Revised (WAIS-R) was 126, with a Verbal IQ of 117 and a Performance IQ of 132. Despite his high level of intellectual function, B.Z. was severely amnesic. On the Wechsler Memory Scale (WMS), his MQ was 87, with scores of 0, 4, and 1 on delayed tests of logical memory, visual reproduction, and hard paired associates, respectively. On a 1-hour delayed test of picture recognition, he correctly classified as "old" 6 of 16 previously presented items and incorrectly classified as "old" 3 of 16 distractor items. A computed tomography (CT) scan showed damage in frontal regions and in the anterior cerebral artery.

The second patient (H.D.) was a 33-year-old woman with a high school education who became amnesic after contracting herpes simplex encephalitis in June 1980. Neuropsychological assessment revealed low-average intelligence (WAIS-R Full Scale IQ = 84; Verbal IQ = 79, Performance IQ = 95) and severe amnesia (WMS MQ = 65; 0 recall on delayed tests of logical memory, visual reproduction, and hard associates; 9 of 16 hits and 9 of 16 false alarms on delayed picture recognition). A CT scan revealed that significant neuropathology was largely restricted to the left temporal lobe.

To assess awareness of deficit, three questionnaires were developed. The *General Self-Assessment Questionnaire* requires patients to rate, on a 7-point scale, the degree to which they are experiencing difficulty with various aspects of memory compared to before their illness (e.g., Compared to before your illness, how much difficulty do you have remembering your recent experiences?). The patients' spouses were also asked to assess patients' functioning on this scale. The *Everyday Memory Questionnaire* comprised ten *specific* everyday situations that require remembering different types of information. Patients rated on a 7-point scale the likelihood that they would remember the target information in these hypothetical situations after delays of 10 minutes, 1 hour, 1 day, and 1 week (e.g., How likely would you be to remember a telephone conversation with a friend [10 minutes, 1 hour, 1 day, 1 week] after it occurred?). In addition, patients used the same scale to rate the likelihood that they would have been able to remember the target information *before* their illness and to rate the likelihood that their *spouse* would remember this information. The logic underlying this procedure is straightforward: If patients rate their current likelihood of remembering in the same way that they rate their memory prior to illness and their spouse's current memory, there would be converging evidence of unawareness of memory deficit. Patients' predictions with respect to the four delay intervals provide information about their general knowledge of how memory normally functions: If patients are aware of how memory normally works, they make increasingly lower predictions as a function of the length of retention interval. This questionnaire was also given to spouses, who rated their own likelihood of remembering in the ten everyday situations as well as the patient's likelihood both now and prior to illness.

The third questionnaire, the *Item Recall Questionnaire,* requires patients to predict how many items they would be able to remember (both now and prior to illness) if they were shown lists consisting of ten items of various kinds (e.g., names, paired-associates) and were tested at each of the four delays mentioned above. In addition, one-half of the hypothetical lists were concerned with items that would be considered relatively "easy" to remember (e.g., familiar names) and half involved items that would be considered relatively "difficult" to remember (e.g., unfamiliar names). Comparing predictions for easy and difficult items provided another index of patients' general knowledge of how memory functions: If such knowledge is preserved, patients predict higher recall of the former type of item than of the latter. Patients also predicted their spouses' performance on this task, and spouses predicted patients' performance as well as their own.

The tasks and procedures used in this study allow us to investigate a richer set of questions and comparisons than in previous questionnaire studies. Consider first the results from the ACAA patient B.Z. On the General Self-Assessment Questionnaire, B.Z. consistently indicated that he currently has little or no problem with memory (mean rating 5.2, where 6.0 indicates no difficulty with a particular item), whereas his spouse reported correctly that he has a great deal of difficulty on the various memory items (mean rating = 0.2, where 0 indicates maximal difficulty). The results of the Everyday Memory Questionnaire (Table 8-1) indicated that B.Z. rated himself much more likely to remember in these naturalistic scenarios at all retention intervals than did his wife. No such pattern was observed in B.Z.'s ratings of himself prior to illness or of his wife's current memory abilities; in fact, there was a trend at the longer delays in these conditions for B.Z. to provide lower ratings than his wife. It is also clear that B.Z. knows perfectly well that memory performance decays over time, as indicated by consistent drops in his rating across retention intervals.

On the Item Recall Questionnaire (Table 8-2), B.Z. rated his current memory as no worse than his memory prior to illness or his wife's current memory function. He also substantially overestimated his current recall performance relative to his wife's predictions: He consistently claimed that he would remember four to six items at the short delays and three or four items at the long delays whereas his wife predicted that he would remember zero to two items at the short delays and none at the long delays; these predictions were in fact accurate in

TABLE 8–1 Prediction of Self and Others' Performance by Patients and Their Spouses on the Item Recall Questionnaire as a Function of Item Type (Easy vs. Difficult)

Performance predicted	Person predicting					
	Item type			Item type		
	Easy	Difficult	M	Easy	Difficult	M
	B.Z.			*Spouse*		
B.Z., now	4.5	3.1	3.8	0.9	0.3	0.6
B.Z., before	4.3	3.5	3.9	4.2	2.8	3.5
Spouse	4.3	3.3	3.8	3.7	2.5	3.1
	H.D.			*Spouse*		
H.D., now	1.9	0.8	1.4	2.8	0.6	1.7
H.D., before	4.9	2.0	3.5	6.3	4.1	5.2
Spouse	5.6	3.0	4.2	6.5	4.1	5.3

Note. In the "now" condition, patients and spouses predicted patients' current memory ability; in the "before" condition, they predicted patients' ability prior to the onset of amnesia. Each entry in the table reflects the predicted number of recalled items from a maximum of ten. M = Mean.

relation to our test data on B.Z. However, B.Z.'s "predictions" of his performance prior to illness were virtually identical to those made by his wife, and his assessment of his wife's recall performance was similar to her predictions about her own performance. Finally, B.Z., like his wife, predicted higher recall for easy than difficult items and for short than long delays.

In sharp contrast to B.Z., the encephalitic H.D. expressed acute awareness of her memory problems; her ratings were generally consistent with both her spouse's ratings and objective measures of memory function. Thus she indicated that she was experiencing a great deal of difficulty with memory on the General Self-Assessment Questionnaire (mean rating 1.0), closely matching her spouse's rating (mean rating 1.2). On the Everday Memory Questionnaire, H.D.'s ratings of her performance were comparable to, though slightly higher than, her spouse's ratings of her performance; but in contrast to B.Z., she rated herself as far less

TABLE 8–2 Prediction of Self and Others' Performance by Patients and Their Spouses on the Everyday Memory Questionnaire as a Function of Retention Interval

Performance predicted	Person predicting									
	10 min	1 hr	1 day	1 week	M	10 min	1 hr	1 day	1 week	M
	B.Z.					*Spouse*				
B.Z., now	6.0	5.8	5.3	4.4	5.4	4.7	3.5	0.3	0.0	2.1
B.Z., before	5.9	5.5	4.0	2.2	4.4	6.0	5.9	5.6	4.9	5.6
Spouse	5.9	5.1	5.3	5.0	5.6	6.0	6.0	6.0	5.7	5.9
	H.D.					*Spouse*				
H.D., now	3.2	2.2	1.1	0.7	1.8	2.0	1.0	0.2	0.0	0.8
H.D., before	5.8	5.4	4.6	4.1	5.0	5.8	5.3	5.0	4.5	5.1
Spouse	5.3	4.8	4.0	3.5	4.4	5.9	5.9	5.8	5.0	5.6

Note. Each entry in the table reflects the predicted likelihood of recall in a specific condition, where "6" indicates maximal likelihood of recall and "1" indicates minimal likelihood of recall. M = mean.

likely to remember now than before her illness and far less likely to remember than her spouse (Table 8–1). She also gave generally accurate recall predictions on the Item Recall Questionnaire relative to her spouse's predictions and our test data, and she clearly differentiated between current and prior memory function on this questionnaire (Table 8–2). H.D.'s general knowledge of how memory functions was also generally unimpaired, as indicated by higher predictions for short than long delays and easy than difficult items that closely resembled the ratings of her spouse.

Although these results are preliminary (we are currently collecting further data with other patients), they do highlight several important points. First, the data are consistent with prior evidence that unawareness of memory deficit is related to frontal damage. It is interesting to note in this regard that B.Z. had a much higher IQ than did H.D. (126 versus 84), so his lack of awareness cannot be attributed to generalized intellectual deterioration. Similarly, his memory problems were no more severe than those of H.D., thereby suggesting that he would not be more likely to "forget" that he had a memory problem than would H.D.

The latter observation raises the general question of the relation between level of memory function on the one hand and awareness of memory deficit on the other: How does a densely amnesic patient such as H.D. know that she has a deficit? One possibility that must be considered in H.D.'s case is that such awareness is acquired or learned over time as a function of experiencing repeated episodes of forgetting. H.D. became amnesic in 1980, seven years prior to the McGlynn et al. study, so she would have had many opportunities to learn about her memory deficit. Because it is known that amnesic patients can acquire various kinds of information through extensive repetition (e.g., Milner et al., 1968; Cohen and Squire, 1980; Glisky, Schacter, and Tulving, 1986a,b) and that H.D. shows excellent incremental learning (Glisky and Schacter, 1987, 1989), this possibility must be considered seriously. B.Z., on the other hand, had been amnesic for only 2 years at the time of study and might not have had enough "learning trials" to become aware of his deficit. Although this hypothesis cannot be rejected, the previously mentioned observations on patients with transient global amnesia suggest that it does not suffice as a general explanation of awareness of deficit in amnesia: Transient global amnesia patients are aware of their profound anterograde amnesia almost from the moment of onset.

It is also interesting to consider the *types* of information that might underlie "aware" responding on a memory questionnaire. For example, how does a patient such as H.D. "know" that she would be unlikely to remember a telephone conversation 10 minutes after it occurred? One possibility is that patients are able to remember salient *instances* in which they exhibited pathological forgetting and make use of such instances when judging their memory abilities. However, in view of amnesic patients' well documented difficulties with explicit recall of individual episodes, an instance-based account, at least in simple form, seems implausible. Alternatively, patients may learn a more abstract and general proposition about their memory abilities (i.e., "I have a poor memory")—even though they do not remember any specific instance of memory failure—and respond to questionnaire items on the basis of such abstract knowledge.

Although data that distinguish between these two positions are not available, it seems clear that specification of the mechanisms underlying awareness of memory function in both amnesic patients and normal subjects will facilitate understanding of what has gone wrong in patients who are unaware of their deficit.

The foregoing considerations indicate that a great deal more research is needed that attempts to elucidate the processes by which amnesic patients become aware of their memory deficits, and the kinds of information that underlie such awareness. Research that uses experimental paradigms to investigate awareness may be useful for achieving this objective.

Experimental Investigations

What kinds of experimental paradigms might be useful for studying awareness of memory deficit? One possibility is suggested by cognitive research concerning a phenomenon referred to as *metamemory* or *memory monitoring:* knowledge concerning the characteristics of one's own memory performance. Cognitive psychologists have investigated metamemory with a variety of experimental paradigms, but in most of them people are required to *predict* some aspect of their memory performance. Thus, for example, subjects might predict at the time of study whether they will remember each to-be-remembered item (e.g., Groninger, 1979), predict just prior to a memory test how many items they think they will remember (e.g., Schacter, 1986), or predict the likelihood of recognizing items that they have failed to recall (e.g., Hart, 1965; Nelson, Leonesio, Shimamura, et al., 1982; Schacter, 1983; Nelson, 1984; Schacter and Worling, 1985). With respect to the present concerns, ability to predict memory performance accurately in metamemory paradigms may provide a useful index of awareness of memory deficit. A few experimental studies have investigated metamemory in amnesic patients.

Consider first a study by Shimamura and Squire (1986), who examined the ability of various amnesic patients to predict recognition of unrecalled information in the "feeling-of-knowing" paradigm developed originally by Hart (1965). In experiment 1, subjects were asked general knowledge questions of varying levels of difficulty about different topics (e.g., What is the name of the ship on which Charles Darwin made his scientific voyage? *The Beagle*). For each subject, a set of unrecalled facts was generated from the first 24 questions on which they failed to provide correct answers. Subjects then made feeling-of-knowing ratings about these items in which they indicated how likely they thought they would be to recognize the correct answer if they were given a few choices. A 4-point scale was used, where 1 indicated a high feeling of knowing that they would recognize the answer, 2 indicated a medium feeling of knowing, 3 indicated a low feeling of knowing, and 4 indicated a pure guess. The critical question was whether amnesic patients, like normal subjects, show greater recognition accuracy for unrecalled items given high rather than low feeling-of-knowing ratings. Three groups of amnesic patients participated in the experiment: Korsakoff patients, electroconvulsive therapy patients, and a group of mixed etiology patients [anoxia, ischemia, left diencephalic lesion (patient N.A.)]. Results indicated that only the Korsakoff patients showed impaired feeling-of-knowing accuracy: The correlation between their predictions and recognition performance was significantly lower than the corresponding correlations for control subjects and for the other groups of amnesic patients, who did not differ significantly from controls.

These data suggest that non-Korsakoff amnesics may be able to predict recognition of unrecalled items as accurately as do control subjects. One problem with this interpretation, however, is that the non-Korsakoff patients showed normal performance on the general knowledge test, whereas the Korsakoff patients' recall performance was significantly impaired compared to that of control subjects. It is thus possible that feeling-of-knowing accuracy in amnesic patients is intact only when recall performance is intact; amnesic patients may not show normal feeling-of-knowing accuracy when tested within the domain of their deficit.

To test this idea, Shimamura and Squire examined feeling-of-knowing accuracy for newly learned items in experiment 2. The reasoning was that recall of newly learned items is impaired in all amnesic patients, so it should be possible to determine if intact feeling-of-knowing accuracy can be observed in non-Korsakoff amnesics even when recall performance is impaired. Subjects in this experiment studied sentences (e.g., "Patty's garden was full of marigolds"), were later given the sentence frame as a recall cue (e.g., "Patty's garden was full of _____"), and then made feeling-of-knowing ratings for unrecalled items on the same 4-point scale as was used in experiment 1. Amnesic patients were tested after a 5-minute retention interval; controls were tested either at this delay or at a 1- to 7-day delay when recall performance was about equal to that of amnesic patients at the 5-minute delay. The feeling-of-knowing predictions of non-Korsakoff amnesics were significantly correlated with recognition performance; the magnitude of the correlation was similar to control subjects' accuracy at the long delay and somewhat lower than control subjects' accuracy at the short delay. For Korsakoff patients, in contrast, there was no correlation between feeling-of-knowing predictions and recognition performance.

The general pattern of results from this study, then, indicates that Korsakoff amnesics have severe difficulty monitoring and predicting their memory performance, whereas non-Korsakoff patients do not. In view of previously mentioned data indicating that Korsakoff patients show signs of frontal lobe pathology, this finding is consistent with, and extends the generality of, the idea that impaired awareness of memory function is observed in patients with frontal signs.

A study that used a somewhat different type of metamemory pradigm was reported by Schacter, McLachlan, Moscovitch, and Tulving (1986). They examined the performance of three groups of memory-disordered patients—those with closed head injuries, those with ruptured ACAAs, and patients in the early stages of Alzheimer's disease—as well as matched control groups on a task that required prediction of free recall performance. The experiment consisted of three phases: study, prediction, and testing. All subjects studied two 20-item categorized lists, each consisting of four items from each of five categories (e.g., fruit: lemon, grape, apple, banana). One list was oraganized in a *blocked* manner; the four members of a given category were presented successively for 5 seconds each, followed by the four members of a second category, and so forth. A second list was presented in an *unblocked* manner; the 20 list items appeared in a random order. The unblocked list was always studied and tested before the blocked list. After the final list item was presented, subjects were told that they would be asked shortly to recall as many list items as possible. They were then instructed that they should first try to predict how many of the 20 items they thought they could recall during the 5 minutes that would be allotted to them. After they made their recall predictions, subjects were given 5 minutes for free recall.

Data concerning recall and prediction performance are presented in Table 8–3. Not surprisingly, the results indicate that free recall performance for each of the three patient groups was significantly lower than for their corresponding controls on both blocked and unblocked lists. The recall prediction data, however, indicate that the head-injured and ACAA patients were about as accurate as their controls in predicting the number of items they would recall: Predictions were, on average, within one or two items of actual performance, with a general trend toward modest overprediction of performance. Alzheimer patients, in contrast, predicted that they would recall many more items than they did; on average, they overpredicted performance by about seven items on both blocked and unblocked lists.

The fact that Alzheimer patients showed impaired ability to predict their recall performance is consistent with other data indicating that such patients are unaware of their deficits (McGlynn and Schacter, 1989; see also Chapter 6) and are characterized by extensive frontal lobe pathology (Kaszniak, 1986). It is perhaps more surprising that the head-injured and ACAA patients showed relatively normal recall predictions because, as noted earlier, these patients are often characterized by unawareness of deficit and frontal signs. This point is discussed later in the chapter.

Prediction of recall performance was also used in a study that examined if awareness of deficit could be increased through appropriate training (McGlynn, Schacter, and Glisky, in preparation; see also Schacter, Glisky, and McGlynn, 1990). This study focused on the ACAA patient B.Z., whose unawareness of deficit was documented on the General Self-Assessment, Everyday Memory, and

TABLE 8-3 Prediction of Recall Performance on Blocked and Unblocked Categorized Lists by Patients and Controls

Subjects	Blocked list		Unblocked list	
	PR	RC	PR	RC
ACAA	7.6	5.7	8.5	6.3
Controls	12.5	13.5	13.1	12.0
CHI	5.8	4.3	4.8	4.5
Controls	16.3	15.5	12.4	11.0
DAT	8.9	1.8	9.2	1.9
Controls	11.6	10.4	10.9	8.8

Note. ACAA = anterior communicating artery aneurysm patients; CHI = closed head injury patients; DAT = dementia of the Alzheimer type patients. PR = predicted number of items recalled; RC = actual number of items recalled (maximum possible predicted/recalled = 20).

Item Recall Questionnaires described previously. B.Z. was required to predict his performance on two tasks: free recall of a 16-word list, and free recall of eight simple actions that B.Z. performed in the laboratory (e.g., putting a cup on a desk). For both tasks, B.Z. was first exposed to the appropriate list, was then asked to predict how many list items he thought he could recall after a 15-minute delay, and then attempted recall after a filled retention interval. B.Z. was then provided with extensive feedback and discussion concerning the discrepancies between his predicted and actual performance. The general idea was that with repeated feedback of this kind B.Z. would be able to become aware of his memory problem. Awareness was assessed by examining the relation between his predicted and actual performance on the recall tasks and by his responses on the General Self-Assessment and Everyday Memory questionnaires described previously. In addition, a further questionnaire was used that required B.Z. to rate the likelihood that he would be successful if he returned to his former job (a manager in a government office). This Job Performance Questionnaire included a variety of job scenarios in which intact memory function was required in order to perform adequately. Two interventions were conducted, each involving two prediction-feedback sessions per day; the first intervention lasted for three consecutive days, the second for five consecutive days. Long-term follow-up sessions were conducted 1, 2, and 6 weeks after the conclusion of the second intervention.

The most interesting outcome of the study was that the intervention appeared to have different effects on different indices of awareness. For example, whereas B.Z. initially grossly overpredicted recall performance on both the word and action recall tasks, his predictions became somewhat more realistic within each day. However, his predictions returned to baseline at the beginning of subsequent days of training in both the first and second intervention. By contrast, his response to a general question about his memory function on the General Self-Assessment Questionnaire (i.e., Compared to before your illness, how much difficulty are you currently having with your memory?) showed consistent improvement that was retained across days during the second intervention: At the beginning of the final day of the intervention, B.Z. indicated that he was having considerable difficulty with his memory. Moreover, B.Z. continued to rate himself as having substantial memory difficulties at the 1-, 2-, and 6-week follow-up sessions. Yet his response to several of the more specific items on this questionnaire (e.g., Compared to before your illness, how much difficulty do you have remembering conversations with members of your family?) showed no consistent change at any point in the intervention. His ratings on the specific, hypothetical scenarios of the Everyday Memory Questionnaire showed some improvement within-days but no consistent evidence of change across days or at long-term follow up. On the Job Performance Questionnaire, B.Z. also showed some small improvements within-days but none across-days. The between-day and long-term follow-up data suggest that B.Z. had acquired through feedback an isolated bit of new knowledge (e.g., "I have problems with my memory") that he did not apply flexibly to all appropriate situations. These data suggest that conclusions about awareness of memory deficit may depend on how awareness is assessed.

Summary of Research on Awareness of Memory Deficit

It is possible to identify at least three significant issues in the foregoing discussion. The first concerns the role of memory impairment itself in awareness/ unawareness of memory deficits. The data from clincial observations, questionnaire studies, and experimental paradigms concerning temporal lobe and other nonfrontal amnesics indicate that the existence of amnesia does not preclude awareness of deficit: Even a profoundly amnesic patient such as H.M. is to some extent aware of his memory disorder. Nevertheless, it is possible that in many cases amnesia *initially* produces unawareness, and awareness of deficit is acquired slowly over time. The fact that many of the temporal lobe cases reported in the literature were not probed concerning awareness until years after onset is consistent with this possibility. However, observations of intact awareness in transient global amnesia (TGA) patients almost immediately after the onset of an amnesic episode indicate that unawareness of deficit is not an inevitable consequence of amnesia, even when the opportunity for gradual "acquisition" of awareness has been excluded. Thus although memory disorder alone does not appear to be a sufficient condition for producing unawareness (and observations of anosognosia in nonamnesic populations indicate that it is not a necessary condition of unawareness), memory disorder likely contributes to *sustaining* unawareness. In the training study discussed previously, for example, patient B.Z. showed enhanced awareness of his memory problems on various measures immediately after appropriate feedback but failed to "retain" awareness on most of these measures the next day. A similar point is made by an incident that occurred in a naturalistic study in which I observed the memory functions of a densely amnesic Alzhemier patient during two rounds of golf (Schacter, 1983). This patient believed that he had a "slight" memory problem but expressed no awareness of its severity. After completing play on one hole, we walked off the green and proceeded to the next tee, which was only a few feet from the green. While waiting to tee off, I asked M.T. if he could remember where he had just putted on the adjacent green. He was unable to do so, expressed shock and disbelief that he could have forgotten the event so quickly, and stated that his memory must be "a complete mess" for such a thing to have occurred. By the time we hit our drives and proceeded down the fairway, however, M.T. had forgotten this incident and acknowledged only that he might have a slight memory problem. Clearly, amnesia contributed to sustaining unawareness in this case, and it seems reasonable to assume that similar processes occur in other patients.

A second, related issue concerns the role of frontal lobe damage in unawareness of memory deficit. There is some evidence from each of the three types of study considered—clinical, questionnaire, and experimental—that impaired awareness of memory deficit is associated with signs of frontal lobe dysfunction. One major source of support for this conclusion is provided by the finding that Korsakoff amnesics have exhibited impaired awareness in every study that has examined these patients' awareness of their memory deficit. A second source of support is that there have been no documented instances in which a patient with amnesia attributable to restricted temporal lobe pathology has shown seriously defective awareness of memory deficit. These observations reinforce the idea that unawareness of memory disorder is not a necessary consequence of the same lesions that produce amnesia itself.

How might frontal lobe pathology contribute to unawareness of memory deficit? Two related possibilities are worth considering. The first is suggested by evidence linking the frontal lobes with such functions as integration of information and monitoring of responses (e.g., Luria, 1976; Stuss and Benson, 1986; Schacter, 1987c.) It seems reasonable to suggest that an amnesic patient could become aware of his or her deficit if (1) retrieval of information (i.e., a recent experience) were attempted, (2) the desired information was not retrieved; (3) the patient realized that a person with intact memory would have successfully remembered the target information; and (4) the patient could integrate and evaluate this sequence of events. It is precisely this sort of "on-line" monitoring that appears to result in awareness of (and distress about) memory disorder in TGA patients (e.g., Evans, 1966). To the extent that intact frontal lobe function is needed for such on-line evaluation, amnesic patients with frontal lobe damage would be expected to show impaired awareness. A second, related idea is that frontal lobe damaged patients often have difficulty inhibiting strong, though currently inappropriate, response tendencies and have problems as well making temporal discriminations (e.g., Luria, 1976; Milner, Petrides, and Smith, 1985; Schacter, 1987c; Moscovitch, 1989). If a patient with frontal lobe damage is asked about his or her memory function, the "strongest" available response may be based on the patient's knowledge of his or her *premorbid* memory function. If in addition the patient does not have access to temporal information regarding the appropriateness of the response (i.e., that the information concerns "then" and not "now"), unawareness of memory deficit would be a natural consequence.

Although the foregoing considerations suggest an important role for frontal lobes in awareness of memory deficit, the literature is not entirely free of potential counterexamples. For instance, patients with amnesia attributable to ruptured ACAAs typically show evidence of damage to frontal regions or to structures intimately linked with the frontal lobes, such as the basal forebrain (Alexander and Freedman, 1984). Yet there have been clinical reports of intact awareness in ACAA patients (Luria, 1976; Volpe and Hirst, 1983), and, as noted earlier, ACAA patients as a group showed intact memory monitoring in the recall prediction paradigm of Schacter et al. (1986). (Later in the chapter the case of a head-injured patient with extensive frontal lobe damage who is aware of his deficit is presented.)

The latter considerations are related to a third theme that is suggested by a few of the reviewed studies: Conclusions about whether a patient is "aware" of his or her memory deficit may depend on the way in which awareness is assessed (see Chapter 6 for a similar observation). Thus even though clinical and questionnaire studies suggest that ACAA and head-injured patients are unaware of their deficits, these patients made reasonably accurate recall predictions in the Schacter et al. (1986) study. (Of course, it must be determined if the *same patients* who showed realistic predictions in this study also show signs of unawareness on a questionnaire.) Similarly, patient B.Z. showed improved awareness of his memory problems on some but not all measures in the McGlynn et al. training study.

These observations, though preliminary, raise the possibility that simply describing patients as "aware" or "unaware" of their memory deficits may be too broad a description to be useful in many cases. That is, awareness of memory deficit may not be a monolithic, all-or-none entity that a patient either "has" or "lacks." It is entirely conceivable that there are different aspects or components of awareness that can be tapped by different measures and tasks. Thus the processes that underlie "aware" responding on a memory questionnaire may not be identical to the processes that underlie "aware" responding on a recall prediction or feeling-of-knowing task. A generally accepted principle in the analysis of memory function is that conclusions about the nature of underlying processes and representations depend on the way in which memory performance is tested (e.g., Tulving, 1983); the same principle may hold with respect to metamemory or awareness of memory function. An important objective for future research is to evaluate systematically the viability of the idea that awareness/unawareness of memory deficit can be fractionated into distinct components (see Chapter 14 for further discussion).

UNAWARENESS OF DEFICIT AND UNAWARENESS OF KNOWLEDGE: WHAT KIND OF RELATION?

As noted at the outset of the chapter, the performance of amnesic patients on certain kinds of tests can be facilitated by information acquired during a specific learning episode, even though they do not consciously remember the study episode at the time of the test. This dissociation between implicit and explicit memory (Graf and Schacter, 1985; Schacter, 1987b) was known to early clinical observers (e.g., Korsakoff, 1889; Claparede, 1911) but has been studied systematically and intensively since the early 1970s (for reviews, see Shimamura, 1986; Schacter, 1987a,b). Perhaps the most striking feature of implicit memory in amnesia is the patients' lack of awareness that they have been influenced by a recent event. An interesting question that has not yet been addressed concerns what relation exists, if any, between the kind of "unawareness" that characterizes implicit memory phenomena and unawareness of memory deficit.

Let us consider first two rather extensively studied implicit memory phenomena: skill learning and repetition priming. Early work by Milner and her colleagues demonstrated that patient H.M. could learn pursuit rotor and other motor skills, even though he did not explicitly remember the prior learning trials and sessions: H.M. was "unaware" that he had acquired any new skills (Milner et al., 1968). It has since been demonstrated that various types of amnesic patient can acquire perceptual and motor skills in normal or near-normal manner. Thus, for example, Brooks and Baddeley (1976) found that head-injured and other types of amnesic patients learned to solve puzzles more quickly with practice; Cohen and Squire (1980) reported that Korsakoff amnesics, patients who have undergone electroconvulsive therapy, and patient N.A. learned the skill of reading mirror-inverted script at a normal rate; Eslinger and Damasio (1985) observed intact motor skill learning in Alzheimer patients; and Nissen and Bullemer (1987) demonstrated normal learning of a repeated spatiotemporal pattern in Korsakoff patients. In related studies, Glisky et al. (1986a) and Glisky and Schacter (1989) reported that amnesic patients of diverse etiologies were able to learn (albeit much more slowly than normal subjects) and retain, across delays of 7 to 9 months, knowledge and skills necessary to interact with and program a microcomputer. Although these and other studies have demonstrated beyond dispute that various kinds of memory-disorderd patients can learn new skills, only some of them have reported data indicating that patients are "unaware" that they have acquired a new skill. Nissen and Bullemer (1987), for instance, showed that their Korsakoff patients were unaware of the existence of the repeated pattern that had a demonstrable influence on their performance, and Glisky et al. (1986a) noted that one of their densely amnesic patients (C.H.) did not remember ever having worked on a microcomputer—even though he had participated in close to 100 computer training sessions—and in that sense was unaware of the knowledge and skills he had acquired.

Similar phenomena have been produced by studies of repetition priming. In these studies, a single presentation of a stimulus facilitates the performance of amnesic patients on subsequent implicit memory tests that do not require conscious recollection of a prior episode. This phenomenon was first demonstated clearly in the well known studies of Warrington and Weiskrantz (1968, 1974), who found that after studying a list of familiar words (e.g., "table") amnesic patients of mixed etiologies showed an enhanced tendency to complete three-letter stems (e.g., "tab____") with previously presented items. Amnesic patients showed normal priming effects on this task even though their explicit recognition of the prior occurrence of the words was seriously impaired. Subsequent research has revealed that amnesic patients show normal retention on the stem completion task only when implicit memory instructions (e.g., Complete the stem with the first word that comes to mind) are given; when the stem completion task is turned into an explicit memory task by asking subjects to try to *remember* study list words, amnesic patients of various kinds are seriously impaired (Graf et al., 1984). Robust priming effects have also been observed in amnesic patients with diverse etiologies on various other implicit memory tasks, including free association (Shimamura and Squire, 1984; Schacter, 1985), perceptual identification (Cermak, Talbot, Chandler, and Wolbarst, 1985), homophone spelling (Jacoby and Witherspoon, 1982), category instance production (Gardner, Boller, Moreines, and Butters, 1973; Graf, Shimamura, and Squire, 1985), reading degraded words (Moscovitch, Winocur, and McLachlan, 1986), and solving sentence puzzles (McAndrews, Glisky, and Schacter, 1987). All of these studies have found that amnesic patients' recall or recognition of previously presented words is severely impaired, thereby suggesting that many patients are "unaware" that they acquired any knowledge during the study episode.

The main question for the present concerns whether the kind of unawareness of knowledge revealed in skill learning and priming studies is produced by similar mechanisms as, or is in any way related to, unawareness of memory deficit. A simple hypothesis is that the two phenomena are produced by a deficit in the same underlying mechanism and hence that unawareness of knowledge is observed only in those patients who are also unaware of their deficits. One difficulty in attempting to evaluate this hypothesis is that few of the foregoing studies have provided any information on awareness/unawareness of deficit in their patient populations. Nevertheless, enough information is available to suggest that unawareness of deficit and unawareness of knowledge are not simply different manifestations of the same underlying deficit. As noted earlier, unawareness of memory deficit is observed primarily in patients with frontal lobe damage; patients with restricted temporal lobe damage seem to be well aware of their deficits. Yet both skill learning and priming effects have been observed in amnesic patients with temporal lobe damage and no reported frontal lobe pathology. For example, the temporal lobe patient H.M. shows "unawareness of knowledge" in skill learning and repetition priming (Corkin, 1984) paradigms, yet is reported to be aware of his deficit. Similarly, several of Warrington and Weiskrantz's patients had temporal lobe encephalitis and were thus likely aware of their deficits; another profoundly amnesic encephalitic patient (S.S.) who is reported to be aware of his deficit shows unawareness of knowledge in various priming paradigms (Cermak, Blackford, O'Conner, and Bleich), 1988). The only suggestive link between the two classes of phenomena is provided by the finding that source amnesia tends to occur most frequently in patients with frontal lobe damage (e.g., Schacter, Harbluk, and McLachlan, 1984).

A dissociation between unawareness of deficit and unawareness of knowledge is also illustrated by a profoundly amnesic head-injured patient who has participated in a number of studies conducted by my colleagues and me. (This patient has been referred to in various papers as C.H., N.N., and K.C.; I use the latter initials here.) As noted above, K.C. was able to learn and retain computer knowledge and skills despite his inability to remember that he had ever worked on a computer (Glisky et al., 1986a; Glisky and Schacter, 1989; Schacter and Glisky, 1986). K.C. also showed robust priming effects on free association (Schacter, 1985), word completion (Schacter and Graf, 1986b), and sentence puzzle tasks (McAndrews et al., 1987), despite his lack of explicit memory for target items and the study episode itself. Particularly impressive evidence of this kind was provided by the McAndrews et al. (1987) experiment, in which subjects were initially exposed to ambiguous sentences (e.g., The haystack was important because the cloth ripped) (Auble and Franks, 1979), given a minute to try to think of a word that would make the sentence comprehensible, and then provided with a disambiguating cue (e.g., parachute). When re-presented with the ambiguous sentences after delays ranging from 1 minute to 1 week, K.C., like normal subjects, showed a strong priming effect: He came up with the disambiguating cue word more much frequently on the second presentation of a sentence than on the first, even at the 1-week delay. Yet on a Yes/No recognition test, K.C. failed to remember any of the sentences or cues at all delays, including the 1-minute retention interval. We have also found that K.C. exhibits priming of knowledge acquired prior to his head injury (Tulving, Schacter, McLachlan, and Moscovitch, 1988).

The foregoing data demonstrate clearly that K.C. was entirely unaware of recent experiences that influenced his test performance. In sharp contrast, K.C.

showed excellent awareness of his memory deficit. For example, on the General Self-Assessment Questionnaire described earlier, K.C. consistently rated himself as having a great deal of difficulty with his memory: Mean response to the nine items probing current memory function was 0.3 (where 0 indicates maximal difficulty), compared to a mean of 5.7 for nonmemory items. These ratings were similar to corresponding ratings of K.C.'s function made by his mother, with whom he lives (0.1 for memory and 5.6 for nonmemory items). K.C.'s awareness of the nature of his memory deficit is clearly revealed in the following conversation with the author.

D.S.:   How is your memory doing these days?

K.C.:   Pretty lousy, I guess.

D.S.:   Why do you say that?

K.C.:   It's just not there.

D.S.:   What do you mean it's not there?

K.C.:   I have no memory of things that just happened.

D.S.:   How do you know?

K.C.:   I try to remember and I can't.

Interestingly, when asked to provide an everyday example that illustrates his memory problem, K.C. was unable to recall a single relevant incident.

Although further research must be done to evaluate systematically the relation between unawareness of deficit and unawareness of knowledge, the foregoing considerations indicate that it is unlikely that the two phenomena are in any simple sense manifestations of the "same" underlying deficit. This conclusion is not particularly surprising for at least two reasons. First, as discussed earlier, unawareness of deficit itself may not be a unitary phenomenon: Patients may be more or less "aware" of their deficits depending on the way in which awareness is assessed, and different types of unawareness may be produced by various kinds of brain damage (McGlynn and Schacter, 1989). Second, different implicit memory phenomena may be produced by distinct mechanisms (Schacter, 1987b; Richardson-Klavehn and Bjork, 1988), thereby suggesting that "unawareness of knowledge" in amnesic patients is not a unitary phenomenon. In the next section of the chapter, these points are elaborated by discussing them in the context of some theoretical ideas.

Unawareness of Deficits and the DICE Model

To bring the foregoing issues into sharper focus, a highly condensed sketch of a descriptive model is provided that was put forward to accommodate implicit/explicit dissociations (Schacter, 1989) and that has also been applied to unawareness of deficits (McGlynn and Schacter, 1989). A major motivation for this model is the accumulating evidence that patients with various kinds of neuropsychological deficit show preserved implicit knowledge within the specific domain in which they are impaired on explicit tasks: Patients can demonstrate knowledge in task performance that they are not aware they possess. Thus, for example, it has been shown that prosopagnosic patients, who lack the ability to consciously recognize familiar faces, show implicit or covert recognition when familiarity is assessed through GSR measures (Bauer, 1984; Tranel and Damasio, 1985) or various kinds of priming techniques (DeHaan, Young, and Newcombe, 1987; Young and DeHaan, 1988). Similarly, Wernicke's aphasics show associative priming effects for semantic relations that are not explicitly comprehended (e.g., Blumstein, Milberg, and Schrier, 1982); blindsight patients can "guess" the location of visual stimuli they do not consciously perceive (Weiskrantz, 1986; see Campion, Latto, and Smith, 1983, for critique); and alexic patients can make reasonably accurate lexical decisions and category judgments about words they fail to identify explicitly (Shallice and Saffran, 1986). The foregoing and other implicit/explicit dissociations are reviewed and discussed in detail by Schacter, McAndrews, and Moscovitch (1988).

These kinds of dissociations suggest that the processes that mediate conscious identification and recognition must be distinguished from the modular systems that operate on linguistic, perceptual, and other kinds of information. This general idea has been endorsed by a number of theorists (e.g., Posner, 1978; Johnson-Laird, 1983; Marcel, 1983; Gazzaniga, 1985; Kihlstrom, 1987; Moscovitch, 1989) and forms the basis of the model I proposed (Schacter, 1989). This model, referred to by the acronym DICE (dissociable interactions and conscious experience), takes as a starting point the idea that conscious experiences of perceiving, knowing, and remembering require the activation of a *conscious awareness system* (CAS) that normally interacts with, but can become disconnected from, modular-level processors. Activation at the modular level alone produces a change in performance or behavior (i.e., priming effects) but is not sufficient to result in awareness of the activated information (for more detailed discussion of the nature of CAS, see Schacter, 1989). CAS in turn has an output link to an *executive system* that is necessary for initiation and monitoring of strategic responding.

With respect to memory, it was suggested that CAS can be activated by the outputs of a declarative or episodic memory system that represents newly acquired information about recent experiences or by the outputs of various knowledge modules—processors that represent familiar or overlearned information of different kinds, such as lexical, conceptual, or autobiographical knowledge. When CAS is activated by outputs from the episodic module, the result is a conscious or "aware" reexperiencing of a recent event; when CAS is activated by output from a knowledge module, the result is a conscious experience of knowing a particular bit of information. The model also postulates that acquisition of skills is mediated by a procedural or habit memory system that does not have an input connection to CAS, thus reflecting the idea that one cannot become aware of procedural knowledge (Johnson-Laird, 1983; Kihlstrom, 1987).

Turning to the data on implicit memory in amnesic patients discussed in the preceding section, the model allows three main types of implicit memory phenomenon. First, normal perceptual/motor skill learning is attributed to preservation of the procedural memory system (Cohen, 1984; Squire, 1987). Because this system does not have an input link to CAS, preserved skill learning in amnesia would be expected to occur without any awareness of the prior experiences that produced skill acquisition. Second, some priming effects can be attributed to the activation of preexisting representations in a knowledge module. Thus, for example, presentation of the word "table" on a study list activates a lexical representation of it; when the patient is later asked to complete the stem "tab_____" the recently activated word may "pop to mind" or, in the terms of the model, gain access to CAS. However, if the declarative/episodic memory system is compromised in amnesic patients, the patients are unable to remember the episode in which the word was presented, thereby resulting in the expression of knowledge without awareness of the experiential basis of it. Third, it was suggested that in some instances a relatively intact episodic memory system may be disconnected from CAS. In this scenario, patients can show long-lasting priming effects that reflect preservation of context-specific information about an episode, even though they are unaware of the episode at the time of the test. Although some results are suggestive of such a possibility, stronger data demonstrating implicit access to contextual features of episodes are needed to support the idea unequivocally (for fuller discussion, see Schacter, 1989).

We are now in a position to consider the implications of the foregoing for the unawareness of deficit issue. Within the context of the model, there are several ways in which unawareness of deficit can be produced (McGlynn and Schacter, 1989). However, in view of the data linking frontal lobe dysfunction and unawareness of memory deficit, and the fact that the executive system in the model is held to be frontally based (Schacter, 1989), the most likely locus of unawareness of memory deficit is disruption of the executive system. Such disruption would produce the sort of monitoring, integrative, and temporal discrimination deficits that, as discussed earlier, could underlie unawareness of memory deficit. An important implication of this idea for the preceding discussion of implicit memory phenomena is that the locus of the disruption that produces unawareness of deficit is different from the locus of most of the various disruptions that lead to unaware expressions of memory. Accordingly, one would not expect any necessary relation between unawareness of deficit and unawareness of knowledge in amnesic patients.

It is also worth discussing briefly another way in which unawareness of deficit can be produced in this model: selective disconnection of CAS from a specific module. In the model, CAS normally takes as input highly activated outputs of a specific module; that is, strongly activated outputs from a module result in conscious awareness, whereas weakly activated outputs do not. If CAS were disconnected from a particular module, it would no longer receive these highly activated outputs and hence would have no information about the module's damaged condition: The disconnected module would have the same status as a normally functioning module that is in a "baseline" state of low activation. As McGlynn and Schacter (1989) suggested, such a disconnection could produce unawareness of deficit because the patient would not have information about the module's damaged condition.

The most interesting aspect of this idea with respect to the present discussion is that it leads to the following prediction: Patients in whom unawareness of knowledge can be attributed to a disconnection between CAS and a specific module should also be unaware of their deficit. This prediction applies not only to amnesic patients but also to the other patients noted earlier who exhibit implicit/explicit dissociations. Unfortunately, the evidence needed to attribute disconnection from CAS as the basis of a particular disorder is thus far equivocal (see Schacter et al., 1988, for discussion). Nevertheless, attempts to evaluate the validity of this prediction will likely provide useful information concerning the relation between unawareness of deficit and unawareness of knowledge in various neuropsychological syndromes.

ACKNOWLEDGMENT

This chapter was supported by an NIH biomedical research support grant. I thank John Kihlstrom and Susan McGlynn for useful discussion of issues addressed in the chapter and Mindy Tharan for help in preparation of the manuscript.

REFERENCES

Alexander, M. R., and Freedman, M. (1984). Amnesia after anterior communicating artery aneurysm rupture. *Neurology* 34:752–757.

Auble, P. M., and Franks, J. J. (1979). Effort toward comprehension: elaboration or "aha"? *Memory Cogn.* 7:426–434.

Bauer, R. M. (1984). Autonomic recognition of names and faces in prosopagnosia: a neuropsychological study. *Neuropsychologia* 22:457–469.

Bennett-Levy, J., Polkey, C. E., and Powell, G. E. (1980). Self-report of memory skills after temporal lobectomy: the effect of clinical variables. *Cortex* 16:543–557.

Blumstein, S. E., Milberg, W., and Shrier, R. (1982). Semantic processing in aphasia: evidence from an auditory lexical decision task. *Brain Lang.* 17:301–315.

Boake, C., Freedland, J., Ringholz, G. M., Nance, M., and Edwards, K. E. (1987). Awareness of memory loss after severe head injury. *J. Clin. Exp. Neuropsychol.* 9:53 (abstract).

Brooks, D. N., and Baddeley, A. D. (1976). What can amnesic patients learn? *Neuropsychologia* 14:111–122.

Brooks, N., and Lincoln, N. B. (1984). Assessment for rehabilitation. In *Clinical Management of Memory Problems,* London: Aspen.

Butters, N., and Cermak, L. S. (1980). *Alcoholic Korsakoff's Syndrome.* New York: Academic Press.

Byer, J. A., and Crowley, W. J. (1980). Musical performance during transient global amnesia. *Neurology* 30:80–82.

Campion, J., Latto, R., and Smith, Y. M. (1983). Is blindsight an effect of scattered light, spared cortex, and near-threshold vision? *Behav. Brain Sci.* 6:423–486.

Cermak, L. S., Blackford, S. P., O'Conner, M., and Bleich, R. P. (1988). The implicit memory ability of a patient with amnesia due to encephalitis. *Brain Cogn.* 7:312–323.

Cermak, L. S., Talbot, N., Chandler, K., and Wolbarst, L. R. (1985). The perceptual priming phenomenon in amnesia. *Neuropsychologia* 23:615–622.

Claparede, E. (1951). Recognition and "me-ness." In D. Rapaport (ed.), *Organization and Pathology of Thought*. New York: Columbia University Press. (Reprinted from *Arch. Psychol.* 11:79–90, 1911.

Cockburn, J., Wilson, B., and Baddeley, A. (1986). How well do people with memory problems recognize their difficulties? Unpublished manuscript.

Cohen, N. J. (1984). Preserved learning capacity in amnesia: evidence for multiple memory systems. In L. R. Squire and N. Butters (eds.), *Neuropsychology of Memory*. New York: Guilford Press, pp. 83–103.

Cohen, N. J., and Squire, L. R. (1980). Preserved learning and retention of pattern-analyzing skill in amnesia: dissociation of "knowing how" and "knowing that." *Science* 210:207–209.

Corkin, S. (1984). Lasting consequences of bilateral medial temporal lobectomy: clinical course and experimental findings in H.M. *Semin. Neurol.* 4:249–259.

DeHaan, E. H. F., Young, A., and Newcombe, F. (1987). Face recognition without awareness. *Cogn. Neuropsychol.* 4:385–415.

Eslinger, P. J., and Damasio, A. R. (1985). Preserved motor learning in Alzheimer's disease: implications for anatomy and behavior. *J. Neurosci.* 6:3006–3009.

Evans, J. H. (1966). Transient loss of memory, an organic mental syndrome. *Brain* 89:539–548.

Fisher, C. M. (1982). Transient global amnesia. *Arch. Neurol.* 39:605–608.

Gardner, H., Boller, F., Moreines, J., and Butters, N. (1973). Retrieving information from Korsakoff patients: effects of categorical cues and reference to the task. *Cortex* 9:165–175.

Gazzaniga, M. S. (1985). *The Social Brain*. New York: Basic Books.

Glisky, E. L, and Schacter, D. L. (1987). Acquisition of domain-specific knowledge in organic amnesia: training for computer-related work. *Neuropsychologia* 25:893–906.

Glisky, E. L., and Schacter, D. L. (1989). Extending the limits of complex learning in organic amnesia: computer training in a vocational domain. *Neuropsychologia* 27:107–120.

Glisky, E. L., Schacter, D. L. and Tulving, E. (1986a). Computer learning by memory-impaired patients: acquisition and retention of complex knowledge. *Neuropsychologia* 24:313–328.

Glisky, E. L., Schacter, D. L., and Tulving, E. (1986b). Learning and retention of computer-related vocabulary in memory-impaired patients: method of vanishing cues. *J. Clin. Exp. Neuropsychol.* 8:292–312.

Graf, P., and Schacter, D. L. (1985). Implicit and explicit memory for new associations in normal and amnesic subjects. *J. Exp. Psychol.* [*Learn. Mem. Cogn.*] 11:501–518.

Graf, P., Shimamura, A. P., and Squire, L. R. (1985). Priming across modalities and priming across category levels: extending the domain of preserved function in amnesia. *J. Exp. Psychol.* [*Learn. Mem. Cogn.*] 11:385–395.

Graf, P., Squire, L. R., and Mandler, G. (1984). The information that amnesic patients do not forget. *J. Exp. Psychol.* [*Learn. Mem. Cogn.*] 10:164–178.

Groninger, L. D. (1979). Predicting recall: the "feeling-that-I-will-know" phenomenon. *Am. J. Psychol.* 92:45–58.

Hackler, E., and Tobis, J. S. (1983). Reintegration into the community. In M. Rosenthal, R. Griffith, M. R. Bond, and J. D. Miller (eds.), *Rehabilitation of the Head Injured Adult*. Philadelphia: Davis, pp. 421–424.

Hart, J. T. (1965). Memory and the feeling-of-knowing experience. *J. Educ. Psychol.* 56:208–216.

Hart, T., and Hayden, M. E. (1986). The ecological validity of neurospychological assessment and remediation. In B. Uzzell and Y. Gross (eds.), *Clinical Neuropsychology of Intervention*. Boston: Martinus Nijhoff, pp. 21–50.

Hermann, D. J. (1982). Know the memory: the use of questionnaires to assess and study memory. *Psychol. Bull.,* 92:434–452.

Jacoby, L. L., and Witherspoon, D. (1982). Remembering without awareness. *Can. J. Psychol.* 36:300–324.

Jarho, L. (1973). Korsakoff-like amnesic syndrome in penetrating brain injury. *Acta Neurol. Scand.* 49:44–67.

Jensen, T. S., and Olivarius, B. F. (1981). Transient global amnesia: its clinical pathophysiological basis and prognosis. *Acta Neurol. Scand.* 63:220–230.

Johnson-Laird, P. N. (1983). *Mental Models.* Cambridge, MA: Harvard University Press.

Kaszniak, A. (1986). The neuropsychology of dementia. In J. Grant and K. M. Adams (eds.), *Neuropsychological Assessment of Neuropsychiatric Disorders.* New York: Oxford University Press, pp. 172–220.

Kaushall, P. I., Zetin, M., and Squire, L. R. (1981). A psychosocial study of chronic, circumscribed amnesia. *J. Nerv. Ment. Dis.* 169:383–389.

Kihlstrom, J. F. (1987). The cognitive unconscious. *Science* 237:1445–1452.

Korsakoff, S. S. (1889). Etude medico-psychologique sur une forme des maladies de la memoire. *Rev. Philos.* 5:501–530.

Luria, A. R. (1976). *The Neuropsychology of Memory.* New York: Wiley.

Marcel, A. J. (1983). Conscious and unconscious perception: experiments on visual masking and word recognition. *Cogn. Psychol.* 15:197–237.

McAndrews, M. P., Glisky, E. L., and Schacter, D. L. (1987). When priming persists: long-lasting implicit memory for a single episode in amnesic patients. *Neuropsychologia* 25:497–506.

McGlynn, S. M., and Schacter, D. L. (1989). Unawareness of deficits in neuropsychological syndromes. *J. CLin. Exp. Neuropsychol.* 11:143–205.

McGlynn, S. M., Schacter, D. L., and Glisky, E. L. (1989). Unawareness of deficits in organic amnesia. *J. Exp. Clin. Neuropsychol.* 11 (abstract), 50.

Milner, B., Corkin, S., and Teuber, H. L. (1968). Further analysis of the hippocampal amnesic syndrome: 14 year follow-up study of H.M. *Neuropsychologia* 6:215–234.

Milner, B., Petrides, M., and Smith, M. L. (1985). Frontal lobes and the temporal organization of memory. *Hum. Neurobiol.* 4:137–142.

Moscovitch, M. (1982). Multiple dissociations of function in amnesia. In L. S. Cermak (ed.), *Human Memory and Amnesia.* Hillsdale, NJ: Lawrence Erlbaum Associates, pp. 337–370.

Moscovitch, M. (1989). Confabulation and the frontal system: strategic vs. associative retrieval in neuropsychological theories of memory. In H. L. Roediger and F. I. M. Craik (eds.), *Varieties of Memory and Consciousness: Essays in Honor of Endel Tulving.* Hillsdale, NJ: Lawrence Erlbaum Associates.

Moscovitch, M., Winocur, G., and McLachlan, D. (1986). Memory as assessed by recognition and reading time in normal and memory-impaired people with Alzheimer's disease and other neurological disorders. *J. Exp. Psychol. [Gen.]* 115:331–347.

Nelson, T. O. (1984). A comparison of current measures of the accuracy of feeling-of-knowing predictions. *Psychol. Bull.* 95:109–133.

Nelson, T. O., Leonesio, R. J., Shimamura, A. P., Landwehr, R. F., and Narens, L. (1982). Overlearning and the feeling-of-knowing. *J. Exp. Psychol. [Learn. Mem. Cogn.]* 8:279–288.

Nissen, M. J., and Bullemer, P. (1987). Attentional requirements of learning: evidence from performance measures. *Cogn. Psychol.* 19:1–32.

Pansford, J. L., and Donnan, G. A. (1980). Transient global amnesia—a hippocampal phenomenon. *J. Neurol. Neurosurg. Psychiatry* 43:285–287.

Parkin, A. J., Bell, W. P., and Leng, N. R. C. (in press). A study of metamemory in amnesic and normal adults. *Cortex*

Posner, M. (1978). *Chronometric Exploration of Mind.* Hillsdale, NJ: Lawrence Erlbaum Associates.

Prigatano, G. P., and others (1986). *Neuropsychological Rehabilitation after Brain Injury.* Baltimore: Johns Hopkins University Press.

Richardson-Klavehn, A., and Bjork, R. A. (1988). Measures of memory. *Annu. Rev. Psychol.* 39:475–543.

Rimel, R. W., Giordani, B., Barth, J. T., Boll, T. J., and Jane, J. A. (1981). Disability caused by minor head injury. *Neurosurgery* 9:221–228.

Roman-Campor, G., Poser, C. M., and Wood, F. B. (1980). Persistent retrograde memory deficit after transient global amnesia. *Cortex* 16:509–518.

Rose, F. C., and Symonds, C. P. (1960). Persistent memory defect following encephalitis. *Brain* 83:195–212.

Schacter, D. L. (1983). Amnesia observed: remembering and forgetting in a natural environment. *J. Abnorm. Psychol.* 92:236–242.

Schacter, D.L. (1985). Priming of old and new knowledge in amnesic patients and normal subjects. *Ann. N.Y. Acad. Sci.* 444:41–53.

Schacter D. L. (1986). Feeling-of-knowing ratings distinguish between genuine and simulated forgetting. *J. Exp. Psychol. [Learn. Mem. Cogn.]* 12:30–41.

Schacter, D. L. (1987a). Implicit expressions of memory in organic amnesia: learning of new facts and associations. *Hum. Neurobiol.* 6:107–118.

Schacter, D. L. (1987b). Implicit memory: history and current status. *J. Exp. Psychol. [Learn. Mem. Cogn.]* 13:501–518.

Schacter, D. L. (1987c). Memory, amnesia, and frontal lobe dysfunction. *Psychobiology* 15:21–36.

Schacter, D. L. (1989). On the relation between memory and consciousness: dissociable interactions and conscious experience. In H. L. Roediger and F. I. M. Craik (eds.), *Varieties of Memory and Consciousness: Essays in Honor of Endel Tulving.* Hillsdale, NJ: Lawrence Erlbaum Associates, 355–389.

Schacter, D. L. (1990). Toward a cognitive neuropsychology of awareness: implicit knowledge and anosognosia. *Journal of Clinical and Experimental Neuropsychology* 12:155–178.

Schacter, D. L., and Glisky, E. L. (1986). Memory remediation: restoration, alleviation, and the acquisition of domain-specific knowledge. In B. Uzzell and Y. Gross (eds.), *Clinical Neuropsychology of Intervention.* Boston: Martinus Nijhoff, pp. 257–282.

Schacter, D. L, and Graf, P. (1986a). Effects of elaborative processing on implicit and explicit memory for new associations. *J. Clin. Exp. Neuropsychol.* 12:432–444.

Schacter, D. L., and Graf, P. (1986b) Preserved learning in amnesic patients: perspectives from research on direct priming. *J. Clin. Exp. Neuropsychol.* 8:727–743.

Schacter, D. L, and Worling, J. R. (1985). Attribute information and the feeling-of-knowing. *Can. J. Psychol.* 39:467–475.

Schacter, D. L., Glisky, E. L., and McGlynn, S. M. (1990). Impact of memory disorder on everyday life: awareness of deficits and return to work. In D. Tupper and K. Cicerone (eds.), *The Neuropsychology of Everyday Life. Vol. I: Theories and Basic Competencies.* Boston: Kluwer Academic Publishers, pp. 231–298.

Schacter, D. L., Harbluk, J. L., and McLachlan, D. R. (1984). Retrieval without recollection: an experimental analysis of source amnesia. *J. Verbal Learn. Verbal Behav.* 23:593–611.

Schacter, D. L., McAndrews, M. P., and Moscovitch, M. (1988). Access to consciousness: dissociations between implicit and explicit knowledge in neuropsychological syndromes. In L. Weiskrantz (ed.), *Thought Without Language.* Oxford: Oxford University Press, pp. 242–278.

Schacter, D. L., McLachlan, D. R., Moscovitch, M., and Tulving, E. (1986). Monitoring of recall performance by memory-disordered patients. *J. Clin.Exp. Neuropsychol.* 8:103 (abstract).

Shallice, T., and Saffran, E. (1986). Lexical processing in the absence of explicit word identification: evidence from a letter-by-letter reader. *Cogn. Neuropsychol.* 3:429–448.

Shimamura, A. P. (1986). Priming effects in amnesia: evidence for a dissociable memory function. *Q. J. Exp. Psychol.* 38A:619–644.

Shimamura, A. P., and Squire, L. R. (1984). Paired-associated learning and priming effects in amnesia: a neuropsychological study. *J. Exp. Psychol.* 113:556–570.

Shimamura, A. P., and Squire, L. R. (1986). Memory and metamemory: a study of the feeling-of-knowing phenomenon in amnesic patients. *J. Exp. Psychol.* [*Learn. Mem. Cogn.*] 12:452–460.

Squire, L. R. (1987). *Memory and Brain.* New York: Oxford University Press.

Stuss, D. T., and Benson, D. F. (1986). *The Frontal Lobes.* New York: Raven Press.

Sunderland, A., Harris, J. E., and Baddeley, A. D. (1983). Do laboratory tests predict everyday memory? A neuropsychological study. *J. Verbal Learn. Verbal Behav.* 22:341–357.

Sunderland. A., Harris, J. E., and Baddeley, A. I. (1984). Assessing everyday memory after severe head injury. In J. E. Harris and P. E. Morris (eds.), *Everyday Memory, Actions and Absent-Mindedness.* New York: Academic Press, pp. 191–206.

Talland, G. A. (1965). *Deranged Memory.* New York: Academic Press.

Tranel, D., and Damasio, A. R. (1985). Knowledge without awareness: an autonomic index of facial recognition by prosopagnosics. *Science* 228:1453–1454.

Tulving, E. (1983). *Elements of Episodic Memory.* Oxford: Clarendon Press.

Tulving, E., Schacter, D. L., McLachlan, D. R., and Moscovitch, M. (1988). Priming of semantic autobiographical knowledge: a case study of retrograde amnesia. *Brain Cogn.* 8:3–20.

Victor, M., Adams, R. D., and Collins, G. N. (1971). *The Wernicke-Korsakoff Syndrome.* Philadelphia: Davis.

Vilkki, J. (1985). Amnesic syndromes after surgery of anterior communicating artery aneurysms. *Cortex* 21:431–444.

Volpe, B. T., and Hirst, W. (1983). Amnesia following rupture and repair of an anterior communicating artery aneurysm. *J. Neurol. Neurosurg. Psychiatry.* 46:704–709.

Warrington, E. K., and Weiskrantz, L. (1968). New method of testing long-term retention with special reference to amnesic patients. *Nature* 217:972–974.

Warrington, E. K., and Weiskrantz, L. (1974). The effect of prior learning on subsequent retention in amnesic patients. *Neuropsychologia* 12:419–428.

Weiskrantz, L. (1986). *Blindsight.* New York: Oxford University Press.

Whitlock, F. A. (1981). Some observations on the meaning of confabulation. *J. Med. Psychol.* 54:213–218.

Young, A. W., and DeHaan, E. H. F. (1988). Boundaries of covert recognition in prosopagnosia. *Cogn. Neuropsychol.* 5:317–336.

Zangwill, O. L. (1966). The amnesic syndrome. In C. W. M. Whitty and O. L. Zangwill (eds.), *Amnesia.* London: Butterworth, pp. 104–117.

9
Three Possible Mechanisms of Unawareness of Deficit

ELKHONON GOLDBERG
AND WILLIAM B. BARR

Unawareness of deficit may take a variety of forms. It is a common feature of many neuropsychological syndromes (McGlynn and Schacter, 1989), and it is unlikely to reflect a single cause. One has to consider a variety of possible mechanisms of unawareness of deficit from a cognitive and a neuroanatomical standpoint. To understand the mechanisms of the awareness of deficit and its disintegration, a more basic question must be asked first. *What are the mechanisms of one's cognitive acts—their operational composition and content in normal cognition?* Conceptually, there may be three fundamental reasons why deficits of awareness of cognitive impairment are selectively associated with certain lesion sites but not with others. One of these explanations implies, metaphorically speaking, the existence of an "aware homunculus," and the other two do not.

Intact awareness of deficit implies an intact process of error monitoring (Zaidel, 1987). The breakdown of the awareness of deficit reflects the breakdown of the error monitoring process. Schematically, the process of error monitoring rests on three components: (1) the internal representation of the desired cognitive product; (2) feedback regarding one's own output; and (3) comparison between the content of the feedback and the representation of the desired cognitive product. This tripartite control loop has been the basic element of neural cybernetics (Miller, Galanter, and Pribram, 1960; Bernstein, 1967). It can also be applied as the basis for understanding the awareness of deficit. To be aware of a specific cognitive deficit, the subject must have (1) an internal representation of the desired cognitive product or cognitive operations, (2) the feedback regarding his actual output when these operations are applied, and (3) an intact mechanism responsible for comparing the actual output with the internal representation of the desired cognitive product. Breakdowns of different elements of this tripartite mechanism may account for different types of compromised awareness of deficit.

Both postmorbid (caused by the disease) and premorbid (related to some limitations inherent in normal cognition and antedating the disease onset) factors may play a role in the mechanisms of impaired awareness of deficit, even when the deficit itself is clearly disease-related. We review here three types of impaired awareness of deficit that represent different types of interaction between the factors outlined above.

First, a brain lesion may interfere with the *mechanism* of awareness. In terms of our tripartite error-monitoring system, this possibility implies the existence of a localized "aware homunculus" in charge of comparing the feedback content with the internal representation. This point of view explains deficits of awareness through the postmorbid breakdown of the "awareness mechanism" as a direct consequence of brain disease. It implies that if a lesion affects the "aware homunculus" site, awareness will be impaired for *any* associated cognitive deficit. If a lesion produced a cognitive deficit of which the subject is unaware, it is inferred that the lesion affected regions that contain the locus of the function in question and the locus of awareness. If a lesion produced a cognitive deficit of which the subject is aware, it is inferred that the lesion affected the locus of the function in question but not the locus of the "aware homunculus."

Second, it is possible that the selectivity of awareness of deficit is a direct reflection of the selectivity of awareness of normal cognitive operations in an intact organism. This explanation does not invoke the notion of a localizable "aware homunculus," but it does imply certain premorbid limitations of awareness. It is based on the assumption that an intact individual is normally aware of some of his cognitive processes but not others; or to put it more cautiously, normal cognition is characterized by varying degrees of awareness of the operational content of cognitive processes. Then, if a lesion produces a cognitive deficit of which the subject is unaware, it is inferred that the lesion disrupted those cognitive processes whose cognitive composition is not readily available to awareness even under normal circumstances. If a lesion produces a cognitive deficit of which the subject is aware, it is inferred that the lesion disrupted those cognitive processes whose cognitive composition is readily available to awareness under normal conditions. Awareness of deficit is therefore viewed as an extension of the awareness of the underlying intact cognitive process. It is assumed that to be aware of the loss of function the subject must first be aware of the operational content of the function itself while it is intact. In terms of our tripartite error-monitoring scheme, it means that the subject may be unaware of a cognitive deficit because even premorbidly the internal representation of the corresponding intact cognitive functions was rather "fuzzy."

Third, the patient's awareness of deficit may be diminished not because of a flawed "comparator" or premorbidly "fuzzy" representations, but because of the degradation of sensory feedback of his or her own cognitive output or of internal representations of desired cognitive output as a direct result of brain disease. In this case, the impaired awareness of deficit is due to the postmorbid impairment (rather than premorbid vagueness) of the first or second element of our tripartite error-monitoring scheme. For instance, if the patient suffers simultaneously from a higher-order cognitive disorder *and* a sensory deficit in a relevant modality, his or her awareness of the higher-order deficit may be compromised for the simple reason that the feedback is degraded owing to the sensory deficit, even if the "comparator" and the internal representations are intact.

We believe that all three mechanisms may play a role in affecting the patient's awareness of his deficit, leading to three distinctly different classes of syndrome. We propose that the first class of syndromes, associated with damage to the elements of the "mechanisms of awareness," is seen following lesions of the prefrontal and related upper brain stem systems. "Frontal syndromes" are characterized by a notorious lack of awareness of associated cognitive deficits and lack of concern for their consequences. We believe, on the other hand, that some phenomena of anosognosia caused by lesions of the right hemisphere are best explained by the premorbid selectivity of the subject's awareness (and lack of awareness) of his or her cognitive deficits.

If one were to design a formal test to distinguish between these two mechanisms of unawareness of deficit in brain disease, the following solution comes to mind. If the lack of awareness is due to the damage to the *aware homunculus,* a diffuse lesion that simultaneously affects site A of the "aware homunculus" and far-removed sites B, C, and D results in the lack of awareness for the loss of functions mediated by area A as well as by areas B, C, and D, no matter how removed the latter are from area A. Assuming that the frontal disregard for the cognitive deficit is produced by this mechanism, a diffuse cortical atrophy affecting both frontal and posterior cortex must be associated with the lack of awareness of both sequential motor (anterior) and perceptual (posterior) difficulties. If, on the other hand, the lack of awareness is a reflection of the *premorbid limitations of awareness,* a diffuse lesion affecting areas A, B, C, and D and producing many cognitive deficits results in the awareness of the loss of those cognitive functions that enjoyed a substantial degree of awareness premorbidly but lack of awareness of the loss of those functions that enjoyed little awareness premorbidly. For instance, if it is true—as we argue—that the functions mediated by the left hemisphere enjoy a greater degree of premorbid awareness than those mediated by the right hemisphere, a diffuse lesion disrupting the functions of both hemispheres must be associated with the awareness of the loss of the "left hemispheric functions" but lack of awareness (or, more prudently, less awareness) of the loss of "right hemispheric functions."

Finally, we believe that the lack of awareness associated with certain forms of aphasia, cortical blindness, and cortical deafness can be best understood in terms of the postmorbid disruption of the sensory basis of feedback, internal cognitive representations, or both. We now turn to a discussion of the various mechanisms of the lack of awareness of cognitive deficit.

DAMAGE TO THE MECHANISMS OF AWARENESS: FRONTAL SYNDROMES

Damage to prefrontal (both dorsolateral and orbitofrontal) systems is known to produce a massive, devastating cognitive deficit of which the patient is often completely oblivious. The lack of the patient's insight into and awareness of his deficit has been noted by many authors (Hécaen and Albert, 1978; Luria, 1980; Stuss and Benson, 1986; Goldberg, Bilder, Hughes, et al., 1989; McGlynn and Schacter, 1989). This lack of awareness usually takes two forms, which often co-occur. They correspond to the breakdown of "local" versus "global" error detection described by Zaidel (1987).

"Local" Error Monitoring

First, it is the lack of awareness of specific errors in one's own performance, the "local" error monitoring deficit, in Zaidel's (1987) terminology. This lack of awareness is present despite the fact that the patient knows the correct answers. Examples of such unawareness of specific errors can be found in perseveration and field-dependent behavior.

Perseveration can be elicited in a "frontal" patient by asking him to draw easily nameable symbols following a rapid sequence of verbal commands (Goldberg and Tucker, 1979; Luria, 1980). Early in the sequence the patient is able to draw correct symbols, but as the sequence continues these symbols become degraded by the properties of intervening stimuli, and graphical perseverations develop (Goldberg and Tucker, 1979). As the patient continues to perseverate, he is completely unperturbed by his errors. This indifference to errors cannot be attributed to the lack of knowledge (internal representation) of what the correct outputs should be, as earlier in the sequence the patient was drawing the same symbols correctly, and he will continue to draw them correctly again as soon as the intervals between the verbal instructions in the sequence are increased. Likewise, the patient's errors cannot be attributed to faulty sensory feedback mechanisms, as the patient is able to identify the symbols correctly in a multiple choice format.

A similar dissociation between the preserved knowledge of correct responses and the inability to use this knowledge to monitor one's own output can be demonstrated in "frontal" patients' field-dependent behavior. Motor field-dependent behavior can be elicited by the technique described by Luria (1980). Two gestures are introduced (e.g., a finger and a fist), and the patient is instructed to watch the examiner and to do opposite to what he is doing ("When I raise my finger, raise your fist; and when I raise my fist, raise your finger"). In a rapid alternation of gestural instructions, the patient initially gives correct responses but then slips into echopraxic imitation of the examiner's postures. This pattern is often accompanied by his own correct verbalizations, such that in response to the examiner's fist the patient says, "I raise my finger" but in fact raises his fist and vice versa. Here too the patient's indifference to his errors cannot be attributed to the lack of knowledge (internal representation) of the correct response or to faulty sensory feedback. Indeed, he can do the task correctly early in the sequence, can verbalize the correct responses even as his actual motor output becomes echopractic, is able to resume correct responses as soon as the intervals between instructions are increased, and can tell a finger from a fist in a multiple choice situation. It appears to be a genuine instance of an error-monitoring breakdown in self, despite the relatively intact knowledge of the correct response.

A similar phenomenon can be demonstrated in a "frontal" patient's verbal behavior. When asked to listen to a story and then recall it, the patient often embellishes it with totally irrelevant statements whose sources are in the external environment. The following example is from Goldberg and Costa (1986, p. 55).

> A patient with a bilateral prefrontal trauma and subsequent removal of the fractured frontal bone and frontal pole resection bilaterally listens to the story "A hen and golden eggs," which reads as follows: "A man owned a hen which was laying golden eggs. The man was greedy and wanted to get more gold at once. He killed the hen and cut it open hoping to find a lot of gold inside, but there was none."

> The patient's recall proceeds as follows: "A man was living with a hen . . . or rather the man was the hen's owner. She was producing gold. . . . The man . . . the owner . . . wanted more gold at once . . . so he cut the hen into pieces but there was no gold. . . . No gold at all . . . he cuts the hen more, . . . no gold . . . the hen remains empty. . . . So he searches again and again. . . . No gold . . . he searches all around in all places. The search is going on with a tape-recorder . . . they are looking here and there, nothing new around. They leave the tape-recorder turned on, something is twisting there . . . what the hell are they recording there . . . some digits . . . 0, 2, 3, 0 . . . so, they are recording all these digits . . . not very many of them . . . that's why all the other digits were recorded . . . turned out to be not very many of them either . . . so, everything was recorded. . . ." (monologue continues).

The introduction of the "tape-recorder" theme into the recall is an example of verbal field-dependent behavior. Instead of selectively staying with the actual plot, the patient describes what he sees in the environment, as the examiner (E.G.) was sitting in front of the patient with a tape-recorder in his lap, recording the monologue presented here. As in the previous example, the deficit appears to be a lack of selectivity of one's own behavior and the lack of the on-line monitoring of his own behavior.

Perseveration can be conceptualized as the impairment of behavioral plasticity, of the ability to switch from one cognitive element to another. Field-dependent behavior, on the other hand, can be conceptualized as the impairment of behavioral stability, of the ability to maintain a cognitive set despite incidental, environmental, or internal-associative distractors. These two types of deficit—behavioral stability and behavioral plasticity—appear to be the two fundamental components of the "executive" syndrome caused by prefrontal dysfunction. Both are characterized by the patient's impaired awareness of his own errors in on-line situations, even when the knowledge of correct responses can be elicited.

Unfortunately, there is a shortage of systematic studies of the unawareness of errors in frontal patients. It is not clear, for instance, whether the lack of awareness is limited to on-line monitoring of self or the patient fails to detect errors even when monitoring somebody else's performance or his own on a videotape. Konow and Pribam (1970) demonstrated, in a single case study of a female patient with a prefrontal tumor, that the ability to detect errors in another person, or even in herself, was more preserved than the ability to actually correct her own errors. A similar single-case study by Luria, Pribram, and Homskaya

(1964) produced inconclusive results. Our own clinical observations are also inconclusive, with the frontal patients often but not always displaying a better ability to monitor errors off-line (when shown the record of their own output later) or in a third party than on-line in themselves.

"Global" Error Monitoring

In addition to the lack of awareness of errors in specific cognitive situations ("local" error monitoring deficit), patients with massive prefrontal damage are notorious for their general lack of appreciation of, and concern about, their diminished position in life and their devastating cognitive, vocational, and personal handicaps (Blumer and Benson, 1975; Luria, 1980; Goldberg, Bilder, Hughes, et al., 1989). In Zaidel's (1987) terminology, it represents a "global" error monitoring deficit. Such general, profound, and almost existential oblivion sets it apart from virtually every other type of brain damage. It is particularly conspicuous in the orbitofrontal syndrome, with its euphoric, unconcerned, happy-go-lucky attitude, which is completely out of line with the patient's devastating debility (Goldberg, Bilder, Hughes, et al., 1989). This attitude is often combined with the patients' technical knowledge of the changes in their lives consequent to the brain damage.

Cognitive self-monitoring and the comparison of the outcome of one's cognitive operations with the objective at hand are central elements of the "executive control" provided by the prefrontal cortex (Luria, 1980; Stuss and Benson, 1986; Goldberg and Bilder, 1987). We propose that the breakdown of these controls impairs the machinery of self-awareness, which accounts for the cognitive manifestations described above, in both the small frame of specific, "local" error self-detection and the large, "global" frame of personal insight.

PREMORBID LIMITATIONS OF AWARENESS: ANOSOGNOSIA OF THE RIGHT HEMISPHERE

Unawareness of deficit is more commonly associated with right hemisphere damage than with left hemisphere damage (for the most up-to-date review, see McGlynn and Schacter, 1989). Anosognosia of the right hemisphere has two distinct components. First is the lack of awareness of the disruption of higher-order perceptual and cognitive functions, which are presumed to be mediated largely by the right hemisphere but manifest symmetrically with respect to input lateralization. Unawareness of facial agnosia or amusia are examples of this aspect of anosognosia. Right hemisphere damage, either by itself or in the context of a bilateral lesion, is critical for these deficits. However, when these deficits are present, they are not limited to the input presented to the left visual hemifield or left ear; rather, they affect any stimulus that falls within the category of faces (or music) regardless of its position within the stimulus field.

The second aspect of anosognosia is a persistent left hemispace/hemifield neglect or inattention secondary to a right hemisphere lesion. It is unawareness for a sensory, perceptual, and, as Bisiach and Luzzatti (1978); Bisiach, Luzzatti, and Percani (1979) have demonstrated, imaging deficit lateralized to the left half of the stimulus field.

We do not discuss left hemispace/hemiinattention in this chapter. Although the mechanisms of the latter deficits are far from clear, we believe that the right hemisphere arousal hypothesis formulated by Heilman, Watson, and Valenstein (1985) or some modification thereof provides the most promising approach among the current attempts to understand these phenomena. We limit our discussion to the lack of awareness of deficit with respect to higher-order functions mediated by the right hemisphere. Traditionally, this form of anosognosia has been explained in terms of a deranged body scheme, presumably residing in the right hemisphere (Roth, 1949), sensitivity and position sense (Nielsen, 1938), or as a disconnection syndrome (Geschwind, 1965). These hypotheses regarding anosognosia of the right hemisphere have been critically reviewed by McGlynn and Schacter (1989). Our account of this form of the unawareness of deficit is radically different from these approaches.

"Linguistic Determinism" Revised

We propose that even with normal cognition the operational content of the processes controlled by the right hemisphere is less available to introspection and awareness than those of the left hemisphere. This premise is based on the assumption that the cognitive tasks mediated by well articulated, routinized representational systems are more easily accessible by introspection than those cognitive tasks that do not rely on such codes. The subject is more aware of the content of the former type of tasks under normal circumstances and consequently more aware of their disintegration following brain damage. The cognitive composition of the latter type of task is more obscure to the subject under normal conditions, and its disintegration in pathology is less apparent. In terms of the tripartite scheme of error-monitoring mechanisms, it implies that even under the normal, premorbid conditions the internal representations of cognitive operations rendered by the right hemisphere are somewhat "fuzzy," which makes it difficult for the subject to note if they have changed as a result of brain disease.

This viewpoint is in the tradition of linking the content of intrapsychic processes with external, culturally determined symbolic systems. This position is often associated with "linguistic determinism," articulated by Sapir (1921) and Whorf (1956), who suggested that the internal experience of the world is structured by the symbolic components of language. Vygotsky (1962) also thought that intrapsychic cognitive processes are in large measure determined by the categorizations implicit in natural language. This position implied the necessity for verbal access to the content of cognitive processes in order for them to reach consciousness.

In the brain-behavioral context, this position led to the postulate that consciousness, or at least its higher forms such as self-awareness, is mediated by the left hemisphere and is available only for the content of the left hemisphere-mediated processes (DeWitt, 1975; Popper and Eccles, 1977; Gazzaniga and LeDoux, 1978; Brown, 1988).

The main difference between these earlier formulations and our position is in the scope of what we regard as well articulated representational systems. Unlike Gazzaniga and LeDoux (1978) and Brown (1988), we do not limit them to those requiring verbal mediation in the sense of natural language. Also unlike Sapir (1921) and Vygotsky (1962), we do not limit them to those representational systems that preexisted in culture in a crystallized, external form.

We believe in the multiplicity of representational systems operative in human cognition, of which the natural language and its derivatives are but a subset. Furthermore, only some (certainly not all) of such representational systems are acquired by an individual through explicit learning of preexisting, external cultural devices. A well articulated representational system may develop intrapsychically as a result of continuous exposure to a particular class of cognitive situations. The existence of many representational systems, not all of them easily reducible to natural language, has been emphasized by many authors (Posner, 1972, 1978; Goldberg, Vaughan, and Gerstman, 1978; Goldberg and Costa, 1981; Warrington, 1982; Zaidel, 1986; Kosslyn, 1987).

Not all such representational systems can be reduced to natural language. Cultural-anthropological and evolutional considerations support this view. Mathematical languages, musical notation, and so on simply would not have survived in culture had they not held some advantage over natural languages in encoding certain types of information. Furthermore, well developed ways of categorizing the world and identifying unique stimuli as members of generic categories clearly antedate the emergence of natural languages in evolution. The breakdown of such nonlinguistic categorizing processes in humans leads to associative agnosias, which are discussed later in the chapter.

It can be further argued that not all such representational systems are the result of explicit learning—of internalization of preexisting external cultural devices. Goldberg and Costa (1981) provided the following classification of representational systems from a cultural-anthropological standpoint.

1. Natural languages form the first type of representational system. They are characterized by the strongest invariants across language users. However, even within the natural language domain, specialized subsystems exist that are not shared by all language users, e.g., scientific and professional terminologies. Therefore the multiplicity of representational systems is seen even within the domain of natural language.

2. Representational systems that are outside natural language but explicitly exist in culture form the second type of representational system. They include mathematical formalisms, musical and dance notations, and games with special notations, e.g., chess. Each of these systems is utilized by only a relatively small group of people, and the concepts communicated by these systems are not always well (or compactly) definable by means of natural language. The first and second types of representational system are similar in the sense that they are acquired by an individual as the internalization of preexisting external cultural devices, through explicit learning.

3. Representational systems that develop intrapsychically as the result of an individual's continuous exposure to a new class of stimuli or cognitive demands constitute the third type of representational system. These systems develop idiosyncratically rather than by way of explicit learning of a preexisting cultural device.

We believe that *any* of such representational systems, *regardless* of its relation to the natural language or culture at large, is mediated predominantly by the left hemisphere. The left hemispheric dominance for language is but a special case of this more general rule.

In this chapter, we argue that the reliance of a cognitive process on *any* well developed representational system, regardless of its relation to natural language, facilitates the availability of this process for consciousness and awareness. Consequently, we argue that, following Gazzaniga and LeDoux (1978) and Brown (1988), left hemisphere-controlled cognitive processes are more readily available to self-awareness than those controlled by the right hemisphere but for reasons that transcend natural language and are more fundamental than the ones implied by these authors.

Ultimately, this general proposition can be best tested through the experiments on normal subjects by accessing the subjects' differential ability to give account of the operational composition of the tasks showing the left hemispheric advantage (both linguistic and nonlinguistic) versus those showing the right hemispheric advantage. We predict that the former will reveal a much greater degree of the subjects' awareness of the ways they do the task than the latter, regardless of the presence or absence of a linguistic component. We are not aware of such experiments in the literature, but hopefully this chapter will provide the impetus for designing and conducting them.

However, even in the absence of a direct assessment of the lateralization of awareness, relevant, albeit indirect, data exist, based on the experiments with intact and split-brain subjects. They have been extensively reviewed by Zaidel (1987), and we discuss here only some of these findings.

In a task of perceptual matching (the board version of The Raven Colored Progressive Matrices), the left hemisphere benefits more than the right hemisphere from self-correction through a trial-and-error approach in patients with complete commissurotomy (Zaidel, 1978; Zaidel, Zaidel, and Sperry, 1981). It was demonstrated by comparing the accuracy of the patients' initial solutions of the problems with those chosen after several successive attempts. Zaidel noted that "it is as if the right hemisphere does not have access to an internal model of its own solution process which it can interrogate to update intermediate steps. . . . The left hemisphere, on the other hand, had benefited substantially from error correction" (1987, p. 258).

Golding, Reich, and Wason (1974) reported similar results in normal subjects asked to solve nonverbal problems through unilateral palpation by one or the other hand with lateralized correction items. The right hand benefited more from such error correction than did the left hand.

Landis, Graves, and Goodglass (1981) compared the accuracy of verbal self-correction in two tasks involving lateralized stimulus presentation to normal subjects. In one task the subject had to make category judgments of objects and in the other of facial expressions. The first task is known to show a right hemi-field advantage and is presumed to be mediated more efficiently by the left hemi-sphere. The second task is known to show a left hemifield advantage and is pre-sumed to be mediated more efficiently by the right hemisphere. The study was designed to ensure equal levels of performance in the two tasks, and the total number of verbal self-corrections (right and wrong added together) was also equal, but the number of correct verbal self-corrections was substantially higher for the object than for the facial expression task.

Taken together, the results of these studies indicate that the functions of error monitoring, detecting discrepancies between the desired cognitive product and actual output, and utilizing the outcome of such comparison for optimizing one's own performance are more effective in the processes controlled by the left than by the right hemisphere. This conclusion seens to be the case not only for verbal but also for nonverbal tasks.

We believe that such findings in non-brain-injured subjects can be best explained in terms of the differential access to consciousness of right versus left hemisphere-mediated processes. However, the "right hemisphere arousal" hypothesis (Heilman et al., 1985) can possibly also account for these findings by postulating competition between cognitive and arousal processes for the same neural circuitry. One could then say that normal people are less aware of their right hemisphere-mediated processes because such processes interfere with the right hemisphere's function of arousal. In other words, the right hemisphere can-not control its unique cognitive processes and provide arousal for the rest of the brain at the same time.

To apply these considerations to the issue of the patient's awareness of cog-nitive deficit, we must first specify the types of cognitive deficit differentially seen following left and right hemispheric lesions. We then review the (unfortunate-ly sparse) evidence of the patients' differential degree of awareness of these def-icits.

Agnosias and Awareness

Among the cognitive deficits following left hemispheric lesions, language deficits are the most prominent. We address them later in the chapter. Meanwhile, we concentrate on the nonverbal deficits associated with lateralized cerebral lesions and on the differences in the degrees of patients' awareness of these deficits.

Following the argument developed by Goldberg (in press), we propose that the perceptual deficits caused by lesions of the left hemisphere are dominated by *associative agnosias,* whereas the perceptual deficits caused by lesions of the right hemisphere are dominated by *apperceptive agnosias.*

Warrington (1982) proposed that object recognition is characterized by two distinct processes. The first type involves physical object identification, the rec-ognition of an object as its own self, invariant across various sensory conditions of observation. The breakdown of such processes is termed *apperceptive agnosia.* The second type of processes involves the identification of specific objects as members of generic categories and is therefore essentially semantic, though not necessarily verbal (for the simple reason that animals are also capable of generic

recognition). The breakdown of such processes is termed *associative agnosia.*
The two types of agnosia can occur separately and independently of one another.

Physical object identification emphasizes the processing of features or attributes that are specific to the object. Semantic object identification involves processing features that are common across many objects. Facial recognition is, by definition, a task of physical identification, as its purpose is to identify one specific person as being different from another. Object recognition is fundamentally different because its emphasis is on processing those features that are common—or in some sense equivalent, or interchangeable—across whole classes of objects. A hierarchical relation exists between these two aspects of perception in terms of the cognitive generalizations that are involved as well as from a developmental standpoint. Generic identification appears to rely on more compact, invariant, and generalized codes than does physical identification.

It may be possible that generic identification, because of its reliance on compact and generalized representations, is directly based on the accessibility to stable memory representations, whereas physical identification always requires de novo computations. In other words, physical identification entails the processing of features that are characterized by a much greater degree of stimulus variability (and often on a continuous scale) than generic identification, and therefore cannot simply rely on preexisting templates or fixed perceptual criteria. Every case of physical identification requires substantial transformation and recomputation of the stimulus pattern before it can be compared to the preexisting memory traces of the "original." For generic identification, this connection can be made in a more immediate fashion, with less reliance on the intermediate steps of mental transformation.

This distinction is consistent with Kosslyn's (1987) distinction between "categorical" representations (related to the left hemisphere) and "coordinate" representations (related to the right hemisphere). It is also consistent with Bernstein's (1967) earlier distinction between "topological" and "metric" representations. The former are more generalized and can be stated in terms of the presence or absence of certain necessary and sufficient qualitative features. The latter are usually characterized in terms of quantitative variations, as they are too informationally complex to afford any explicit account of every possible stimulus variation.

We presume that each hemisphere is capable of both types of processing, but the right hemisphere is more efficient for physical stimulus identification and is dominant for it under the normal circumstances. The left hemisphere is more efficient for categorical object identification and is dominant for it under normal circumstances (Goldberg, in press).

The comparative neuroanatomy of apperceptive agnosias (impairment of physical object identification) and associative agnosias (impairment of generic object identification) supports this assertion. Although apperceptive agnosias are often caused by bilateral posterior cortical lesions (Damasio et al., 1982; Damasio, 1985b), they can be seen following unilateral right but not left cortical lesions (Warrington and James, 1988). It is particularly true with deficits of facial recognition, a variant of apperceptive agnosia (Warrington and James, 1967; Benton and Van Allen, 1968; Warrington and Taylor, 1973; Meadows, 1974; Damasio et al., 1982).

Conversely, associative agnosias can be seen following bilateral posterior cortical damage or left hemispheric damage but not after right hemispheric damage. This occurrence has been demonstrated for all three main modality-specific forms of associative agnosia: *visual object agnosia, pure astereognosia, and semantic associative auditory agnosia.* Table 9–1 summarizes the comparative neuroanatomy of associative and apperceptive agnosias as revealed by the studies reviewed in this chapter.

Visual associative ("object") agnosia was described by Lissauer (1890), Hécaen and Angelergues (1963), DeRenzi and Spinnler (1966), Rubens and Benson (1971), Hécaen et al. (1974), Albert, Reches, and Silberberg (1975), War-

TABLE 9–1. Neuroanatomy of Associative and Apperceptive Agnosias: Literature Review

	References, by lesion site		
Type of agnosia	Left	Bilateral	Right
Associative agnosias			
Visual object	Bauer & Rubens (1985)	Hécaen & Albert (1978)	
	Hécaen & de Ajuriaguerra (1956)	Hoff & Potzl (1935)	
	Hécaen et al. (1974)	von Stauffenberg (1918)	
	Nielsen (1937, 1946)		
Pure astereognosia	Foix (1922)		
	Goldstein (1916)		
	Lhermitte & de Ajuriaguerra (1938)		
Semantic associative auditory	Faglioni et al. (1969)		
	Kleist (1928)		
	Spinnler & Vignolo (1966)		
	Vignolo (1982)		
Apperceptive agnosias			
Visual		Damasio (1985a)	Benton & Van Allen (1968)
		Damasio et al. (1982)	Meadows (1974)
		DeRenzi et al. (1968)	Warrington (1982)
			Warrington & James (1967, 1988)
			Warrington & Taylor (1973)
Auditory			Faglioni et al. (1969)

rington (1975), Hécaen and Albert (1978), and Luria (1980). While visually examining the object, the patient can accurately describe its perceptual components and copy it by drawing but is unable to identify it as a member of a generic category through either language or imitation (Rubens and Benson, 1971; Hécaen and Albert, 1978). Additional testing reveals that the patient's perceptual processing, in terms of basic visuosensory or pattern analysis, is essentially intact. Luria (1980, p. 161) described a patient who identified eyeglasses as "a circle, then another circle, and then some sort of crossbar . . . it may be a bicycle."

Visual object agnosia is not a linguistic deficit. When the patient incorrectly names an object (as in the case of "bicycle" for glasses), the incorrect name is consistent with the incorrect functional description of the object offered by the patient. This pattern of response is opposite to the one observed in anomia, where the description is consistent with the true function of the object rather than with its incorrectly assigned name. The patient's deficit is limited to the visual modality. As soon as he is allowed to examine the object through other sensory modalities, he can immediately name the object and give its correct verbal description. Defective categorical identification due to a disrupted access to nonverbal semantic memory appears to be the underlying deficit in visual object agnosia (Warrington, 1975).

Visual object agnosia is caused by an isolated left occipital or left occipitotemporal lesion (Nielsen, 1937, 1946; Hécaen and de Ajuriaguerra, 1956; Hécaen et al., 1974) or a bilateral posterior lesion most prominent in the left occipital or occipitotemporal areas (von Stauffenberg, 1918; Hoff and Potzl, 1935; Hécaen and Albert, 1978). Left mesial occipital damage therefore appears to be mandatory in this syndrome (Nielsen, 1937; Bauer and Rubens, 1985).

A tactile form of associative agnosia is known as "pure astereognosia" (Hécaen and Albert, 1978) or "tactile asymbolia" (Wernicke, 1894). The patient is unable to identify the object by touch, although he can readily identify it with reliance on other sensory systems. The deficit does not appear to be linguistic. "Pure astereognosia" is an inability to make tactile identification of objects as members of meaningful generic classes, even though the ability to describe separate tactile properties of the stimulus is intact. The deficit is bilateral but results from unilateral lesions affecting temporoparietal aspects of the left hemisphere (Goldstein, 1916; Foix, 1922; Lhermitte and de Ajuriaguerra, 1938).

The auditory form of associative agnosia has also been described (Kleist, 1928; Spinnler and Vignolo, 1966; Faglioni, Spinnler, and Vignolo, 1969; Vignolo, 1982). It involves an inability to understand the "meaning" of nonverbal sounds and associate them with correct sources. Purely auditory perceptual aspects of analysis are, however, intact. The syndrome is caused by a left posterior lesion.

Although associative agnosias often co-occur with language disorders (DeRenzi, Peiczulo, and Vignolo, 1968; Warrington, 1975; Vignolo, 1982), it is by far not always the case, as asymbolias without aphasia have been described (De Renzi et al., 1968; Rubens and Benson, 1971; Albert et al., 1975; Humphreys and Riddoch, 1987). Because the converse situation is also observed (aphasias without associated symbolic agnosias), one can argue that a double dissociation exists between the aphasias and the above-described symbolic disorders. This fact supports the notion that associative agnosias represent a disruption of various, distinct, modality-specific, nonverbal representational systems.

We now contrast the two forms of agnosias—associative and apperceptive—with respect to the patients' awareness of these deficits. Following right hemisphere lesions it has been noted that patients with apperceptive visual agnosias are often unaware of their nature and appear unconcerned by their presence (Rubens, 1979). It has also been noted that some patients with prosopagnosia fail to complain of their problem of recognizing faces (Bogen, 1979). Conversely, patients with visual associative agnosias are commonly described as being aware of their deficits as evidenced by their dissatisfaction with their responses, resulting in prolonged attempts to identify the object by alternative strategies (Frederiks, 1969; Gassell, 1969). Gassell (1969, p. 656) described patients with Brodmann area 19 lesions of the left occipital lobe: "Patients with visual agnosia frequently act in an uncertain and hesitant manner when viewing objects and may complain of difficulty in recognition."

Paradoxical as it may sound, we propose that the right hemisphere lesions are associated with the lack of awareness of higher order deficit not because the right hemisphere is normally critical for awareness but because the individual is not good at being aware of the processes mediated by it to begin with, and "what you don't know doesn't hurt you" (when it is lost). Because unawareness of deficit is known to be asymmetrical and is more likely to be caused by right than by left cerebral lesions, it is often assumed that the mechanisms of awareness—or some elements or precursors thereof, such as arousal—are mediated by the right hemisphere, and the damage to these mechanisms accounts for the asymmetrical nature of anosognosia (Heilman et al., 1985). Although it may well be true with respect to persistent left hemifield/space neglect and inattention, we propose that other mechanisms may play a role in the patients' differential lack of awareness of higher-order cognitive deficits caused by left versus right hemispheric lesions.

The reports of the patients' uneven degrees of awareness for left and right hemisphere-lateralized, nonverbal syndromes is important because these findings indicate that the verbal-nonverbal dimension is not the sole determinant of the cognitive processes' availability to awareness. The notion of nonverbal representational systems also serving as mediators to awareness may be a useful one.

The hypothesis that the differential premorbid availability to awareness of different cognitive domains accounts for postmorbid differences in the awareness of deficit is radically different from the "right hemisphere arousal" hypothesis (Heilman et al., 1985). However, the latter hypothesis can also account for the differences in the awareness of the loss of higher-order functions. One can say that compromised arousal leads to impaired awareness of any cognitive loss. Then if the assumption is made that arousal is mostly controlled by the right hemisphere, it follows that lateralized lesions of the right hemisphere produce the deficit of certain specific, "right hemispheric" cognitive functions *and* the deficit of arousal—and therefore the deficit of awareness of the cognitive loss. On the other hand, lateralized lesions of the left hemisphere produce the deficit of certain specific, "left hemispheric" cognitive functions but no (or less) deficit of arousal—and therefore preserved awareness of the cognitive loss.

The two hypotheses—that of premorbid differences in the access to awareness and of the right hemispheric control of arousal—are not mutually exclusive on either logical or empirical grounds and may both play a role in the asymmetrical nature of awareness of deficit. One way of assessing the relative roles of these two putative mechanisms is to examine the relations between specific cognitive deficits and the awareness of them in patients with diffuse, bilateral lesions that produce impairment of both left and right hemispheric functions. If such patients are equally (un)aware of their right and left hemispheric functional losses, the "right hemisphere arousal" hypothesis is supported. If, however, such patients are proved to be more aware of the left than the right hemispheric functional loss, the "uneven premorbid access to awareness" hypothesis is supported.

Greater awareness of verbal than of visuospatial deficit has been reported for Korsakoff's syndrome and Alzheimer-type dementia (Riesberg, Ferris, Borenstein, et al., 1986; Parsons, 1987). Because these diseases are usually (but not always) bilateral, they satisfy the requirements of the comparison. However, a mere comparison of verbal and visuospatial awareness is not exciting or informative, as it is commonly assumed that subjects are more conscious of their language-mediated cognitive processes. It would be much more informative to compare the patients' awareness with respect to their deficits of nonverbal, left hemisphere-mediated and nonverbal, right hemisphere-mediated cognitive processes. This exercise may be a rather tall order. In effect, such a comparison must be made in cases with bilateral lesions and complex agnosias, combining both associative and apperceptive features. Sophisticated structured interviews are required to assess differentially the patients' awareness of the associative (left hemisphere) and apperceptive (right hemisphere) components of their agnosias.

UNAWARENESS OF DEFICIT DUE TO POSTMORBID DEGRADATION OF SENSORY FEEDBACK OR INTERNAL REPRESENTATIONS

Aphasias and Awareness

Aphasic patients are often keenly aware of their deficit and try to correct it. When present, the aphasic patients' awareness of deficit can be profound and characterized by a severe grief reaction over the loss of their language and motor functions (Benson and Geschwind, 1985). Furthermore, Goldstein's (1952) classic descriptions of "catastrophic reactions" in the context of cerebral impairment stated that they were attributed primarily to the loss of language functions following left hemisphere lesions, which implies the patients' keen awareness of their deficit. However, it is known that aphasias may also be associated with the lack of awareness of the deficit.

A systematic review of awareness of language deficits reveals a remarkably consistent picture. For those aphasias that do not disrupt phonemic perception (e.g., Broca's and anomic aphasias), the patients are usually aware of their deficit (Brown, 1972; Benson, 1979; Kertesz, 1984; Zaidel, 1987). Conversely, a lack of awareness of deficit is associated with those aphasias where the disruption of phonemic perception is at the core of the deficit, e.g., Wernicke's and sensory aphasias (Alajouanine, 1956; Heilman and Scholes, 1976; Benson and Geschwind, 1985).

We can therefore conclude that the degree of an aphasic patient's awareness of deficit stands in direct relation with the condition of the sensory, or rather phonemic, input processing that enables the patient to receive feedback about his or her own output. This feedback mechanism corresponds to the second element of our tripartite scheme of error monitoring.

The aphasic patient's awareness of deficit appears to be also influenced by the condition of the internal representations of lexicon. Although we are not aware of any study directly assessing "global" awareness of deficit as a function of the patients' semantic competence, the study by Gainotti, Silveri, Giampiero, and Miceli (1986) offers a glimpse into their "local" awareness of error. Gainotti et al. (1986) compared anomic patients with and without lexical comprehension disorder. In the first group the deficit was presumed to affect the core of semantic competence, whereas in the second group it affects the output stage of lexical selection when the selected lexical item has to be phonologically encoded. The two groups differed on measures of "tacit knowledge" of words that the patients failed to name properly and on the "editorial comments" revealing the patients' awareness of their naming errors, e.g., "It is not a. . . ." The patients *without* comprehension deficits revealed more preserved tacit knowledge and were more likely to make editorial comments than the patients *with* comprehension deficits.

Because the two groups in the Gainotti et al. (1986) study did not differ on a test of phonemic discrimination, the authors concluded that the differences in performance had to be attributed solely to the differences in lexical competence, i.e., the integrity of their internal semantic representations. The integrity of their internal lexical representations is also likely to account for the differences in the level of awareness of errors. Although it is logically possible that the two groups differ in the condition of the "comparator," it is highly unlikely. We can therefore conclude that the patients' awareness of errors is affected by the integrity of or access to internal representations of the desired cognitive outputs (or both). This point corresponds to the first element of the tripartite scheme of error monitoring.

Robinson and Benson (1981) have found that the severity and frequency of depression is greater in nonfluent aphasias characterized by more anterior lesions of the dominant hemisphere and more intact comprehension than in fluent aphasias characterized by more posterior lesions and more impaired comprehension. Furthermore, a direct relation was present between the severity of depression and the lesion size in the first group but an inverted one in the second group. One of the several possible hypotheses offered by the authors to account for these findings is that the presence and severity of depression is a direct consequence of the extent to which the subjects are aware of their deficit. The nonfluent, anterior aphasics are more aware of their deficit because their comprehension is relatively spared, and they are better able to "hear" their own output. Conversely, the fluent, posterior aphasics are less aware of their deficit because their comprehension is more impaired, and they are less able to "hear" their own output. Furthermore, Robinson and Benson considered the possibility that the paradoxical, inverse relation between the lesion site and the severity of depression in the posterior, fluent group may be due to the fact that smaller lesions are associated with more spared comprehension and therefore greater awareness of deficit.

These findings are important for understanding the mechanisms and limitations of awareness in aphasias, as they imply that so long as the aphasic patient hears his actual output and has an adequate internal representation of the desired output, he is aware of his deficit. For the aphasic patient to be unaware of his deficit, the disorder must literally interfere with the ability to hear his own output or with the integrity of, or access to, the internal semantic representations and therefore with the ability to *know* that the uttered word is a wrong one (or a nonword). In this regard, aphasic patients are drastically different from patients with prefrontal lesions who may both *know* what the output should be and *see* and *hear* what their actual output is, yet fail to note the discrepancy at least in an operational sense.

We propose that the lack of awareness of deficit in aphasias can be accounted for by phonemic feedback disruption or by the degradation of, or impaired access to, internal semantic representations (or both), i.e., by the damage to the first two elements of our tripartite scheme of error detection. There does not seem to be an additional, surplus deficit of awareness in aphasics, which would necessitate postulating an additional breakdown of the comparator itself, the third element of the tripartite scheme. "Kleist's dynamic aphasia," caused by lateralized prefrontal lesions of the dominant hemisphere, may be the only exception to this rule. However, it has been proposed that this syndrome can be best understood as a variant of a partial executive deficit limited to the domain of language, rather than as a form of aphasia per se (Luria, 1980; Goldberg, 1989).

The unawareness of linguistic deficit caused by disorders of phonemic hearing and the degradation of, or impaired access to, internal semantic representations is regarded here as entirely postmorbid. By this statement we mean that it is completely accounted for by the effects of brain damage rather than by a relative (compared to other cognitive processes) unavailability of the impaired processes for introspection even premorbidly, when these processes were intact. In this respect, the unawareness of deficit in aphasias is different from the anosognosias of the right hemisphere discussed in the previous section.

Cortical Blindness and Awareness

Instances of cortical blindness and cortical deafness of which the patients are unaware may constitute examples of combined impairment of sensory input processing *and* internal representations of the physical world in the corresponding sensory modality. They provide another set of examples of postmorbid effects of damage to the first two elements of the tripartite scheme of error monitoring. Degradation of internal representations of the world in the corresponding modality may constitute the major reason these patients are unaware of the interruption of sensory input.

Here cortical blindness/deafness is different from peripheral blindness/deafness, where the internal representations are presumably spared (remember Beethoven composing his greatest music while deaf). Lack of sensory input in combination with the intact knowledge of what it ought to be and, more importantly, *that* it ought to be leads to a blatant discrepancy between the internal representations (invested with distinct content) and the actual sensory input (zero) in peripherally, noncongenitally blind/deaf individuals and hence to keen awareness of deficit.

When, on the other hand, sensory inputs *and* the internal representation of the world are simultaneously damaged in the same modality, the ability to compare the actual sensory experiences with the anticipated ones is impaired because both elements of comparison are degraded. This situation may result in the deficit of "local" error monitoring in Zaidel's (1987) terminology—in other words, in the ability to conclude that a specific percept is distorted or incomplete. If the damage to internal representations in the given modality is profound, a situation may arise that the patient loses not only the precision of internal representations of specific objects—the whole sensory dimension of the multi(sensory) dimensional image of the world is lost. This situation may result not only in the loss of knowledge of *what* the subject is supposed to see/hear in a particular situation but also in the loss of knowledge *that* he is supposed to see/hear. The internal experiential knowledge base for the concept of seeing/hearing is destroyed, and the patient loses the ability to appreciate the loss of the whole sensory modality.

If this reasoning is correct, the cases of cortical blindness/deafness with *unawareness* of deficit must involve bilateral damage to both primary sensory cortical projection areas and the secondary, association areas in the corresponding modality. By contrast, in the cases of cortical blindness/deafness with *preserved awareness* of deficit, damage is limited to the primary cortical sensory projection areas bilaterally but spares secondary, association areas. These neuroanatomical considerations are based on the assumption that the integrated images of the physical world are dimensionalized according to sensory modalities. The "total" representations are viewed as distributed on the cortical level across secondary sensory and association cortices according to the corresponding modalities (Goldberg, 1989; in press).

Indeed, cortical blindness is usually associated with bilateral lesions involving primary visual areas, including the striate cortices and geniculocalcarine pathways (Bergman, 1957; Lessell, 1975). In most cases, patients demonstrate awareness of their acquired blindness (Teuber, Battersby, and Bender, 1960; Aldrich, Alessi, Beck, and Gilman, 1987). However, a variant of cortical blindness characterized by unawareness of deficit also exists. The original description of this syndrome was provided by and subsequently named after Anton (1898), who studied a patient exhibiting an acute denial of blindness. Postmortem examination revealed a bilateral softening in parietooccipital areas (Anton, 1898). Although no systematic neuroanatomical reviews have been conducted, several authors have commented that this disorder most likely results from more widespread cerebral lesions extending from the primary visual areas to adjacent parietal and temporal association cortices (Von Monakow, 1905; DeAjuriaguerra and Hécaen, 1960; Teuber et al., 1960; Joynt, Honch, Rubin, and Trudell, 1984;

Damasio, 1985a) or by lesions disrupting connections between the sensory cortex and the thalamus (Redlich and Dorsey, 1945).

It has been demonstrated that, despite their severe sensory loss, patients with more circumscribed lesions and lucid awareness of deficit usually have preserved visual memory and visual elements of dreaming (Magitot and Hartmann, 1927). We are not aware of any studies of visual memory and visual dreaming (or imaging, for that matter) in patients with Anton's syndrome (cortical blindness with an unawareness of deficit caused by a more extensive lesion). It is likely, however, that these functions are severely impaired in Anton's syndrome. Such a double dissociation between awareness of cortical blindness and the ability to evoke visual images would strongly support the notion that the unawareness of deficit in Anton's syndrome is due to the degradation of, or lack of access to, visual representations.

Cortical deafness results from bilateral lesions in the primary auditory regions (Mott, 1907; Goldstein, Brown, and Hollander, 1975). The pure form of this syndrome has been reported infrequently and is considered somewhat controversial. This fact comes as no surprise, as its presence requires circumscribed and unusually placed lesions that would simultaneously affect two mutually distant regions of the two temporal lobes. (By comparison, the primary visual projection areas of the two hemispheres are relatively close to each other and are therefore more likely to be simultaneously affected by a single vascular event). Furthermore, it is often difficult to distinguish between cortical deafness and pure word deafness and auditory associative agnosia (Hécaen and Albert, 1978; Kertesz, 1984; Bauer and Rubens, 1985).

One form of this disorder, dominated primarily by symptoms consistent with word deafness, is caused by bilateral lesions in the anterior portions of the superior temporal gyri with some sparing in the left Heschl's gyrus (Auerbach, Allard, Naeser, et al., 1982; Bauer and Rubens, 1985). In these cases, patients are aware of the deficit and complain that speech sounds are muffled or sound like a foreign language (Kanshepolsky, Kelley, and Waggener, 1973; Auerbach et al., 1982; Kertesz, 1984; Bauer and Rubens, 1985).

In other forms of the disorder, with more extensive lesions and lesser degrees of awareness, patients fail to attend to auditory stimuli (Earnest, Monroe, and Yarnell, 1977; Rubens, 1979) or exhibit complete denial of their deafness (Anton, 1898). It has been suggested that these more complete forms of cortical deafness combined with the unawareness of deficit arise only after combined damage to the primary auditory regions and the adjacent auditory association areas (Earnest et al., 1977; Mesulam, 1985).

CONCLUSIONS

The purpose of this chapter has been to highlight the multiplicity of factors contributing to patients' normal awareness of their cognitive functions and of their impairment in the presence of brain disease. Consequently, we emphasized the heterogeneity of mechanisms leading to a deficient awareness of one's cognitive loss. When considering these various factors, it is useful to distinguish between premorbid limitations of awareness of one's cognitive functions and postmorbid impairments of various components of the "awareness machinery." Among the latter, it may be useful to distinguish between the metacognitive monitoring functions, to which we referred humorously as the "aware homunculus," and two kinds of information that must be "fed" into such a metacognitive processor: the internal representations of the desired cognitive output and the feedback regarding the actual output.

Although it is reasonably clear that diverse lesion loci may produce cognitive deficits of which the patient is poorly aware, our understanding of the underlying mechanisms is tentative at best. Furthermore, our theorizing about these mechanisms is limited to rather macroscopic descriptions both neuroanatomically and cognitively. We do not know what the fine neurophysiological machinery of awareness is, nor do we know whether the postulated, putative elements of awareness correspond to distinct neural processes or their utility is limited to heuristic but metaphorical diagram drawing.

REFERENCES

Alajouanine, T. (1956). Verbal realization in aphasia. *Brain* 79:1–28.

Albert, M. L., Reches, A., and Silberberg, R. (1975). Associative visual agnosia without alexia. *Neurology* 25:322–326.

Aldrich, M. S., Alessi, A. G., Beck, R. W., and Gilman, S. (1987). Cortical blindness: etiology, diagnosis, and prognosis. *Ann. Neurol.* 21:149–158.

Anton, G. (1898). Ueber Herderkrankungen des Gehirnes, welche von Patienten selbst nicht wahrgenommen werden. *Wien. Klin. Wochnschr.* 11:227–229.

Auerbach, S. H., Allard, T., Naeser, M., Alexander, M. P., and Albert, M. L. (1982). Pure word deafness: analysis of a case with bilateral lesions and a defect at the prephonemic level. *Brain* 105:271–300.

Bauer, R. M., and Rubens, A. (1985). Agnosia. In K. M. Heilman and E. Valenstein (eds.), *Clinical Neuropsychology.* 2nd Ed. New York: Oxford University Press.

Benson, D. F. (1979). *Aphasia, Alexia, and Agraphia.* New York: Churchill Livingstone.

Benson, D. F., and Geschwind, N. (1985). Aphasia and related disorders: a clinical approach. In M. Mesulam (ed.), *Principles of Behavioral Neurology.* Philadelphia: Davis.

Benton, A. L., and Van Allen, M. W. (1968). Impairment in facial recognition in patients with cerebral disease. *Cortex* 4:344–358.

Bergman, P. S. (1957). Cerebral blindness. *Arch. Neurol. Psychiatry* 78:568–584.

Bernstein, N. A. (1967). *Coordination and Regulation of Movements.* New York: Pergamon Press.

Bisiach, E., and Luzzatti, C. (1978). Unilateral neglect of representational space. *Cortex* 14:129–133.

Bisiach, E., Luzzatti, C., and Perani, D. (1979). Unilateral neglect, representational schema and consciousness. *Brain* 102:609–618.

Blumer, D., and Benson, D. F. (1975). Personality changes with frontal and temporal lobe lesions. In D. F. Benson and D. Blumer (eds.), *Psychiatric Aspects of Neurologic Disease.* New York: Grune & Stratton, pp. 151–170.

Bogen, J. E. (1979). The callosal syndrome. In K. M. Heilman and E. Valenstein (eds.), *Clinical Neuropsychology.* New York: Oxford University Press.

Brown, J. W. (1972). *Aphasia, Apraxia, Agnosia.* Springfield, IL: Charles C Thomas.

Brown, J. W. (1988). *The Life of the Mind: Selected Papers.* Hillsdale, NJ: Lawrence Erlbaum Associates.

Damasio, A. R. (1985a). Disorders of complex visual processing: agnosias, achromatopsia, Balint's syndrome, and related difficulties of orientation and construction. In M. Mesulam (ed.), *Principles of Behavioral Neurology.* Philadelphia: Davis.

Damasio, A. R. (1985b). Prosopagnosia. *Trends Neurosci.* 8:132–135.

Damasio, A. R., Damasio, H., and Van Hoesen, G. W. (1982). Prosopagnosia: anatomic basis and behavioral mechanisms. *Neurology* 32:331–341.

DeAjuriaguerra, J., and Hécaen, H. (1960). *Le Cortex Cerebral.* Paris: Mason & Cie.

DeRenzi, E., and Spinnler, H. (1966). Visual recognition in patients with unilateral cerebral disease. *J. Nerv. Ment. Dis.* 142:513–525.

DeRenzi, E., Pieczulo, A., and Vignolo, L. A. (1968). Ideational apraxia: a quantitative study. *Neuropsychologia* 6:41–52.

DeWitt, L. (1975). Conscious mind and self. *British Journal of Philosophical Sciences* 26:41–47.

Earnest, M. P., Monroe, P. A., and Yarnell, P. R. (1977). Cortical deafness: demonstration of the pathologic anatomy by CT scan. *Neurology* 27:1172–1175.

Faglioni, P., Spinnler, H., and Vignolo, L. A. (1969). Contrasting behavior of right and left hemisphere-damaged patients on a discriminative and a semantic task of auditory recognition. *Cortex* 5:366–389.

Foix, C. (1922). Sur une variété de troubles bilatéraux de la sensibilité par lesion unilatérale de cerveau. *Rev. Neurol. (Paris)* 29:322–331.

Frederiks, J. A. M. (1969). The agnosias: disorders of perceptual recognition. In P. J. Vinken and G. W. Bruyn (eds.), *Handbook of Clinical Neurology.* Vol. 4. Amsterdam: North Holland.

Gainotti, G., Silveri, M. C., Giampiero, V., and Miceli, G. (1986). Anomia with and without lexical comprehension disorders. *Brain Lang.* 29:18–33.

Gassell, M. M. (1969). Occipital lobe syndromes. In P. J. Vinken and G. W. Bruyn (eds.), *Handbook of Clinical Neurology.* Vol. 2. Amsterdam: North Holland.

Gazzaniga, M. S., and LeDoux, J. E. (1978). *The Integrated Mind.* New York: Plenum.

Geschwind, N. (1965). Disconnexion syndromes in animals and man. *Brain* 88:237–294, 585–644.

Goldberg, E. (1989). The gradiental approach to neocortical functional organization. *J. Clin. Exp. Neuropsychol.* 11:489–517.

Goldberg, E. (in press). Associative agnosias and the function of the left hemisphere. *J. Clin. Exp. Neuropsychol.*

Goldberg, E., and Bilder, R. M., Jr. (1987). The frontal lobes and hierarchical organization of cognitive control. In E. Pereceman (ed.), *Frontal Lobes Revisited.* New York: JRBN Press, pp. 159–187.

Goldberg, E., Bilder, R. M., Hughes, J. E. O., Antin, S. P., and Mattis, S. (1989). A reticulo-frontal disconnection syndrome. *Cortex* 25:687–695.

Goldberg, E., and Costa, L. D. (1981). Hemisphere differences in the acquisition and use of descriptive systems. *Brain Lang.* 14:144–173.

Goldberg, E., and Costa, L. D. (1986). Qualitative indices in neuropsychological assessment: an extension of Luria's approach to executive deficit following prefrontal lesions. In I. Grant and K. M. Adams (eds.), *Neuropsychological Assessment of Neuropsychiatric Disorders.* New York: Oxford University Press, pp. 48–64.

Goldberg, E., and Tucker, D. (1979). Motor perseveration and long-term memory for visual forms. *J. Clin. Neuropsychol.* 1:273–288.

Goldberg, E., Vaughan, H. G., and Gerstman, L. J. (1978). Nonverbal descriptive systems and hemispheric asymmetry: shape versus texture discrimination. *Brain Lang.* 5:249–257.

Golding, E., Reich, S. S., and Wason, P. C. (1974). Interhemispheric differences in problem solving. *Perception* 3:231–235.

Goldstein, K. (1916). Uber kortikale Sensibilitatsstorungen, *Neurol. Zentralblat.* 19:825–827.

Goldstein, K. (1952). The effect of brain damage on the personality. *Psychiatry* 15:245–260.

Goldstein, M. N., Brown, M., and Hollander, J. (1975). Auditory agnosia and cortical deafness: analysis of a case with three-year follow-up. *Brain Lang.* 2:324–332.

Hécaen, H., and Albert, M. L. (1978). *Human Neuropsychology.* New York: Wiley.

Hécaen, H., and Angelergues, R. (1963). *Le Cecite Psychique.* Paris: Masson et Cie.

Hécaen, H., and de Ajuriaguerra, J. (1956). *Les Troubles Mentaux au Cours du Tumeurs Intracraniennes.* Paris: Masson et Cie.

Hécaen, H., Goldblum, M. C., Masure, M. C., and Ramier, A. M. (1974). Une nouvelle observation d'agnosic d'object: deficit de l'association, ou 2 de la categorisatien, specifique de la modalite visuelle? *Neuropsychologia* 12:447–464.

Heilman, K. M., and Scholes, R. (1976). The nature of comprehension errors in Broca's, conduction, and Wernicke's aphasics. *Cortex* 12:228–265.

Heilman, K. M., Watson, R. T., and Valenstein, E. (1985). Neglect and Related Disorders. In K. M. Heilman and E. Valenstein (eds.), *Clinical Neuropsychology,* 2nd ed. New York: Oxford University Press, pp. 243–293.

Hoff, H., and Potzl, O. (1935). Uber ein neues parieto-occiptaler syndrom (Seelenlahmung des Schauens Storung des korperschemas Wegfall de Zentralen Schens). *J. Psychiatr. Neurol.* 52:173–218.

Humphreys, G. W., and Riddoch, M. J. (1987). *To See But Not To See. A Case Study of Visual Agnosia.* London: Lawrence Erlbaum Associates.

Joynt, R. J., Honch, G. W., Rubin, A. J., and Trudell, R. G. Occipital lobe syndromes. In J. A. M. Frederiks (ed.), *Handbook of Clinical Neurology, Vol. 1 (45): Clinical Neuropsychology.* Amsterdam: Elsevier.

Kanshepolsky, J., Kelley, J. J., and Waggener, J. D. (1973). A cortical auditory disorder: clinical, audiologic, and pathologic aspects. *Neurology* 23:699–705.

Kertesz, A. (1984). Aphasia. In J. A. M. Frederiks (ed.), *Handbook of Clinical Neurology, Vol. 1 (45): Clinical Neuropsychology.* Amsterdam: Elsevier.

Kleist, K. (1928). Gehirnpathologische und Lokalisatorische Ergebuisse uber Hornstorungen, Gerausch-Taubheiten und Amusien. *Monatsschr. Psychiatr. Neurol.* 68:853–860.

Konow, A., and Pribram, K. H. (1970). Error recognition and utilization produced by injury to the frontal cortex in man. *Neuropsychologia* 8:489–491.

Kosslyn, S. M. (1987). Seeing and imagining in the cerebral hemispheres: a computational approach. *Psychol. Rev.* 94:148–175.

Landis, T., Graves, R., and Goodglass, H. (1981). Dissociated awareness of manual performance on two different visual associative tasks: a "split-brain" phenomenon in normal subjects? *Cortex* 17:435–440.

Lessell, S. (1975). Higher disorders of visual function: negative phenomena. In J. S. Glaser and J. L. Smith (eds.), *Neuro-ophthalmology.* Vol 8. St. Louis: Mosby.

Lhermitte, J., and de Ajuriaguerra, J. (1938). Asymbolic tactile et hallucinations du toucher: etude anatomoclinique. *Rev. Neurol. (Paris),* 19, 492–495.

Lissauer, H. (1890). Ein fall von Seelenblindheit nebst einem Beitrag zur Theorie derselben. *Archiv für Psychiatrie und Nervenkrankheiten* 21:222–270.

Luria, A. R. (1980). *Higher Cortical Functions in Man.* 2nd Rev. Ed. New York: Basic Books.

Luria, A. R., Pribram, K. H., and Homskaya, E. D. (1964). An experimental analysis of the behavioral disturbance produced by a left frontal arachnoidal endothelioma (meningioma). *Neuropsychologia* 2:257–280.

Magitot, F. A., and Hartmann, E. (1928). La cecite corticale. *Rev. Otoneuroocul.* 5:81–114.

McGlynn, S. M., and Schacter, D. L. (1989). Unawareness of deficits in neuropsychological syndromes. *J. Clin. Exp. Neuropsychol.* 11:143–205.

Meadows, J. C. (1974). The anatomical basis of prosopagnosia. *J. Neurol. Neurosurg. Psychiatry* 37:489–501.

Mesulam, M. (1985). Patterns in behavioral neuroanatomy: association areas, the limbic system, and hemispheric specialization. In M. Mesulam (ed.), *Principles of Behavioral Neurology.* Philadelphia: Davis.

Miller, G. A., Galanter, E., and Pribram, K. H. (1960). *Plans and the Structure of Behavior.* New York: Holt.

Mott, F. W. (1907). Bilateral lesion of the auditory cortical centre: complete deafness and aphasia. *Br. Med. J.* 2:310–315.

Nielsen, J. M. (1937). Unilateral cerebral dominance as related to mind blindness: minimal lesion capable of causing visual agnosia for objects. *Arch. Neurol. Psychiatry* 38:108–135.

Nielsen, J. M. (1938). Disturbances of the body scheme: the physiologic mechanism. *Bull. Los Angeles Neurol. Soc.* 3:127–135.

Nielsen, J. M. (1946). *Agnosia, Apraxia, Aphasia: Their Value in Cerebral Localization.* 2nd Ed. New York: Hoeber.

Parsons, O. A. (1987). Neuropsychological consequences of alcohol abuse: many questions—some answers. In O. A. Parsons and N. Butters (eds.), *Neuropsychology of Alcoholism.* New York: Guilford Press.

Popper, K., and Eccles, J. C. (1977). *The Self and Its Brain.* New York: Springer.

Posner, M. I. (1972). Coordination of internal codes. In W. G. Chase (ed.), *Visual Information Processing.* New York: Academic Press, pp. 35–73.

Posner, M. I. (1978). *Chronometric Explorations of Mind.* Hillside, NJ: Erlbaum.

Redlich, F., and Dorsey, J. F. (1945). Denial of blindness by patients with cerebral disease. *Arch. Neurol. Psychiatry* 53:407–417.

Riesberg, B., Ferris, S. H., Borenstein, J., Sianaiko, E., DeLeon, M. J., and Buttinger, C. (1986). Assessment of presenting symptoms. In L. Poon (ed.), *Memory Assessment in Older Adults.* Washington, DC: American Psychological Association Press.

Robinson, R. G., and Benson, D. F. (1981). Depression in aphasic patients: frequency, severity, and clinical pathological correlations. *Brain Lang.* 14:282–291.

Roth, M. (1949). Disorders of the body image caused by lesions of the right parietal lobe. *Brain* 72:89–111.

Rubens, A. B. (1979). Agnosia. In K. M. Heilman and E. Valenstein (eds.), *Clinical Neuropsychology.* New York: Oxford University Press.

Rubens, A. B., and Benson, D. F. (1971). Associative visual agnosia. *Arch. Neurol.* 24:305–316.

Sapir, E. (1921). *Language.* New York: Harcourt Brace.

Spinnler, H., and Vignolo, L. A. (1966). Impaired recognition of meaningful sounds in aphasia. *Cortex* 2:337–348.

Stuss, D. T., and Benson, D. F. (1986). *The Frontal Lobes.* New York: Raven Press.

Teuber, H. L., Battersby, W. S., and Bender, M. B. (1960). *Visual Field Defects after Penetrating Missile Wounds of the Brain.* Cambridge, MA: Harvard University Press.

Vignolo, L. A. (1982). Auditory agnosia. *Philos. Trans. R. Soc. Lond.* [*Biol.*] 298:49–57.

Von Monakow, C. (1905). *Gehirnpathologie.* 2nd Ed. Vienna: Alfred Holder.

von Stauffenberg, W. (1918). Klinische und Anatomische Beitrage für kenntnis der aprax-
ischen, agnosischen, und apraletischen Symptome. *Zeitschrift für die Gesamte Neurologie und Psychiatrie* 93:71.

Vygotsky, L. S. (1962). *Thought and Language.* Cambridge, MA: MIT Press.

Warrington, E. K. (1975). The selective impairment of semantic memory. *Q. J. Exp.
Psychiatry* 27:635–657.

Warrington, E. K. (1982). Neuropsychological studies of object recognition. *Philos.
Trans. R. Soc. Lond.* [*Biol.*] 298:16–33.

Warrington, E. K., and James, M. (1967). An experimental investigation of facial recognition in patients with cerebral lesions. *Cortex* 3:317–326.

Warrington, E. K., and James, M. (1988). Visual apperceptive agnosia: a clinical-anatom-
ical study of three cases. *Cortex* 24:13–31.

Warrington, E. K., and Taylor, A. M. (1973). The contribution of the right parietal lobe
to object recognition. *Cortex* 9:152–164.

Wernicke, C. (1894). *Grundriss der Psychiatrie.* Psychophysiologische Einleitung.

Whorf, B. L. (1956). *Language, Thought, and Reality: Selected Writings of Benjamin Lee
Whorf* (edited by J. B. Carroll). New York: Wiley.

Zaidel, D. W. (1986). Memory for scenes in stroke patients. *Brain* 109:547–560.

Zaidel, E. (1978). Auditory language comprehension in the right hemisphere following
commissurotomy and hemispherectomy: a comparison with child language and
aphasia. In A. Caramazza and E. B. Zurif (eds.), *Language Acquisition and Language
Breakdown: Parallels and Divergencies.* Baltimore: Johns Hopkins University Press.

Zaidel, E. (1987). Hemispheric monitoring. In D. Ottoson (ed.), *Duality and Unity of the
Brain.* London: Macmillan, pp. 247–281.

Zaidel, E., Zaidel, D. W., and Sperry, R. W. (1981). Left and right intelligence: case studies of Raven's Progressive Matrices following brain bisection and hemidecortication.
Cortex 17:167–186.

10

Reality Monitoring: Evidence from Confabulation in Organic Brain Disease Patients

MARCIA K. JOHNSON

This chapter addresses the problem of reality monitoring (Johnson and Raye, 1981; Johnson, 1988a) in the context of a general framework for memory research (Johnson, 1983, 1989; Johnson and Hirst, in press). Issues and findings from studies of confabulation in organic brain disease patients are considered within this framework.

MULTIPLE-ENTRY MODULAR MEMORY SYSTEM

The framework I find useful for thinking about cognition and memory is called a Multiple-Entry Modular Memory System, or MEM (Johnson, 1983, 1989; Johnson and Hirst, in press). According to MEM, memory is created by an intricate interplay of processes that are organized at the most global functional level into perceptual and reflective systems. The *perceptual system* records information that is the consequence of perceptual processes, such as seeing and hearing. The *reflective system* records information that is the consequence of internally generated processes, such as planning, comparing, speculating, and imagining. Each of these systems comprises more specific functional subsystems that in turn are made up of yet more specific functional components.

The perceptual system consists of two subsystems, P-1 and P-2; and the reflective system consists of two subsystems, R-1 and R-2 (Fig. 10–1). P-1 processes develop connections or associations involving perceptual information of which we are often unaware, such as the invariants in a speech signal that specify a particular vowel or the aspects of a moving stimulus that specify when it is likely to reach a given point in space. P-2 processes are involved in learning about the phenomenal perceptual world of objects and events such as chairs,

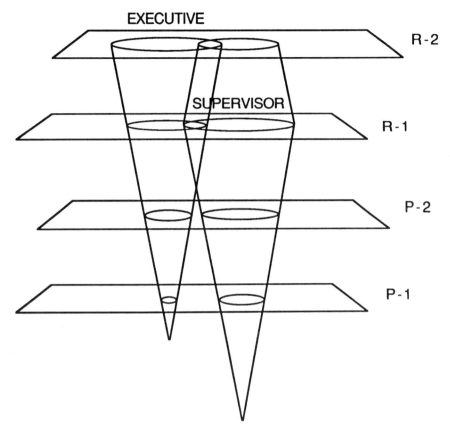

Figure 10–1. Multiple-Entry Modular Memory System, consisting of two reflective subsystems (R-1 and R-2) and two perceptual subsystems (P-1 and P-2). Reflective and perceptual subsystems interact through control and monitoring processes (supervisor and executive processes of R-1 and R-2, respectively), which have relatively greater access to and control over reflective than perceptual subsystems.

people, hearing your name, and catching a ball. A number of findings are consistent with a functional division between P-1 and P-2 processes (Johnson, 1983; Johnson and Hirst, in press). For example, "blindsight" patients may claim they cannot see a stimulus yet may be able to point to its location in space (Weiskrantz, 1986), a phenomenon that could occur if P-2 were disrupted but P-1 intact.

In contrast to perceptual processes, reflective processes occur independently of sensory stimulation. They are sometimes initiated by perception, but reflective processes allow one to go beyond external cues. They are generative; they allow us to manipulate information and memories of events, imagine possible alternatives, compare these alternatives, and so forth. As shown in Figure 10–2, both R-1 and R-2 involve component processes that allow people to sustain, organize, and revive information. Some of these component processes in R-1 are noting, shifting, refreshing, and reactivating. Analogous processes in R-2 are dis-

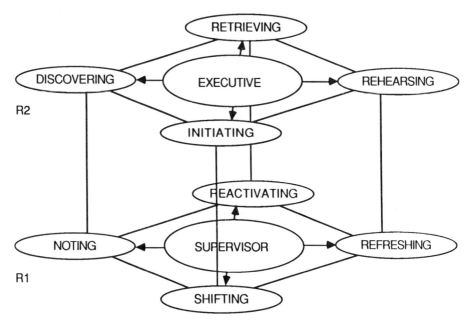

Figure 10-2. Some component processes of reflection. Basic reflective processes (noting, shifting, refreshing, reactivating, and supervisor functions) are represented on the bottom of the cube; and corresponding but more deliberate or strategic reflective functions (discovering, initiating, rehearsing, retrieving, and executive functions) are represented on the top of the cube.

covering, initiating, rehearsing, and retrieving [see Johnson (1989) and Johnson and Hirst (in press) for a discussion of these component processes].

The R-1 and R-2 subsystems also include control and monitoring component processes. For R-1 these processes are collectively referred to as *supervisor processes* and for R-2 as *executive processes.* Supervisor and executive processes set up goals and agendas and monitor or evaluate outcomes with respect to these agendas (Miller, Galanter, and Pribram, 1960; Stuss and Benson, 1986; Nelson and Narens, in press). Furthermore, they recruit other reflective component processes for these purposes. The difference between supervisor and executive processes is something like the difference between "tactical" and "strategic" control and monitoring processes or the difference between habitual and deliberate reflective processes. There is more control, effort, or will (e.g., Shiffrin and Schneider, 1977; Hasher and Zacks, 1979; Norman and Shallice, 1986) associated with executive than with supervisory processing. R-2 can handle more complex tasks than R-1. For example, under the guidance of an R-1 intention to *listen attentively to a story* told by your dinner companion, you might generate tacit implications of sentences, notice relations between one part of the story and an earlier part of which you are reminded, and so forth. Under guidance of an R-2 agenda to *critically evaluate the story,* you might generate objections to the logic of events in the story, actively retrieve other stories for comparison, and so forth. Normal cognitive functioning draws on different component processes of reflection as needed. Disruption of various combinations of component processes results in various patterns of cognitive deficit, including amnesia (Johnson and Hirst, in press) and, as discussed below, confabulation.

P-1, P-2, R-1, and R-2 activities may go on simultaneously, and they produce corresponding changes in memory. At some future time, exactly which of these records are activated depends on the kind of task probing memory (e.g., Jacoby and Dallas, 1981). A task in which you had to identify random syllables spoken by your dinner companion presented in white noise would draw primarily on representations formed by P-1. A recognition task in which you had to discriminate pictures of people who were and were not at the party draws primarily on representations formed in P-2. Recalling your dinner companion's story would draw on R-1 and R-2 records.

Under ordinary circumstances, subsystems interact with each other, although exactly how they interact needs further investigation. During remembering, representations from one subsystem may directly activate related representations from another, or interactions between perceptual and reflective memory may take place through supervisor and executive components. For example, an agenda initiated by the R-2 executive, e.g., *look for a restaurant,* might activate relevant perceptual schemas from perceptual memory (e.g., look for a building with a ground level window, tables visible, menu in window). It might also activate reflective plans adapted to the current situation (e.g., check the restaurant guide for this part of town).

Supervisor and executive processes are depicted in Figure 10–1 as cones passing through planes representing different subsystems. The sizes of the ellipses at the intersects of cones and planes reflect the relative degree of involvement of supervisor and executive processes in each subsystem's activities. Typically, executive functions have greater access to reflective memory than to perceptual memory and greater access to P-2 than to P-1 subsystems. An especially important aspect of reflection is that the supervisor and executive processes in R-1 and R-2 can recruit and monitor each other, as depicted by their overlap in Figure 10–1. For example, an R-2 agenda to *check the restaurant guide* can initiate an R-1 goal to *note the number of stars by each entry.* Interaction between R-1 and R-2 provides a mechanism for sequencing subgoals. It also gives rise to the phenomenal experience of reflecting on reflection. In addition, access to information about one's own cognitive operations provides a salient cue for identifying oneself as the origin of information. These R-1, R-2 interactions contribute to our concept and sense of self.

This general framework has been useful for organizing empirical facts obtained from cognitive-behavioral studies (Johnson, 1983), as well as for generating new research (Johnson and Kim, 1985; Johnson, Kim, and Risse, 1985; Hirst, Johnson, Kim, et al., 1986; Weinstein, 1987; Hirst, Johnson, Phelps, and Volpe, 1988; Johnson, Peterson, Chua-Yap, and Rose, 1989; see also Johnson, 1989). As well as being heuristic, the division between perceptual and reflective memories may capture functional organizations within the nervous system. Several behavioral dissociations support this claim. For example, memory for reflective processing develops later than memory for perceptual processes (e.g., Perlmutter, 1984; Schacter and Moscovitch, 1984; Flavell, 1985; Moscovitch, 1985);

and it appears that P-2 develops later than P-1 and R-2 later than R-1. Moreover, memories for reflective processing are disrupted more easily by stress, depression, aging, and the use of alcohol and other drugs than are memories for perceptual processes (Eich, 1975; Hasher and Zacks, 1979, 1984; Craik, 1986; Hashtroudi and Parker, 1986). Furthermore, the breakdown in memory functioning found in patients with anterograde amnesia appears to fall disproportionately on reflective memory (Johnson, 1983, 1989; Johnson and Hirst, in press; Cermak, 1982).

REALITY MONITORING

Because humans have a cognitive system that takes in information from a number of perceptual sources and that can itself internally generate information as well, one of the mind's most critical cognitive functions is discriminating the origin of information. We constantly use this ability in considering ongoing experience (Is what I see now "out there," or am I only imagining it?) and the products of past experience (Is my memory for an event that happened when I was 5 years old a memory for an actual event or an event I imagined as a child?) (Johnson, 1985). I have suggested we use the term *reality testing* for the processes by which people make such discriminations during ongoing experience (e.g., Perky, 1910) and the term *reality monitoring* for the processes by which people discriminate between memories derived from perception and those that were reflectively generated via thought, imagination, dreams, and fantasy (Johnson, 1977, 1988a; Johnson and Raye, 1981).

Reality monitoring refers not only to monitoring the origin of memories for events but also to discriminating the origin of knowledge, attitudes, and beliefs (e.g., Slusher and Anderson, 1987). Also, within the class of externally derived information we make discriminations (external source monitoring) among alternative sources (Did I see this or hear/read about it? (e.g., Loftus, 1979; Lindsay and Johnson, 1989). Within the class of internally generated information, self-monitoring discriminations are also made (Did I tell Joe or only imagine telling Joe? (e.g., Foley, Johnson, and Raye, 1983). Such self-monitoring discriminates intentions from actions. Although the discussion here and most of our empirical work to date focus on reality monitoring, many of the same factors are important for all of these discriminations, and the current framework provides the beginning of a systematic, integrated approach for considering relations among reality testing, reality monitoring, external source monitoring, and self-monitoring as they apply to either events or knowledge and beliefs (Lindsay and Johnson, 1987; Johnson, 1988a, Hashtroudi, Johnson, and Chrosniak, 1989).

Consistent with MEM, our approach to the issue of reality monitoring assumes that the memory system preserves both the results of perceptual processing and the results of more self-generated or reflective processing (Johnson and Raye, 1981). Reality monitoring failures occur when people confuse the origin of information, misattributing something that was reflectively generated to perception or vice versa. That is, reality is not directly given in perception or remembering but is an attribution that is the outcome of judgment processes.

Confusions can be understood by considering the phenomenal characteristics of memories for perceived and imagined events along with the decision processes people apply to activated information. We proposed that memories for perceived and imagined events differ in average value along a number of dimensions. Memories originating in perception typically have more perceptual information (e.g., color, sound), contextual time and place information, and more meaningful detail, whereas memories originating in thought typically have more accessible information about cognitive operations, i.e., those perceptual and reflective processes that took place when the memory was established. Differences between externally and internally derived memories in average value along these dimensions or attributes form one basis for deciding the origin of a memory. For example, a memory with little information about cognitive operations and a great deal of perceptual information would likely be judged to have been externally derived.

A second type of decision process is based on reasoning: Such processes may include, for example, retrieving additional information from memory and considering if the target memory could have been perceived (or self-generated) given these other specific memories or general knowledge. For example, I might have a memory of telling Ronald Reagan what I think of his policies, but I can correctly attribute it to a fantasy on the basis of the knowledge that I am not acquainted with him. In addition, judgments are affected by people's opinions or "metamemory" assumptions about how memory works. For example, I might believe that something that comes to mind quickly is likely to be an accurate memory of an actual event. Thus reality monitoring most likely produces errors when perceived and imagined events are similar along dimensions that normally provide a discriminative cue (e.g., if the imaginations in question are particularly rich in perceptual and contextual detail), when reasoning fails, when the relevant background knowledge is not retrieved or unknown, or when metamemory assumptions are inaccurate.

A number of experimental findings support this reality monitoring framework. For example, the more imaginations are like perceptions in perceptual detail, the more subjects confuse imaginations with perceptions. In one experiment (Johnson, Raye, Wang, and Taylor, 1979), we varied the number of times subjects saw pictures and the number of times they imagined each picture. Later, we asked subjects how many times they saw each picture. The more often the subjects saw the pictures, the higher their frequency judgments. More important, the more often the subjects imagined the pictures, the more often they thought they had seen them. Furthermore, compared to poor imagers, good imagers were more affected by the number of times they had imagined a picture. In another experiment (Johnson, Foley, and Leach, 1988a) subjects imagined themselves saying some words and heard a confederate say other words. Later, the subjects were good at discriminating the words they had thought from the words the confederate had actually said. In another condition, the procedure was the same except that subjects were asked to think in the confederate's voice; in this case subjects later had much more difficulty discriminating what they had heard from what they had thought. The results of both the good/poor imager study and the think-in-another-person's voice study are consistent with the idea that the more perceptual overlap there is between memories derived from perception and memories generated via imagination, the greater is the confusion between them.

According to the reality monitoring framework, remembered cognitive operations can also be a cue to the origin of a memory. In one experiment (Durso and Johnson, 1980), subjects saw an acquisition list consisting of some words and some line drawings of common objects. We then asked subjects to indicate whether each item had appeared as a word or a picture. We varied how the subjects processed the items initially. At acquisition, some subjects indicated the function of the referent of each item. For example, if they saw a picture of a knife (or the word knife) they might say "you cut with it." Still other subjects identified a particularly relevant feature of each object, for example, *blade* for knife. Other subjects had an artist time judgment task: If a picture was presented, they rated how long it took the artist to draw it. If a word was presented, they constructed an image of a line drawing of the referent and then rated how long it would take the artist to draw the imagined picture.

One important difference between the first two tasks and the last one is that the artist time judgment task involves intentional imagery, whereas the function and relevant feature tasks are likely to involve spontaneous, or incidental, imagery. That is, to answer a question about an object's relevant features, a person might think of a visual representation of the object and "pick out" a relevant feature. Intentional images are under voluntary, reflective control and thus the memories for them should contain more information about cognitive operations than the memories for spontaneous images. If so, people should later be better able to discriminate memories of voluntarily constructed images from memories of pictures than memories of spontaneous images from memories of pictures. Consistent with this prediction, in the artist time judgment condition, subjects rarely said a word had been presented as a picture. In the function and relevant feature conditions, they much more often claimed to have seen pictures of objects that had only been named. Thus spontaneous or incidental images were more likely to be confused with perceptions than were consciously constructed ones.

We have also investigated reality monitoring for naturally occurring, complex events. In one study (Johnson, Kahan, and Raye, 1984) subjects had to discriminate between memories for their own dreams and memories for dreams their roommate, spouse, or lover told them. Two points from this study are especially relevant here. Subjects occasionally misattributed something they dreamed to their partner on the basis of reasoning from general beliefs: "That couldn't have been mine because it is just not the sort of thing I dream." Also, subjects' ability to recall dreams was poor, and if this information was all we had, we might be tempted to conclude that dreams quickly fade away. However, recognition memory for dreams was high. The recognition results suggest that dreams persist in memory for some time and are a potential source of images and ideas.

In another series of studies, we investigated reality monitoring for various kinds of naturally occurring, autobiographical events. In one study (Johnson, Foley, Suengas, and Raye, 1988b) we asked subjects to remember an event from their own experience (a trip to the library, a social occasion, a trip to the dentist, a dream, a fantasy, an unfulfilled intention), and then we asked them how they knew that the event actually had (or had not) taken place. The explanations or justifications used most often were different for actual and imagined events. For actual events, subjects were likely to refer to characteristics of the target memory itself, such as temporal information (e.g., time of the school year), location information ("I know exactly where it happened."), or perceptual detail ("I remember the exact color of his shirt"). Also for actual perceptions subjects were likely to refer to supporting memories. Actual events are embedded in anticipations before the fact (e.g., buying something to wear) and consequences after the fact (e.g., later conversations about the event or later regrets). People frequently refer to these supporting memories to justify their belief that an event really happened. For imaginations, the subjects referred to characteristics of the target memories or to supporting memories much less often. Rather, the overwhelmingly most frequent response for imaginations involved reasoning, such as pointing out inconsistencies between the memory and their general knowledge of the world (e.g., "I was a doctor but really I was too young to be a doctor, so it must be only a fantasy" or "the event breaks physical laws about time and space").

Reality Monitoring and MEM

Reality monitoring processes can be described more specifically in terms of the MEM framework. Reality monitoring requires people to discriminate memories generated by R-1 and R-2 processes from memories derived from P-2 and perhaps P-1 processes. Supervisory and executive processes in R-1 and R-2 are used in judgments about the origin of activated information. For normally functioning adults, most reality monitoring is guided by R-1 supervisory processes; that is, reality monitoring typically takes place rapidly, in a nondeliberative fashion, based on the qualitative characteristics of memories that are activated (e.g., amount or type of perceptual detail). The generally slower, more deliberate retrieval of supporting memories and initiation of reasoning processes (e.g., Does this seem plausible given other things I know?) are R-2 functions and are probably engaged less often. Although less frequently used, they are no less important, of course. Among other things, R-2 processes allow us to look back on ideas we initially accepted and question them.

Using this framework, consider the various ways in which reality monitoring could break down: Disrupted reality monitoring could result from decreases in the difference between phenomenal qualities of perceived and imagined events (disrupted experience or disrupted memory for experience), difficulty retrieving relevant supporting information, failures in reality monitoring judgment processes, or reduced motivation to engage in reality monitoring.

Disrupted Experience

As previously mentioned, if perceptual qualities of imagined events were unusually vivid, they would be more difficult to discriminate from perceived events. It might happen, for example, if reflective processes were especially successful in recruiting perceptual processes during imagination (Kosslyn, 1980) as is evidently the case with good imagers (Johnson et al., 1979). Conversely, if perceptual qualities of perceived events became less vivid, it would also reduce differences between perceived and imagined events. Decreased encoding of perceptual qualities of external events may happen as a consequence of normal aging. Older adults may pay less attention to perceptual aspects of events (Hasher and Zacks, 1988) and the reduced perceptual information in memory could produce an aging deficit in reality monitoring (Hashtroudi, Johnson, and Chrosniak, 1990; Rabinowitz, 1989).

Memories derived from perception typically have more contextual (temporal and spatial) information than memories derived from imagination. Some of this contextual information is inherent in the perception (e.g., perceptual processes spatially organize a face with the nose below the eyes), and some is the product of reflection. For example, the temporal relation between two events is often made salient because we think of the first event at the time of the second, perhaps to compare them (Tzeng and Cotton, 1980; Johnson, 1983). Remembering this reflective activity produces knowledge of temporal order. Anything that differentially reduces the amount of contextual information that usually is associated with perceived events or that differentially increases the contextual information associated with imagined events would make reality monitoring more difficult.

Similarly, any decrease in the cognitive operations information produced during reflection would disrupt reality monitoring. For example, as strategic R-2 reflection becomes a more habitual R-1 function, the resulting reflective entries in memory should be more likely to be confused with perceptual entries. Thus people are especially likely to believe they heard or saw something they only inferred when the inference was a particularly easy or habitual one (e.g., Johnson, Bransford, and Solomon, 1973).

Disrupted Retrieval
Supporting memories for events occurring both before and after a target event are used to help specify the origin of a memory. Anything that would make such supporting information more difficult to retrieve (e.g., disrupted reflective retrieval operations) should disrupt reality monitoring.

Disrupted Judgment
As mentioned above, much of the reality monitoring we do is relatively automatic or nonstrategic and is guided by R-1 processes. Thus if R-1 processes were eliminated or their efficiency or reliability reduced (as indicated by the dotted lines in Figure 10-3A), confusions between perceived and imagined events might be frequent. Some errors could be corrected, however, using R-2 processes to retrieve additional, supporting information or to reason about the plausibility of an event or belief in light of what else is known. On the other hand, if plausible memories were not subjected to a check for perceptual detail, they might be accepted too readily. Thus R-1 processes provide a check on R-2 processes as well as vice versa.

Figure 10-3B shows a situation in which R-1 processes are intact but R-2 processes are eliminated, or their efficiency or reliability is disrupted (indicated by the dotted lines). Reality monitoring judgments guided by R-1 processes and based on such qualitative characteristics as perceptual and contextual detail and

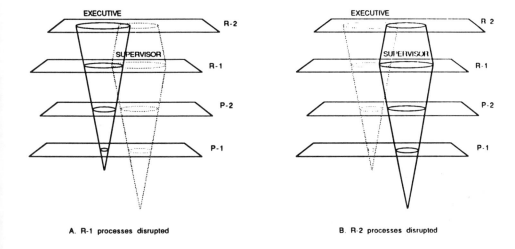

A. R-1 processes disrupted

B. R-2 processes disrupted

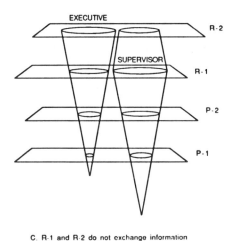

C. R-1 and R-2 do not exchange information
about executive functions

Figure 10–3. Some ways reflective processes could be disrupted.

information about cognitive operations would occur normally. Because of the R-2 deficit, however, there would be less chance of catching R-1 errors on vivid, but implausible, imaginations.

In addition to a global disruption of judgment processes, shifts in the criteria used for R-1 or R-2 processes could increase reality monitoring errors. For example, an increase in the similarity of perceived and imagined information would not necessarily leave a person's decision criteria unchanged. If one were aware that one was encoding less perceptual information than one used to do, one might lower the criterion for the amount of perceptual information required for attributing a remembered event to perception. The consequence of a lower criterion would be to increase the probability of misattributing imagined events to perception (as might occur in some cases of perceptual deficit).

Finally, Figure 10–3C depicts a situation in which both R-1 and R-2 judgment processes are intact but in which R-1 and R-2 supervisor and executive processes no longer exchange information about each other's functioning (compare Figure 10–3C to Figure 10–1). One important consequence of such a disconnection is that it would reduce the availability of cognitive operations as a discriminative cue for origin to either R-2 executive or R-1 supervisor processes.

Reduced Motivation
Any reduction in a person's estimate of the value of accurately reporting events, any decrease in motivation to engage in the effortful processing that is sometimes necessary for accurate reality monitoring, or any lessening of social constraints that promote concern for the truth would increase errors in reality monitoring. The basic underlying mechanisms in these cases, however, most likely are disrupted retrieval and judgment processes resulting from disrupted motivation and not any direct effects of motivation per se.

Summary

Discriminating the origin of information in memory is the outcome of an interplay of input, retrieval, and judgment processes. Reality monitoring involves judgment processes applied to information activated in reflective and perceptual memory systems. For optimal reality monitoring, reflective processes must have access not only to this activated target information but to other potentially relevant supporting information as well. Normally, R-1 processes operate almost continually and R-2 processes more intermittently. There is, furthermore, a critical balance between R-1 and R-2 supervisory and executive processes in that each provides the opportunity to correct errors resulting from the other.

As is the case for other cognitive functions, there are three basic strategies for investigating reality monitoring: studying reality monitoring processes in normal adults, studying the development of these processes in children, and studying the disruption of these processes under special circumstances or in special populations. Discussions drawing largely on the first and second strategies are illustrated elsewhere (Johnson and Raye, 1981; Johnson and Foley, 1984; Johnson, 1985, 1988a; Lindsay and Johnson, 1987; Johnson et al., 1988a,b; Suengas and Johnson, 1988). With respect to the third strategy, the reality monitoring framework can be used to clarify discussions of hallucinations (Bentall, 1990) and delusions (Johnson, 1988a) and to explore potential deficits in monitoring the source of information in older adults (Mitchell, Hunt, and Schmitt, 1986; Rabinowitz, 1989; Hashtroudi, Johnson, and Chrosniak, 1989; Hashtroudi et al., 1990).

CONFABULATION

Reality monitoring deficits that result from brain damage provide a valuable opportunity to evaluate further the usefulness of the present framework; they also provide some intriguing evidence about potential brain mechanisms underlying reality monitoring. To simplify the following discussion I have concentrated on confabulation, although some aspects of related syndromes such as denial of illness and reduplicative paramnesia could be discussed within the present framework as well.

The literature on patients who confabulate contains a number of ideas about mechanisms underlying confabulation that fit within the present framework in that they emphasize either phenomenal characteristics of the information activated during remembering or judgment processes. With respect to characteristics of the information, some investigators have emphasized the context-free and thus incoherent nature of the information retrieved (Kopelman, 1987) or the vividness of the experience (Whitty, 1966). Explanations emphasizing judgment processes include decreased self-monitoring ability (Stuss, Alexander, Lieberman, and Levine, 1978), decreased ability to provide verbal self-corrections (Mercer, Wapner, Gardner, and Benson, 1977), and disruption of a central executive (Baddeley and Wilson, 1986). The present effort attempts to organize these ideas in a larger framework of cognitive processing and memory and to give some of the ideas greater specificity within the context of the MEM and reality monitoring frameworks.

Defining Confabulation

Confabulation is not well understood. Part of the problem is defining what counts as confabulation. Whitlock (1981), for example, pointed out the inconsistent uses of the term in psychiatric textbooks. Most investigators agree that confabulation must be differentiated from lying and from the consequences of delirium and delusions (e.g., Talland, 1961; Whitlock, 1981; Kerns, 1986). That is, confabulations are false statements that are not made to deceive, are typically more coherent than thoughts produced during delirium, and do not reflect underlying psychopathology. These distinctions do not, of course, imply that these various phenomena do not have any processes in common, only that they are identifiable categories that are useful for analytic purposes.

Confabulation varies from relatively subtle alterations of fact to bizarre tales. For example, in a study by Kopelman (1987), subjects heard a story and were asked to recall it. It was a story about a woman who had been robbed and who reported the robbery at the Town Hall police station. One Korsakoff patient said "she asked for help from the Council." This relatively minor distortion would be scored as a confabulation. More dramatic examples of confabulation were reported by Stuss et al. (1978). One hospitalized patient who had frontal lobe damage described how he had played cards the preceding night at a club with his doctor and the head nurse. Another frontal patient fabricated a story of a drowning accident involving one of his children and thought his own head injury occurred in the rescue attempt. Another claimed that during World War II a teenage German girl shot him three times in the head, killing him, but that surgery brought him back to life.

Given this variation in patients' errors and false statements, it has been proposed that there are two distinct confabulatory phenomena (Talland, 1961). Talland suggested that *confabulation* involves a distortion of true events, e.g., misplacement of an event in time, whereas *fabrication* is fantastic and incongruous material involving figments of imagination. Some investigators distinguish between confabulation produced in response to questions (*reactive* confabulation) and *spontaneous* or *fantastic* confabulation (Berlyne, 1972; Stuss et al., 1978; Whitlock, 1981; Kopelman, 1987). Reactive confabulation tends to embellish true memories and to be plausible; spontaneous confabulation tends to be more bizarre, implausible, or fantastic. The distinctions between confabulation and fabrication and between reactive and spontaneous confabulation point to differences in the degree to which confabulation appears to draw on true memories or on imagination. The difference between distorted "true" memories and new fabrications may not, however, be so clear-cut. Even fantastic spontaneous fabrications might draw on accurate memories for premorbid fantasies and imagined horrors (Talland, 1961), reflecting a reality monitoring failure of attributing the products of prior imagination to prior perception. As we saw in our dream study, dreams persist in memory for some time, as do memories of waking fantasies (Johnson et al., 1984).

Relation to Memory Loss

Another issue that has been raised in the literature on confabulation is the extent to which confabulation is associated with or dependent on loss of memory. Confabulation is often found in amnesics, especially alcoholic Korsakoff patients. In fact, confabulation is sometimes defined as false statements made in connection with organic amnesia (Berlyne, 1972, cited in Shapiro, Alexander, Gardner, and Mercer, 1981) and thought to be a direct consequence of memory loss (Barbizet, 1963, cited in Stuss et al., 1978). In this view, confabulation is a gap-filling process (e.g., Wyke and Warrington, 1960) that is not different from the constructive processes found in normal individuals (Kopelman, 1987). Thus amnesics are said to fill in the gaps in memory much as normal individuals do; but because amnesics' gaps are so much more extensive, they show marked confabulation.

According to this constructive, gap-filling view of confabulation, as normal recall after long retention intervals approaches the low level of amnesic recall, normal subjects should show increasing confabulation. Contrary to this expectation, the literature reporting studies of normal memory includes little experimental evidence of anything approaching "florid" distortions in recall even after substantial retention intervals. Investigators looking for constructive recall have often been disappointed by the lack of intrusions in subjects' protocols (Alba and Hasher, 1983). Even in Bartlett's (1932) classic studies, after long retention intervals and repeated recall, subjects tended to produce briefer and increasingly stereotyped reports, not more embellished ones. The fact that normal subjects do not show as much gap-filling as the notion of unchecked constructive processes would lead one to expect suggests that people naturally engage in reality monitoring processes that help them distinguish true recall from their own constructions and reconstructions (Johnson and Raye, 1981). This fact in turn suggests that amnesics show confabulation not because they have memory gaps to fill but because the processes that normally monitor remembering are deficient.

There are several other problems with assuming that confabulation reflects nothing but a normal response to gaps in memory. Confabulation is not a necessary consequence of amnesia because many amnesics do not appear to confabulate. Furthermore, patients may confabulate only in the early stages of amnesia and then settle into a chronic state of profound amnesia with little or no apparent confabulation. Although confabulation is sometimes assumed to be a defining symptom of the Korsakoff syndrome, a number of investigators have pointed out that confabulation does not invariably occur in Korsakoff patients, and when it does it often is a transient component of an acute phase of the disease (Talland, 1961). Another problem with the idea of confabulation as a natural process of gap filling is that many amnesics readily admit to the gaps in their memory and do not appear to be compelled to fill them in. Finally, additional evidence regarding the dissociation of amnesia and confabulation comes from cases in which confabulation is found in the absence of marked amnesia. For example, Whitty and Lewin (1957) studied a group of patients who had undergone anterior cingulectomy for treatment of severe obsessional neurosis. This operation resulted in a striking tendency of patients to spontaneously confabulate, but they otherwise had clarity of consciousness, orientation for place and person, and awareness of the operation. Although some patients showed minor disorientation of time and misplacement of events, they did not have marked memory deficits. Thus, overall, it appears that amnesia and confabulation have different substrates (Stuss et al., 1978).

Although confabulation and amnesia may be distinct phenomena, at a more general level confabulation is itself a type of memory disorder. Confabulation is a failure of reality monitoring, and reality monitoring is a memory function, just as recall and recognition are memory functions (Johnson and Raye, 1981). Although we may want to reserve the term "amnesia" for a particular form of memory disorder, confabulation represents a memory disorder as well. The fact that the memory system can be disordered in the particular way we call confabulation provides evidence regarding normally functioning aspects of the complex, integrated cognitive system of memory.

Confabulation and Awareness

Another interesting issue is whether confabulating patients are aware that they do so. Although a striking feature of confabulation is that patients typically do not realize the absurdity or erroneous nature of their comments (Joseph, 1986), sometimes awareness accompanies or, rather, follows closely on the heels of confabulation. Most of Whitty and Lewin's (1957, 1960) cingulectomy patients were aware that they confabulated, and some of them actually described themselves as having difficulty discriminating fact from fantasy and dreams. ("My thoughts seem to be out of control, they go off on their own—so vivid. I am not sure half the time if I just thought it or it really happened,"—Whitty and Lewin, 1957, p. 73.) Furthermore, on occasion they corrected themselves without prompting, ("I have been having tea with my wife. . . . Oh, I haven't really. She's not been here today,"—Whitty and Lewin, 1957, p. 73.) Such observations provide some clues not only about the mechanisms of reality monitoring but about the nature of awareness.

According to the present view, awareness of confabulation arises as a natural outcome of normally functioning reality monitoring processes. For example, consider a remembered fantasy. The output of R-1 processes assessing the vividness of a memory may indicate that the event really happened. The output of R-2 processes assessing its plausibility may indicate it could not have happened. Awareness of confabulation would arise from the experience of conflict between the output of these two processes. That is, we do not become aware that we are confabulating unless we catch ourselves doing it (or somebody else catches us and we recognize the conflict). Presumably, Whitty and Lewin's cingulectomy patients were aware of their confabulation because R-2 reality monitoring processes that could detect errors from the output of R-1 processes were still intact. If the processes that do the catching break down, so does the awareness. Lack of awareness of confabulation would accompany a more extensive breakdown of reality monitoring processes, in particular perhaps a disruption of R-2 processes.

The more general point is that awareness or consciousness is not a separate system superimposed on other processes; rather, it is the natural outgrowth of certain (but not all) cognitive processes. If a process is disrupted, the awareness it gives rise to is disrupted. Disruptions in awareness can be specific because disruptions in processes can be specific.

Brain Regions Implicated in Confabulation

Available evidence about the brain regions disrupted in confabulating patients provides a reasonably systematic and suggestive picture. The relatively controlled lesions made in anterior cingulectomy patients produce dramatic but temporary confabulation lasting several days (Whitty and Lewin, 1957, 1960). Damage to the basal forebrain region produces confabulation that may last weeks to months (Damasio, Graff-Radford, Eslinger, et al., 1985), and damage to various areas in the frontal lobes produces confabulation that may last months to years (Stuss et al., 1978). Stuss et al. made a persuasive argument for the role of frontal lobe damage in confabulation. They reported five patients with demonstrable frontal lobe lesions who all showed spontaneous, persisting confabulation. At least temporary, and sometimes long-lasting, confabulation is found in Korsakoff patients, who often show prefrontal symptomatology as well as damage to thalamic nuclei that project to prefrontal and anterior cingulate cortex. The fact that confabulators often show perseverative tendencies, difficulty in shifting response sets, and lack of concern about incorrect behavior (all recognized symptoms of frontal damage) suggests frontal involvement.

In sum, disruption of areas immediately adjacent to the frontal lobes produces marked but transient effects. Structural damage to the frontal lobes themselves produces more permanent effects. Thus overall there is a fairly consistent pattern of evidence pointing to confabulation as a potential consequence of disruption of frontal lobe functioning, implicating the frontal lobes in normal reality monitoring processes.

Characteristics of Confabulation and Reality Monitoring Mechanisms

Transient confabulation may be produced by temporary disruption of an intact area either because of loss of some inputs, the presence of unusual inputs, or a metabolic upset that recovers. For example, cingulectomy patients may experience spontaneous activation of information with a high degree of perceptual content. This unusual perceptual input could be a consequence of disruption of reflective processes that normally inhibit access to perceptual entries (e.g., Johnson, 1983) or a consequence of signals from damaged areas that activate cortical areas subserving perceptual information. In either case, the high perceptual value of the information would easily pass the criterion for externally derived information according to the R-1 "fast-guess" reality monitoring judgment process, producing a reality monitoring failure. Alternatively, information activated by signals from a damaged area may not be more vivid perceptually, but it may lack voluntary cognitive operations information, thereby reducing the discriminability between perceived and imagined information. Assuming R-2 processes were still intact, the reality monitoring failures produced by R-1 processes that are most inconsistent with other knowledge (the most bizarre or implausible events) could be corrected with R-2 processes. This corrective process results in awareness of the reality monitoring problem.

Another potential reason confabulation is sometimes temporary is that R-1 and R-2 judgment mechanisms may learn to compensate for disrupted experience or disrupted retrieval either by tightening criteria or invoking R-2 more often. In this case, the patient might experience a period of awareness of confabulation followed by increased ability to withhold confabulated ideas. Thus some patients may not stop having confabulated thoughts but may develop strategies for dealing with them. A person's willingness to claim they remember something is affected by shifts in the criteria used for reality monitoring or shifts in criteria along with metamemory assumptions, and the nature of the criterial shift may be determined by a patient's personality or metamemory beliefs. For example, some amnesics, as they gain insight into their amnesia, may become reluctant to claim they remember something because they do not have the normal ways available for verifying veridicality (e.g., for retrieving additional information). On the other hand, other amnesia patients may react to the same situation by adopting more lax criteria. They might believe, for example, that if they are asked a question and an answer occurs to them, the answer must be correct or otherwise why would they have thought of it? This metamemory assumption would produce a type of reactive confabulation. Assuming that responses would be based on general knowledge or retrieval of fragments of autobiographical experience, most confabulation of this sort would not necessarily be unusual or bizarre. The confabulation seen in Korsakoff patients is often of this type (e.g., Talland, 1961).

Permanent confabulatory tendencies presumably are produced by irreversible damage to structures or mechanisms underlying R-1 or R-2 processes or their interaction. For example, disruption of R-2 processes would result in confabulation whenever particularly compelling but false information passes the R-1 criterion. How frequently this situation occurs should depend on individual differences in the criteria adopted or in the relative richness of memories for perceived and imagined events. Assuming that for most of us, most of the time, reality monitoring largely is a consequence of R-1 processes, the more frequently a patient confabulates, the more we might suspect that the confabulation is a result of unusual informational input (high in perceptual detail or low in cognitive operations), disruption of R-1 processes, or a combination of the two factors. Less frequent but more bizarre confabulations suggest disruption of the R-2 processes.

Of course, memory deficits, superimposed on reality monitoring deficits, compound any reality monitoring problem because patients are not able to remember previous reality monitoring judgments (even if correct) for a particular thought. If these thoughts recur (perhaps because of "priming" processes or more permanent effects of repetition), they may be even more likely to seem to have been initially perceived because of their ease of production. Also, insofar as some reality monitoring processes depend on activation and evaluation of supporting information in memory, anything that disrupts the availability of such information could disrupt reality monitoring.

As we learn more, it should be possible to express observed differences in reality monitoring deficits as specific combinations of disrupted processes (Table 10–1). For example, disrupted experience (e.g., unusually vivid imaginations or reduced intentionality) may underlie the type of confabulation we see in the case of certain drugs, brain stimulation, cingulectomy patients, and Anton's syndrome patients. Disrupted retrieval, especially in combination with lax criteria, could produce filling in of detail and displaced true memories. These sorts of confabulation are not particularly fantastic but are of the reactive type often seen in amnesics, especially Korsakoff patients. Disrupted judgment processes, especially disruption of R-2 processes, would result in less plausible and more fantastic confabulations of the sort characteristic of frontal patients. Various combinations of disruption may produce reality monitoring deficits as people age normally or in delusional patients. Table 10–1 summarizes several working hypotheses about which disrupted functions produce confabulation in various subject groups.

TABLE 10-1 Patterns of Disruption Hypothesized for Various Clinical Syndromes

Syndrome	Aspect of reality monitoring		
	Experience	Retrieval	Judgment
Normal Errors	+	+	+
Cingulectomy	−	+	+
Amnesia	+	−	+
Frontal disorder	+	+	−
Aging	−	−	+
Delusion	−	+	−
Confabulation (with memory deficit)	+	−	−
Global confusion	−	−	−

(+) indicates intact function; (−) indicates disruption in experience, retrieval, or judgment aspect of reality monitoring.

Evaluating such a scheme depends, among other things, on developing a better taxonomy of confabulation based on analyses of patient protocols. A great deal of useful information would result from a systematic and theoretically motivated analysis of the content of confabulations and a specification of conditions under which confabulations of various types are and are not produced. For this purpose, it would be desirable to have more consistency among investigators in the format used to report patients' confabulations. It would also be interesting to have subjective reports from patients about the qualities of their phenomenal experiences while remembering confabulated and actual events as well as while remembering previously imagined events (e.g., Johnson, 1988b). Such studies would give us important sources of converging evidence about the qualitative characteristics of confabulations of various types and etiology.

CONCLUSIONS

Reality monitoring is a fundamental memory function that anchors us in a perceived external world, in a felt past life with an autobiographical quality, and in a network of knowledge and beliefs that we take to be derived from experience in a veridical way. At the same time, reality monitoring produces in us a compelling sense of ownership over our own ideas, fantasies, and hopes. It is only when the boundary between externally derived and internally generated information becomes blurred, as in the case of confabulation or delusions, that we can fully appreciate how central this discrimination is to defining the characteristics of normal mental experience and to functioning effectively in the world.

Reality monitoring is the consequence of the coordinated activity of a number of processes embedded in a complex memory system (MEM). Although some of the components of these processes are shared with other functions (e.g., recall), the facts that reality monitoring deficits can occur in the absence of other memory problems and that other memory problems do not necessarily result in reality monitoring deficits suggest that reality monitoring is based on an identifiable, systematic organization of these components. Furthermore, the pattern of deficits produced by different types of brain damage provides some encouragement for the theoretical account of reality monitoring described here. The evidence is consistent with the idea that reality monitoring involves at least two types of judgment process: One is based on a nondeliberative evaluation of the characteristics of activated information, such as the type and amount of perceptual detail (tentatively identified in MEM as an R-1 function). The other is based on a more deliberate evaluation of the meaningful content of activated information in light of other memories and knowledge (tentatively identified in MEM as an R-2 function). Cingulectomy patients experience reality monitoring failures that appear to be the consequence of errors during the first type of process, produced by either unusually vivid mental experiences or disruption of R-1 judgment processes. Patients with frontal damage who confabulate experience reality monitoring failures that appear to be the consequence of errors during the second type of process, i.e., as a consequence of disruption of R-2 judgment processes. Finally, evidence from brain-damaged patients exhibiting confabulation is consistent in implicating the frontal lobes as critical for normal reality monitoring.

ACKNOWLEDGMENTS

This chapter was partially prepared while I was a Fellow at the Center for Advanced Study in the Behavioral Sciences (1987–1988). I am grateful for financial support provided by the John D. and Catherine T. MacArthur Foundation, Princeton University, and the National Science Foundation (grant BNS-8510633). I would also like to acknowledge the excellent assistance of Margaret Amara and Rosanne Torre from the CASBS library. Comments on an earlier draft from Carol Raye, Don Spence, and especially Carl Olson were extremely helpful in developing and clarifying various ideas.

REFERENCES

Alba, J. W., and Hasher, L. (1983). Is memory schematic? *Psychol. Bull.* 93:203–231.

Baddeley, A., and Wilson, B. (1986). Amnesia, autobiographical memory, and confabulation. In D. C. Rubin (ed.), *Autobiographical Memory.* New York: Cambridge University Press.

Barbizet, J. (1963). Defect of memorizing of hippocampal-mammillary origin: review. *J. Neurol. Neurosurg. Psychiatry* 26:127–135.

Bartlett, F. C. (1932). *Remembering.* Cambridge: Cambridge University Press.

Bentall, R. P. (1990). The illusion of reality: a review and integration of psychological research on hallucinations. *Psychol. Bull.* 107:82–95.

Berlyne, N. (1972). Confabulation. *Br. J. Psychiatry* 120:31–39.

Cermak, L. S. (1982). *Human Memory and Amnesia.* Hillsdale, NJ: Lawrence Erlbaum Associates.

Craik, F. I. M. (1986). A functional account of age differences in memory. In F. Klix and H. Hagendorf (eds.), *Human Memory and Cognitive Capabilities.* NY: Elsevier, pp. 409–422.

Damasio, A. R., Graff-Radford, N. R., Eslinger, P. J., Damasio, H., and Kassell, N. (1985). Amnesia following basal forebrain lesions. *Arch. Neurol.* 42:263–271.

Durso, F., and Johnson, M. K. (1980). The effects of orienting tasks on recognition, recall, and modality confusion of pictures and words. *J. Verbal Learn. Verbal Behav.* 19:416–429.

Eich, J. E. (1975). State-dependent accessibility of retrieval cues in the retention of a categorized list. *J. Verbal Learn. Verbal Behav.* 14:408–417.

Flavell, J. H. (1985). *Cognitive Development.* 2nd Ed. Englewood Cliffs, NJ: Prentice-Hall.

Foley, M. A., Johnson, M. K., and Raye, C. L. (1983). Age-related changes in confusions between memories for thoughts and memories for speech. *Child Dev.* 54:51–60.

Hasher, L., and Zacks, R. T. (1979). Automatic and effortful processes in memory. *J. Exp. Psychol.* 108:356–388.

Hasher, L., and Zacks, R. T. (1984). Automatic processing of fundamental information: the case of frequency of occurrence. *Am. Psychol.* 39:1372–1388.

Hasher, L., and Zacks, R. T. (1988). Working memory, comprehension, and aging: a review and a new view. In G. H. Bower (ed.), *The Psychology of Learning and Motivation: Advances in Research and Theory.* Vol. 22. New York: Academic Press, pp. 193–225.

Hashtroudi, S., and Parker, E. S. (1986). Acute alcohol amnesia: what is remembered and what is forgotten. In H. D. Cappell, F. B. Glaser, Y. Israel, et al. (eds.), *Research Advances in Alcohol and Drug Problems.* Vol. 9. New York: Plenum.

Hashtroudi, S., Johnson, M. K., and Chrosniak, L. D. (1989). Aging and source monitoring. *Psychol. Aging* 4:106–112.

Hashtroudi, S., Johnson, M. K., and Chrosniak, L. D. (1990). Aging and qualitative characteristics of memories for perceived and imagined complex events. *Psychol. and Aging.* 5:119–126.

Hirst, W., Johnson, M. K., Kim, J. K., Phelps, E. A., and Volpe, B. T. (1986). Recognition and recall in amnesics. *J. Exp. Psychol. [Learn. Mem. Cogn.]* 12:445–451.

Hirst, W., Johnson, M. K., Phelps, E. A., and Volpe, B. T. (1988). More on recognition and recall in amnesics. *J. Exp. Psychol. [Learn. Mem. Cogn.]* 14:758–762.

Jacoby, L. L., and Dallas, M. (1981). On the relationship between autobiographical memory and perceptual learning. *J. Exp. Psychol. Gen.* 110:306–340.

Johnson, M. K. (1977). What is being counted none the less? In I. M. Birnbaum and E. S. Parker (eds.), *Alcohol and Human Memory.* Hillsdale, NJ: Lawrence Erlbaum Associates, pp. 43–57.

Johnson, M. K. (1983). A multiple-entry, modular memory system. In G. H. Bower (ed.), *The Psychology of Learning and Motivation.* Vol. 17. New York: Academic Press, pp. 81–123.

Johnson, M. K. (1985). The origin of memories. In P. C. Kendall (ed.), *Advances in Cognitive-Behavioral Research and Therapy.* Vol. 4. New York: Academic Press, pp. 1–27.

Johnson, M. K. (1988a). Discriminating the origin of information. In T. F. Oltmanns and B. A. Maher (eds.), *Delusional Beliefs: Interdisciplinary Perspectives.* New York: Wiley, pp. 34–65.

Johnson, M. K. (1988b). Reality monitoring: an experimental phenomenological approach. *J. Exp. Psychol. [Gen.]* 117:390–394.

Johnson, M. K. (1989). Functional forms of human memory. In J. L. McGaugh, N. M. Weinberger, and G. Lynch (eds.), *Brain Organization and Memory: Cells, Systems and Circuits.* New York: Oxford University Press.

Johnson, M. K., Bransford, J. D., and Solomon, S. K. (1973). Memory for tacit implications of sentences. *J. Exp. Psychol.* 98:203–204.

Johnson, M. K., and Foley, M. A. (1984). Differentiating fact from fantasy: the reliability of children's memory. *J. Soc. Issues* 40:33–50.

Johnson, M. K., and Hirst, W. (in press). Processing subsystems of memory. In R. G. Lister and H. J. Weingartner (eds.), *Perspectives in Cognitive Neuroscience.* New York: Oxford University Press.

Johnson, M. K., and Kim, J. K. (1985). Recognition of pictures by alcoholic Korsakoff patients. *Bull. Psychonom. Soc.* 23:456–458.

Johnson, M. K., Peterson, M. A., Chua-Yap, E., and Rose, P. M. (1989). Frequency judgments and the problem of defining a perceptual event. *J. Exp. Psychol. [Learn. Mem. Cogn.]* 15:126–136.

Johnson, M. K., and Raye, C. L. (1981). Reality monitoring. *Psychol. Rev.* 88:67–85.

Johnson, M. K., Foley, M. A., and Leach, K. (1988a). The consequences for memory of imagining in another person's voice. *Mem. Cogn.* 16:337–342.

Johnson, M. K., Foley, M. A., Suengas, A. G., and Raye, C. L. (1988b). Phenomenal characteristics of memories for perceived and imagined autobiographical events. *J. Exp. Psychol. [Gen.]* 117:371–376.

Johnson, M. K., Kahan, T. L., and Raye, C. L. (1984). Dreams and reality monitoring. *J. Exp. Psychol. [Gen.]* 113:329–344.

Johnson, M. K., Kim, J. K., and Risse, G. (1985). Do alcoholic Korsakoff patients acquire affective reactions? *J. Exp. Psychol. [Learn. Mem. Cogn.]* 11:22–36.

Johnson, M. K., Raye, C. L., Wang, A. Y., and Taylor, T. H. (1979). Fact and fantasy: the roles of accuracy and variability in confusing imaginations with perceptual experiences. *J. Exp. Psychol.* [*Hum. Learn. Mem.*] 5:229–240.

Joseph, R. (1986). Confabulation and delusional denial: frontal lobe and lateralized influences. *J. Clin. Psychol.* 42:507–520.

Kerns, L. L. (1986). Falsifications in the psychiatric history: a differential diagnosis. *Psychiatry* 49:13–17.

Kopelman, M. D. (1987). Two types of confabulation. *J. Neurol. Neurosurg. Psychiatry* 50:1482–1487.

Kosslyn, S. M. (1980). *Image and Mind.* Cambridge, MA: Harvard University Press.

Lindsay, D. S., and Johnson, M. K. (1987). Reality monitoring and suggestibility: children's ability to discriminate among memories from different sources. In S. J. Ceci, M. P. Toglia, and D. F. Ross (eds.), *Children's Eyewitness Memory.* New York: Springer-Verlag, pp. 92–121.

Lindsay, D. S., and Johnson, M. K. (1989). The eyewitness suggestibility effect and memory for source. *Mem. Cogn.* 17:349–358.

Loftus, E. F. (1979). *Eyewitness Testimony.* Cambridge, MA: Harvard University Press.

Mercer, B., Wapner, W., Gardner, H., and Benson, D. F. (1977). A study of confabulation. *Arch. Neurol.* 34:429–433.

Miller, G. A., Galanter, E., and Pribram, K. A. (1960). *Plans and the Structure of Behavior.* New York: Holt, Rinehart & Winston.

Mitchell, D. B., Hunt, R. R., and Schmitt, F. A. (1986). The generation effect and reality monitoring: evidence from dementia and normal aging. *J. Gerontol.* 41:79–84.

Moscovitch, M. (1985). Memory from infancy to old age: implications for theories of normal and pathological memory. *Ann. N.Y. Acad. Sci.* 444:78–96.

Nelson, T. O., and Narens, L. (in press). Metamemory: A theoretical framework and some new findings. In G. H. Bower (ed.), *The Psychology of Learning and Motivation.*

Norman, D. A., and Shallice, T. (1986). Attention to action: willed and automatic control of behavior. In R. J. Davidson, G. E. Schwartz, and D. Shapiro (eds.), *Consciousness and Self-Regulation.* New York: Plenum, pp. 1–18.

Perky, C. W. (1910). An experimental study of imagination. *Am. J. Psychol.* 21:422–452.

Perlmutter, M. (1984). Continuities and discontinuities in early human memory paradigms, processes, and performance. In R. Kail and N. E. Spear (eds.), *Comparative Perspectives on the Development of Memory.* Hillsdale, NJ: Lawrence Erlbaum Associates, pp. 253–284.

Rabinowitz, J. C. (1989). Judgments of origin and generation effects: comparisons between young and elderly adults. *Psychol. Aging* 4:259–268.

Schacter, D. L., and Moscovitch, M. (1984). Infants, amnesics, and dissociable memory systems. In M. Moscovitch (ed.), *Infant Memory.* New York: Plenum Press, pp. 173–216.

Shapiro, B. E., Alexander, M. P., Gardner, H., and Mercer, B. (1981). Mechanisms of confabulation. *Neurology* 31:1070–1076.

Shiffrin, R. M., and Schneider, W. (1977). Controlled and automatic human information processing. II. Perceptual learning, automatic attending, and a general theory. *Psychol. Rev.* 84:127–190.

Slusher, M. P., and Anderson, C. A. (1987). When reality monitoring fails: the role of imagination in stereotype maintenance. *J. Pers. Soc. Psychol.* 52:653–662.

Stuss, D. T., and Benson, D. F. (1986). *The Frontal Lobes.* New York: Raven Press.

Stuss, D. T., Alexander, M. P., Lieberman, A., and Levine, H. (1978). An extraordinary form of confabulation. *Neurology* 28:1166–1172.

Suengas, A. G., and Johnson, M. K. (1988). Qualitative effects of rehearsal of memories for perceived and imagined complex events. *J. Exp. Psychol.* [*Gen.*] 117:377–389.

Talland, G. A. (1961). Confabulation in the Wernicke-Korsakoff syndrome. *J. Nerv. Ment. Dis.* 132:361–381.

Tzeng, O. J. L., and Cotton, B. (1980). A study-phase retrieval model of temporal coding. *J. Exp. Psychol.* [*Hum. Learn. Mem.*] 6:705–716.

Weinstein, A. (1987). Preserved recognition memory in amnesia. Unpublished doctoral dissertation, State University of New York at Stony Brook.

Weiskrantz, L. (1986). *Blindsight.* Oxford: Clarendon Press.

Whitlock, F. A. (1981). Some observation on the meaning of confabulation. *Br. J. Med. Psychol.* 54:213–218.

Whitty, C. W. M. (1966). Some early and transient changes in psychological function following anterior cingulectomy in man. *Int. J. Neurol.* 5:403–409.

Whitty, C. W. M., and Lewin, W. (1957). Vivid day-dreaming: an unusual form of confusion following anterior cingulectomy. *Brain* 80:72.

Whitty, C. W. M., and Lewin, W. (1960). A Korsakoff syndrome in the post-cingulectomy confusional state. *Brain* 83:648–653.

Wyke, M., and Warrington, E. (1960). An experimental analysis of confabulation in a case of Korsakoff's syndrome using a tachistoscopic method. *J. Neurol. Neurosurg. Psychiatry* 23:327–333.

11
Anosognosia, Consciousness, and the Self

JOHN F. KIHLSTROM
AND BETSY A. TOBIAS

Brain damage can lead to profound disruptions of mental function; amnesia, aphasia, agnosia, apraxia, and dementia are just a few of the syndromes produced by insult, injury, or disease of the brain (Heilman and Valenstein, 1985). Perhaps the most disturbing consequence, so far as the patient is concerned, is the sense of cognitive loss: that certain tasks, once routine and effortless, are now difficult or impossible. The actress Patricia Neal wrote in her autobiography (Neal, 1988):

> After a stroke, anger grows with awareness of what you have lost. The fog of unconsciousness that held you prisoner from the outside world was, in fact, a blessing in disguise. First you're like a soul with no body, but the soul is drugged. Then the soul awakens into a body you cannot command. You are a prisoner in a private hell.

Goldstein (1948), in his classic account of the psychological consequences of brain damage, made a similar point in his description of the "catastrophic reaction" in aphasic patients. Apparently, the patient's awareness of cognitive loss, of the fact that he or she cannot do things that were possible before, can precipitate episodes of profound dysphoria (for a review, see Heilman, Bowers, and Valenstein, 1985).

On the other hand, some patients suffer precisely the opposite problem: They do not seem to be aware of their cognitive and behavioral impairments. This phenomenon was originally noticed in cases of left-sided hemiplegia and hemianopia and was called *anosognosia* by Babinski (1914, 1918); it was drawn to the attention of modern workers by Weinstein and Kahn (1955) and later Bisiach (e.g., Bisiach, Vallar, Perani, et al., 1986). Anosognosia, the brain-damaged patient's failure to recognize or appreciate his deficits, raises interesting questions concerning subjective awareness of the mechanisms of consciousness.

The purpose of this chapter is to explore some of these concerns, mostly from a *non*neuropsychological point of view. The goal is to integrate the neuropsychological literature on anosognosia with other work in cognitive psychology that also bears on the nature of consciousness and the relations between conscious and nonconscious mental states (for related treatments of these issues, see Kihlstrom, 1984, 1987, 1989, 1990b).

ANOSOGNOSIA, DENIAL, AND INDIFFERENCE

Let us first comment on some definitional issues. As McGlynn and Schacter (1989) have indicated, terminology here is important, and there is good reason to try to draw some distinctions between anosognosia proper and the related symptoms of defensive denial and indifference (e.g., Weinstein and Kahn, 1955). *Anosognosia,* as defined by Babinski, is a deficit in awareness: The patient appears unaware of any problems in memory, language, perception, voluntary movement, or whatever. Evidence bearing on the claim of unawareness may come in various forms: (1) the person may simply not acknowledge that there is anything wrong; (2) the person may acknowledge some difficulty but attribute it to some source other than disease; or (3) the person may actively deny any difficulty at all.

Denial and Indifference

Denial, as an aspect of behavior, is particularly problematic (Weinstein and Kahn, 1955). One may attribute "denial" to a patient under a variety of circumstances. For example, a patient may merely answer the doctor's query in the negative, as in, "Patient denies alcohol abuse." Alternatively, the patient may fail to acknowledge something that the examiner knows to be true. This situation is closer to the phenomenon that concerns us, but it is still ambiguous as behavior. Thus such denial could reflect lack of awareness, but it could also reflect strategic self-presentation on the part of a patient who is fully cognizant of the problem.

Perhaps the term *defensive denial* should be reserved for those cases where the claim of unawareness appears to be motivated by self-presentational concerns, rather like repression. In this context, it is interesting to reflect on some of the manifestations of denial, broadly construed, anticipated by psychodynamic theory (A. Freud, 1936/1966; Sandler and Freud, 1985). As is well known, Sigmund Freud postulated a number of cognitive maneuvers employed by the ego to deflect, suppress, and disguise unacceptable sexual and aggressive impulses arising from the id. Although classical psychoanalytic theory held that these defense mechanisms served to reduce "neurotic" anxiety stemming from conflicts between instinctual demands and social constraints, there is no reason why similar defenses could not be deployed to reduce "reality" anxiety such as might be aroused by the neurological patient's awareness and acknowledgment of loss of function.

If the psychodynamic mechanism of denial operates in neurological patients, its expression might take a number of forms. We have no idea how often any of these forms of denial are actually observed, but certain possibilities seem intuitively likely. For example, *repression* might yield the characteristics of classic anosognosia: the patient's simple denial that he or she suffers any psychological deficit. Alternatively, the patient might engage in *rationalization,* acknowledging the problem but making reasonable-sounding, plausible excuses for it (e.g., "I'm too tired to move my arm"). On the other hand, a patient might employ a defense mechanism similar to *projection,* in which anxiety is reduced by attributing the deficit to others, instead of oneself. In pure projection, for example, the amnesic patient would attribute memory failure to others while denying it in him- or herself. With shared projection, the patient would acknowledge the deficit but also attribute it to others, as if to say that it is nothing unusual or any cause for concern (e.g., "Everybody forgets things"). With *displacement,* a patient may deny a deficit in one domain but claim a deficit in another, even fabricating a deficit for this purpose. We can even imagine defensive denial taking the form of *reaction formation,* in which the patient, far from acknowledging his or her deficit, claims superior functioning in that domain.

One of Freud's insights was that it is easier to repress something when we can acknowledge something else. For example, he noted that in most individuals autobiographical memory from birth to about 5 to 7 years of age was impoverished (Kihlstrom and Harackiewicz, 1982; Schacter and Kihlstrom, 1989), a phenomenon he attributed to the successful repression of affect-laden memories with the resolution of the Oedipus complex. He also acknowledged, however, that a few early childhood recollections stood out against this background of infantile and childhood amnesia. Freud (1899/1962, 1901/1960) called these surviving recollections "screen memories" and argued that they aided the repression of more threatening material by giving the person something to remember. In an analogous manner, it might occur that patients with multiple deficits acknowledge one—perhaps the least debilitating—while steadfastly denying the other(s).

Indifference is different from denial because it implies a lack of caring on the part of a patient who otherwise acknowledges his or her deficit; this reaction too may be defensive in nature, but at least the defense does not go as far as denial. Perhaps, as with the dementing syndromes, the patient is aware of the deficit but does not fully comprehend it or its significance for functioning. Janet (1901, 1907), of course, remarked on *la belle indifference* in cases of hysteria, now called dissociative or conversion disorder (Kihlstrom, 1984, 1990a): the patient's casual acceptance of, or indifference to, his or her symptom. In neurological cases, this phenomenon is often referred to as anosodiaphoria (Heilman et al., 1985). Although anosodiaphoria may be interesting as an expression of inappropriate or flat affect and may bear importantly on the pathophysiology of emotion, it does not raise the same questions about awareness that are our primary concern in this chapter.

Organic and Functional Anosognosia

The distinctions between unawareness, denial, and indifference are potentially important because they remind us that the term "anosognosia" itself is descriptively neutral. It means, simply, unawareness of deficits and thus carries no etiological connotations. Anosognosia might reflect brain damage, as is plausibly the case in the neurological cases reviewed by McGlynn and Schacter (1989). Thus lesions of the right parietal region have been implicated in anosognosia arising in cases of hemianopia and hemiplegia, whereas frontal lesions seem to be involved when amnesics are unaware of their memory deficits. McGlynn and Schacter suggested a Geschwind-like "disconnection" between a hypothetical cortical center mediating conscious awareness and some other, damaged brain site subserving the lost function.

There might be cases of *functional* anosognosia as well, i.e., cases where there is unawareness of deficits but no sign of the organic brain syndromes commonly associated with the symptom in aphasia (or whatever). One place to look for this problem is in schizophrenia (in making this suggestion there is no implication that schizophrenia is not a genetic-biochemical disorder—just that it does not involve frank insult, injury, or disease in the brain). To what extent are schizophrenics aware of their own symptoms, especially the negative symptoms (Andreason, 1982; Andreason and Olson, 1982), i.e., incoherence of speech, neologisms, loose and clang associations, poverty of speech and content, perseveration, blocking, flat, blunted, or inappropriate affect (for a review, see Chapter 6). Paranoid patients are certainly aware of these symptoms, and in fact there is reason to believe that their delusions stem from their attempts to explain their anomalous experiences (e.g., Kihlstrom and Hoyt, 1988). What about *non*paranoid patients? Do they commonly acknowledge their cognitive and behavioral deficits, so obvious to others? If not, to what extent does this failure reflect lack of awareness, denial, or indifference?

Another domain in which something similar to anosognosia may be seen is hypnosis. Hypnosis is a social interaction in which one person, designated the subject, responds to suggestions offered by another person, the hypnotist, for imaginative experiences involving alterations in perception, memory, or voluntary action (Kihlstrom, 1985a). In the classic case, these responses are accompanied by feelings of subjective conviction bordering on delusion (Kihlstrom and Hoyt, 1988) and of involuntariness bordering on compulsion (the "classic suggestion effect"; see Weitzenhoffer, 1974; K. S. Bowers, 1981; P. G. Bowers, 1982). Many of these suggestions involve perceptual-cognitive deficits that roughly parallel some of the symptoms of organic brain syndrome. For example, it may be suggested that the subject cannot see objects presented in his or her visual field, hear sounds that would otherwise be clearly audible, or feel even fairly intense tactile stimulation. Alternatively, it may be suggested that the subject does not remember, upon termination of hypnosis, the events and experiences that transpired while he or she was hypnotized (Kihlstrom, 1984).

Although to our knowledge there has never been a systematic study of the matter, we do occasionally observe something like anosognosia when subjects respond to such suggestions. For example, upon inquiry many (if not most) subjects with posthypnotic amnesia acknowledge some degree of memory deficit: they assert (or agree) that they did some things while they were hypnotized but state that they cannot remember the details. Some subjects, however, seem to be blithely unaware that they did anything at all: They may acknowledge the induction and termination procedures but nothing in between. The latter subjects appear to be unaware of their memory deficits, in much the same manner as patients with Korsakoff syndrome (for a review see Chapter 8). It is not known to what extent this difference simply reflects the degree of response to the amnesia suggestion: Perhaps our "anosognosic" subjects have simply forgotten that they have forgotten. However, the fact that something like anosognosia occurs with hypnosis, where there is no question of frontal or parietal lobe dysfunction, suggests that the syndrome can be functional as well as organic in nature.

Awareness and Disorientation

Setting aside the conceptual distinction between true anosognosia and defensive denial, and the possibility of functional as well as organic deficits in awareness, there are difficulties here as well. It is impressive that anosognosia commonly appears in the acute stage of neurological disorder and remits as the illness becomes chronic (McGlynn and Schacter, 1989). As we detail later, the possibility must be raised that these acute patients may not yet have had the kinds of exchanges with their environments that would allow them to become aware of their deficits. At an internal, cognitive level of analysis, however, the possibility must also be raised that the anosognosia observed in acute neurological syndromes is secondary to the patients' generalized confusion and disorientation. If a person does not know who he is, where he is, or what time it is, it may not be fair to expect him to know he is impaired.

There is apparently at least one counterexample to this generalization: When anosognosia appears in cases of Alzheimer's disease and other forms of dementia, it occurs relatively late, not early, in the course of the disease (see Chapter 6). This fact of natural history merely underscores the point, however, because it is at the late stages of illness that the Alzheimer patient shows the most disorientation and intellectual deterioration. It is not fair to expect such a patient to be aware of his or her deficits. The point, then, is that when diagnosing and studying anosognosia we must be careful to rule out such contaminating factors as insufficient environmental feedback and general clouding of consciousness. Anosognosia is most interesting when it reflects a specific disorder of awareness, rather than a secondary symptom of dementia, i.e., when the person's awareness of self and world is not otherwise impaired.

CONSCIOUSNESS AND THE COGNITIVE UNCONSCIOUS

At this point, we set aside explicitly neuropsychological issues and try to link the literature on anosognosia to a wider body of work on the nature of conscious awareness and the relations between conscious and nonconscious mental life that is emerging from contemporary cognitive psychology (see also Kihlstrom, 1984, 1987, 1989). As everyone knows, scientific psychology began as the study of consciousness. Wundt, Titchener, and others who founded the earliest psychological laboratories generally assumed that the mind is able to observe its own inner workings. Their research relied on the method of introspection by which trained observers attempted to analyze their own percepts, memories, and thoughts into elementary sensations, images, and feelings. This line of scientific inquiry on conscious mental life was interrupted by the radical behaviorism of Watson and his followers, who argued that consciousness was nonexistent, epiphenomenal, or irrelevant to behavior. One of the most salutary by-products of the "cognitive revolution" and the subsequent development of an interdisciplinary cognitive science has been a revival of interest in consciousness (Hilgard, 1977, 1980, 1987).

Only 20 years ago, a mere decade into the cognitive revolution, the dominant theory was Atkinson and Shiffrin's (1968) multistore model of memory, which was modeled after the modern high-speed computer. True to its name, the multistore model distinguished between three storage structures—sensory memory, primary (or short-term) memory, and secondary (or long-term) memory—and attempted to characterize the properties of these structures and the processes that transferred information between them. In the classic multistore model, consciousness was identified either with attention and rehearsal or with primary memory, the cognitive staging area that holds those percepts, memories, and actions to which attention is being directed.

A somewhat different perspective on conscious mental life is provided by more recent versions of information processing theory, such as Anderson's (1983) ACT*. ACT* assumes a single, unitary memory store, but it classifies the contents of memory into declarative knowledge structures that represent the individual's fund of general and specific factual information, including his or her knowledge of the current environment, and the procedural knowledge repertoire of skills, rules, and strategies that operate on declarative knowledge in the course of perception, memory, thought, and action. Consciousness is identified with working memory, which is similar to the primary memory of the classic model but with a much larger capacity. Working memory contains activated declarative representations of the organism in its current environment, currently active processing goals, and preexisting declarative knowledge structures activated by perceptual inputs or by the operations of various procedures.

This theory is fine as far as it goes, but even the nineteenth century psychologists had recognized that the mental structures and processes that underlie experience, thought, and action were not completely encompassed within the span of conscious awareness; i.e., consciousness is not all there is to the mind. For example, Helmholtz concluded that conscious perception was the product of unconscious inferences based on the individual's knowledge of the world and memories of past experience. Somewhat later, of course, Freud asserted that our conscious mental lives are determined by unconscious ideas, impulses, and emotions, as well as defense mechanisms unconsciously arrayed against them (see Whyte, 1960; Ellenberger, 1970; Bowers and Meichenbaum, 1984).

Perhaps the most forceful advocate of nonconscious mental life was William James (1890; see also Hilgard, 1969; Myers, 1986). This may at first seem paradoxical, because in Chapter 6 of the *Principles* James (1890) listed no fewer than ten refutations of "The Mind-Stuff Theory," which held that conscious experience is composed of elements that were themselves unconscious; he even went so far as to assert that the idea of "unconscious thought" was a contradiction in terms on the grounds of the doctrine of *esse est sentiri* (to be is to be sensed). However, in his later chapters (specifically those on The Relations of Minds to Other Things, The Stream of Thought, The Consciousness of Self, and Attention), James made it clear that mental states could be unconscious in at least two senses. First, a mental event can be excluded from attention or consciousness: "We can neglect to attend to that which we nevertheless feel" (1890, pp. 201 and 455–458). These unattended, unconscious feelings are themselves mental states. Second, and just as important, James drew on the clinical observations of cases of hysteria and multiple personality by Janet, Binet, and Prince, and himself to argue for a division of consciousness into primary and secondary (and, for that matter, tertiary and more) consciousnesses, only one of which is accessible to phenomenal awareness at any point in time. To avoid possible oxymoron in the negation of consciousness, James preferred to speak of "co-conscious" or "subconscious" mental states, rather than "unconscious" ones. Even so, the idea of the "cognitive unconscious" is here to stay (Kihlstrom, 1987, 1989), and we must live with some imprecision of speech.

We have more to say about James' ideas later, but for the present we wish to put him aside and return to our historical account. Of course, the radical behaviorists were no more interested in nonconscious than in conscious mental life, so empirical interest in the kinds of problems that interested Helmholtz and James, not to mention Freud, declined precipitously during the years after World War I. To the extent that the problem was kept alive, it was principally through the efforts of the psychoanalytic ego psychologists such as Klein and Rapaport, who tried to integrate psychoanalysis with clinical psychology, and Jerome Bruner and his kindred souls, who fostered the development of the "New Look" in perception (for a review, see Hilgard, 1987; Kihlstrom, 1990b). Serious theoretical interest in nonconscious mental life, however, again had to await the triumph of the cognitive revolution.

Consider once again the classic multistore model of memory of Atkinson and Shiffrin. By implicitly making consciousness coterminous with attention and primary memory, the multistore model seems to identify nonconscious mental life with early, "preattentive" mental processes, e.g., feature detection and pattern recognition, that occur prior to the formation of a mental representation of an event in primary memory. The implication of this view is that unattended percepts and unretrieved memories make no contact with higher mental processes and thus cannot influence conscious experience, thought, and action. In other words, the classic multistore model of human information processing, by regarding attention and rehearsal as prerequisites for a full-fledged cognitive analysis of an event and implicitly identifying consciousness with higher mental processes, leaves little or no room for the *psychological unconscious*—mental structures and processes that influence experience, thought, and action but that are nevertheless inaccessible to phenomenal awareness.

A rather different perspective on nonconscious mental life is provided by Anderson's (1983) ACT* model of the architecture of cognition. ACT* holds that people can become aware of declarative knowledge (about themselves, their environments and processing goals, and other relevant information), and that this awareness depends on the amount of activation possessed by the representations in question. However, it also holds that procedural knowledge is not available to introspection under any circumstances. Thus procedural knowledge appears to be unconscious in the strict sense of the term. Because unconscious procedural knowledge is the cognitive basis for all higher thought processes, ACT* and similar revisionist models afford a much wider scope for the cognitive unconscious than did the classic statements.

An even larger place for nonconscious mental structures and processes has been created by a variant on information-processing theory known as connectionism or parallel distributed processing (PDP) (McClelland, Rummelhart, and PDP Research Group, 1986; Rummelhart, McClelland, and PDP Research Group, 1986). Whereas ACT* and similar models assume the existence of a single central processing unit (e.g., primary or working memory), PDP models postulate the existence of a large number of processing units, or modules, each devoted to a specific task. PDP models assume that information about an object or event is distributed widely across the processing system, rather than localized in any particular unit. Moreover, the activation of individual processing units can vary continuously rather than discretely. For these reasons it is not necessary for an object to be fully represented in consciousness before information about it can influence experience, thought, and action. In addition, traditional information-processing theories tend to assume that various perceptual-cognitive functions are bound together in a unitary processing system operating under a single set of rules and under the control of a central executive. By contrast, PDP models assume that various systems (e.g., those supporting perception and language) operate independently and under different rules. Only some modules are assumed to be accessible to awareness and subject to voluntary control.

Finally, PDP models abandon the traditional assumption that information is processed in a sequence of stages. Parallel processing permits a large number of activated units to influence each other at any particular moment in time, so that information can be analyzed rapidly. The number of simultaneously active processing units and the speed at which they pass information among themselves may exceed the span of conscious awareness. In contrast to multistore information processing theories that restrict the cognitive unconscious to elementary sensory-perceptual operations, PDP models seem to consider almost all information processing, including the higher mental functions involved in language, memory, and thought, to be unconscious.

Automatic Processing

Theories aside, there is no doubt that a good deal of mental activity is unconscious in the strict sense of being inaccessible to phenomenal awareness under any circumstances. In conversational speech, for example, the listener is aware of the meanings of the words uttered by the speaker but not of the phonological and linguistic principles by which the meaning of the speaker's utterance is decoded. Similarly, during perception the viewer may be aware of two objects in the external environment but not of the mental calculations performed to determine that one is closer or larger than the other. Unconscious procedural knowledge of this sort appears to be innate. However, other cognitive procedures appear to be acquired through experience. A great deal of evidence now indicates that cognitive and motoric skills that are not innate may become routinized through practice and their operations thereby rendered unconscious. Employing a metaphor derived from computer science, this process is described as knowledge compilation, suggesting that the format in which the knowledge is represented has been changed (Anderson, 1982). In this way, both innate and acquired cognitive procedures may be unconscious in the strict sense of the term.

Unconscious procedural knowledge has also been described as automatic rather than controlled or effortful (for reviews, see Kahneman and Triesman, 1984; Shiffrin and Schneider, 1984). Automatic processes are so named because they are inevitably engaged by the presentation of specific stimulus inputs, regardless of any intention on the part of the subject. In addition, automatic processes consume little or no attentional resource. It is a fundamental premise of cognitive psychology that the amount of attention that can be allocated to various activities is limited, producing a bottleneck in information processing. Thus our ability to perform two or more tasks simultaneously is limited by the demands they make on available attentional resources. If attentional demands exceed attentional resources, the tasks interfere with each other. Nevertheless, routinized processes consume little or no attentional capacity. For this reason, it is possible for expert typists to carry on a conversation while transcribing even complicated material or for skilled drivers to negotiate the road while listening to the radio news.

Automaticity is important because it permits a great deal of complex cognitive activity to go on outside of conscious awareness. However, automatization can have negative consequences for conscious awareness (Spelke, Hirst, and Neisser, 1976). In the first place, automaticity may render us unable to describe our skills to others. Just try to get an old salt to teach you how to tie a sailor's knot or an accomplished pianist how to play an arpeggio. Moreover, as golfers and tennis players know, too much attention paid to an automatized skill can actually interfere with its execution. Finally, automatic processes may not leave accessible traces of themselves in memory. Skilled typists often have difficulty describing texts they have transcribed, and skilled drivers may have poor memory for details of their journeys over familiar stretches of road.

Implicit Perception, Memory, and Thought

Although the procedural knowledge structures that guide thought and action are unconscious, the declarative knowledge structures on which they operate are ordinarily thought to be accessible to conscious awareness. Thus we generally assume that people notice and can describe the salient features of an object or event, even if they cannot articulate the way in which those features have been integrated to form certain judgments made about it. However, another implication of automatization is that the processes in question may operate on declarative knowledge structures that are not themselves fully conscious. This point raises the question of subliminal perception: the possibility that stimuli that are not consciously detected nonetheless have an impact on perceptual and cognitive functioning.

Ever since the first demonstration of subliminal perception by Peirce and Jastrow (1884), a variety of methodological critiques have sought to demonstrate that stimuli cannot be analyzed for meaning unless they have been consciously identified and attended to (for a review, see Holender, 1986). However, a number of compelling demonstrations of preconscious processing have now appeared in the literature. For example, Marcel (1983a,b) employed a lexical decision task in which one stimulus word (the prime) is followed by another word (the target), and the subject has to decide if the target is a meaningful word. It is well known that such judgments are facilitated when the prime is also a word and especially when the prime and target are from the same taxonomic category; but most of these demonstrations have involved primes that were consciously detectable by the subject. Marcel arranged to present the prime followed by a second stimulus (called the mask) consisting of randomly arranged letters, before the target appeared. The interval between prime and mask was short, with the result that subjects were unable to reliably detect masked primes. Nevertheless, such primes facilitated performance on the lexical decision task. Because lexical decisions obviously require some degree of semantic processing, it appears that meaning analyses are performed on stimuli that are themselves outside of conscious awareness.

Because preconscious processing appears to be mediated by the activation of relevant mental representations already stored in memory, the question is raised whether analogous effects may be observed in memory itself. That is, just as there are palpable effects on experience, thought, and action of events that cannot be consciously perceived, there may be similar effects of events that cannot be consciously remembered. An early demonstration of the effects of consciously inaccessible memories was provided by Nelson (1978), whose subjects showed significant savings in relearning paired-associates that they were unable to recall or even recognize from a previous learning experience. Other demonstrations have made use of repetition priming effects in which the processing of an item is facilitated by the fact that it had been encountered previously. Similarly, studies of priming in tests involving lexical decision or word identification (e.g., Jacoby and Dallas, 1981) or word-fragment completion (e.g., Tulving, Schacter, and Stark, 1982) have shown that the magnitude of the priming effect is independent of the subject's ability to recognize the item as having been presented in a previous study session (see Schacter, 1987, for a review).

Relearning and priming effects such as the ones just described show that task performance may be affected by available memories of prior experiences, even though those experiences are not accessible to conscious recall. On the basis of such results, Schacter (1987) has drawn a distinction between explicit and implicit memory. Explicit memory involves the conscious reexperiencing of some aspect of the past, whereas implicit memory is revealed by a change in task performance that is attributable to information acquired during a prior episode. An increasing amount of literature derived from reports on both patient and nonpatient populations indicates that people can display implicit memory without having any conscious recollection of the experiential basis of the effect.

Implicit memory effects are conceptually similar to subliminal perception effects, in that both reveal the impact on experience, thought, and action of events that are not accessible to conscious awareness. The term "implicit" perception might be offered as an alternative to "subliminal" perception in an attempt to get away from the unfortunate psychophysical implications of the concept of the *limen*. However, in contrast to implicit perception, the events contributing to implicit memory effects were clearly detectable by the subject at the time they occurred, attention was devoted to them, and they were represented in phenomenal awareness at the time. Arguably, implicit memory should be reserved for those situations where a consciously perceived event is subsequently lost to conscious recollection, leaving implicit perception for instances where stimulus information in the current (or immediately past) environment affects ongoing experience, thought, and action. Because memory is the residual trace of perceptual activity, it stands to reason that implicit percepts can reveal themselves in memory, even if it should turn out that implicit percepts produce only implicit memories. Still, both sets of phenomena illustrate the cognitive unconscious by showing perception and memory outside of phenomenal awareness.

Implicit perception and memory do not exhaust the domain of the psychological unconscious because it appears we can also have implicit *thought*. Consider one of the more interesting and controversial phenomena of problem-solving: "incubation." Subjects are asked to work on a difficult problem: If they fail to achieve the correct solution within a specified period of time, they are given something else to do. Later, when they are confronted again with the original, as-yet unsolved problem, they arrive at the solution fairly readily. Sometimes the solution appears spontaneously, even after the person has consciously abandoned the problem. Sometimes the solution appears in the person's dreams, although the most famous example of problem-solving in dreams, Kekule's discovery of the structure of the benzine molecule, may have been a fabrication (Browne, 1988). One interpretation of incubation is that the person continues to work on the problem subconsciously, after consciously setting the problem aside, and then finds the problem solved or at least considerable progress made when attention is subsequently returned to it.

Although this interpretation of incubation is as controversial as the phenomenon itself, some experiments by Bowers (1984, 1987) and his associates are important. In these experiments, subjects are presented with word triads patterned after those of the Remote Associates Test and are instructed to think of a concept they have in common. A classic example is as follows.[1]

Democrat
Girl
Favor

Two others[2] are shown below, the first semantically convergent (where the meaning of the target word does not change from element to element within the triad)

---

[1] The uniting concept is *party*.
[2] The uniting concepts are *mountain* and *match,* respectively.

and the second semantically divergent (where different senses of the target word must be employed to solve the problem).

Goat	Strike
Pass	Same
Green	Tennis

The trick in Bowers' experiments is that some of the triads are soluble, meaning that there really is some concept, however remote, that unites the individual words. Other triads are insoluble, however, meaning that there is no such uniting concept, except in the minds of subjects with psychotically loose associations. Bowers presented subjects with both kinds of triads simultaneously and asked his subjects to indicate which is which. An example is provided below.[3]

Triad A	*Triad B*
Playing	Still
Credit	Pages
Report	Music

Bowers found that subjects can do this task with some degree of accuracy, even though they have not achieved the solution to the soluble triad. They seem to be responding to some vague "feeling of knowing" analogous to that observed with episodic and semantic memory. The point is that the correct solution influences the subjects' behavior, even though they are not consciously aware of it, in much the same manner as does implicit perception and memory.

So these three reference experiments provide evidence for three aspects of the cognitive unconscious. In Schacter's (1987) work, there is implicit memory: a change in task performance attributable to some past event but in the absence of conscious recollection of that event. In Bowers' (1984, 1987) studies, there is implicit thought: reflections in behavior of problem-solving activity outside phenomenal awareness. In Marcel's (1983a,b) work, there is implicit perception: a change in task performance attributable to some *current* event but in the absence of conscious perception of that event. Note that these sorts of implicit cognition effects are produced under conditions that might be described as *degraded:* stimulus presentations that are too brief to be consciously perceived; encoding conditions, or retention intervals, that produce memories too weak (in some sense) to be retrieved; problems that are too difficult to be solved except by crossword mavens.

Implicit Cognition in Clinical Syndromes and Special States

In other cases, the problem is not in the task environment imposed on the subjects but, rather, with the subjects themselves. For example, some of the most dramatic demonstrations of implicit memory effects come from studies by Schacter (1987) and his associates, among others, on cases of the amnesic syndrome resulting from bilateral damage to the medial temporal lobe (including

[3]Triad A is soluble, and the uniting concept is *card.*

the hippocampus) and diencephalon (including the mamillary bodies). These patients display a gross anterograde amnesia, meaning that they cannot remember events that occurred since the onset of the brain damage; other intellectual functions remain relatively intact. When such patients are asked to study a list of familiar words and to recall them shortly thereafter, they show gross impairments in memory compared to controls. Different results are obtained, however, when the subjects are asked to identify briefly presented words or to complete a word stem or other fragment with a meaningful word. Not surprisingly, intact subjects show superior performance on trials where the correct response is a word that had appeared on the previously studied list compared to those where the correct response is an entirely new word. This advantage of old over new items reflects a sort of priming effect of the previous learning experience. However, amnesic subjects also show normal levels of priming, despite the fact that they cannot remember the words they studied.

Although the available evidence is somewhat controversial, some phenomena analogous to implicit cognition appear to be observed in a variety of other neuropsychological syndromes as well. For example, Weiskrantz (1980) and his colleagues (Weiskrantz, Warrington, Sanders, and Marshall, 1974) have reported a patient, D.B., who had extensive damage to the striate cortex of the occipital lobes. Although the patient reported an inability to see, he was nonetheless able to respond appropriately to some visual stimuli, a phenomenon called *blindsight* (for a review, see Campion, Latto, and Smith, 1983). Similar phenomena have been obtained in other patients. Thus blindsight involves a behavioral response to objects and events of which the person is apparently unaware—a dissociation of visually guided behavior from visual awareness analogous to the implicit perception that occurs with briefly presented stimuli. Similarly, patients with bilateral lesions to the mesial portions of the occipital and temporal cortex are unable to recognize previously encountered faces as familiar, a condition known as *prosopagnosia*. Nevertheless, there are now several reports indicating that prosopagnosic patients show differential behavioral responses to old and new faces (e.g., Tranel and Damasio, 1985; deHaan, Young, and Newcombe, 1987), a dissociation similar to the implicit memory seen in the amnesic syndrome.

Even in the absence of demonstrable brain insult, injury, or disease, conceptually similar effects have been reported with conversion hysteria, functional amnesia and fugue, and multiple personality (for review, see Hilgard, 1977; Kihlstrom, 1984, 1985b). For example, Hilgard (cited in Hilgard and Marquis, 1940) found that a patient with functional anesthesia and paralysis could acquire a conditional finger-withdrawal response in the affected arm, and Brady and Lind (1961) showed that a functionally blind patient nonetheless displayed discriminative responses to visual stimulation. In the domain of learning and memory, experiments by Ludwig and his colleagues (Ludwig, Brandsma, Wilbur, et al., 1972) on a case of multiple personality found some transfer of learning among alter egos, despite the patient's apparent lack of awareness of their experiences.

Setting aside the neurological and psychiatric syndromes, even normal subjects who are asleep (Evans, 1979b), anesthetized for surgery (Kihlstrom and Schacter, 1989), or hypnotized (Kihlstrom, 1984, 1985) can give evidence of perception, memory, and thought outside of awareness. Consider an experiment by Kihlstrom (1980) that was originally construed as bearing on the episodic-semantic distinction in memory. The subjects memorized a list of 15 unrelated words to a strict criterion of learning and then received a suggestion that they would not be able to remember the words they had learned. On an initial test of recall, the hypnotic virtuosos displayed dense posthypnotic amnesia, remembering virtually none of the words they had previously memorized. At this point the subjects were asked to give word associations to various probes: half of them, called critical stimuli, were selected because they had a high a priori probability of eliciting the items from the previously memorized word list; the remaining, neutral stimuli targeted items the subjects had not learned. The most important finding was that the subjects were more likely to give the targeted response to critical than to neutral stimuli. This response represents a kind of priming effect of the earlier learning experience on the word-association task. However, equal amounts of priming were observed in the densely amnesic virtuoso subjects and their nonsusceptible, nonamnesic counterparts.

What we see in these priming results is an effect of episodic memory for a prior experience on subjects' performance on a semantic memory task, despite the fact that the subjects cannot remember the experience that is the source of the priming effect. In other words, the hypnotic subjects displayed implicit memory for their earlier experience, just as amnesic patients do. There is a big difference, however: Amnesic patients have not encoded these memories particularly well, as evidenced by the fact that there are no known circumstances under which they can display explicit memory for them. By contrast, posthypnotically amnesic subjects are able to recall their experiences perfectly after administration of prearranged reversibility cues. Thus for hypnotic subjects the episodic memories remain available for conscious retrieval by virtue of having been adequately encoded at the outset, even if they are temporarily inaccessible.

TOWARD A TAXONOMY OF CONSCIOUSNESS

The clinical and experimental studies described above, conducted in a wide variety of domains and with many types of subject, seem to lead to two general conclusions. First, consciousness is not to be identified with any particular perceptual-cognitive functions such as discriminative response to stimulation, perception, memory, or the higher mental processes involved in judgment or problem-solving. All of these functions can proceed outside of phenomenal awareness. Rather, consciousness is an experiential quality that may accompany any of these functions. The fact of conscious awareness may have particular consequences for psychological function: It seems necessary for voluntary control, for example, as well as for communicating one's mental states to others and for sponsored teaching. It is not necessary, however, for many forms of complex psychological functioning. Second, they lead to a provisional taxonomy of nonconscious mental structures and processes constituting the domain of the cognitive unconscious:

> Unconscious (Proper)
> Preconscious
> Subconscious

There are, within the domain of procedural knowledge, a number of complex processes that are inaccessible to introspection, in principle, under any circumstances. By virtue of routinization (or perhaps because they are innate), such procedures operate on declarative knowledge without conscious intent or conscious awareness in order to construct the person's ongoing experience, thought, and action. Execution of these mental processes, which can be known only indirectly, through inference, is inevitable and consumes no attentional capacity. They may be described as unconscious in the strict sense of that term; in short, they comprise the *unconscious proper*.

In principle, declarative knowledge is available to phenomenal awareness and can be known directly through introspection or retrospection. Traditional information-processing analyses seem to imply that conscious access to declarative knowledge is a matter of activation. If a knowledge structure is activated above some threshold, it is conscious; if not, it is not. There is the further implication that declarative knowledge structures activated at subthreshold levels are essentially latent. However, it is now clear that procedural knowledge can interact with and utilize declarative knowledge that is not itself accessible to conscious awareness. The phenomena of implicit perception and memory, then, suggest a category of *preconscious* declarative knowledge structures. Unlike automatized procedural knowledge, these percepts and memories would be available to awareness under ordinary circumstances. Although activated to some degree by current or prior perceptual inputs and thus able to influence ongoing experience, thought, and action, they do not cross the threshold required for representation in working memory and thus for conscious awareness. These representations, which underlie the phenomena of implicit perception and memory, may be classified as preconscious, implying that, in contrast to unconscious procedural knowledge, these mental representations reside on the fringes of consciousness, and changed circumstances could render them consciously accessible, at least in principle.

In addition to unconscious cognitive procedures operating on declarative representations and preconscious declarative representations that serve as sources of spreading activation, the phenomena of hypnosis and related states seem to exemplify a category of *subconscious* declarative knowledge. These mental representations—fully activated by perceptual inputs or acts of thought above the threshold ordinarily required for representation in working memory and available to introspection and retrospection under some circumstances— seem nevertheless inaccessible to phenomenal awareness.

During the nineteenth century, Janet described such structures as dissociated from conscious awareness, and more recently Hilgard (1977) revived these ideas in the form of his neodissociation theory of divided consciousness. Dissociative phenomena are of theoretical interest because they do not comfortably classify as either unconscious or preconscious. They are not limited to innate or routinized procedural knowledge, their execution is not automatic, and it consumes cognitive capacity. The stimulus input has not been degraded in any way, and the resulting memory traces are fully encoded and available for explicit retrieval. From the point of view of activation notions of consciousness, these phenomena are theoretically interesting because they indicate that high levels of activation, supported by the active deployment of attention and complex mental processing, although presumably necessary for residence in working memory, are not sufficient for conscious awareness.

ANOSOGNOSIA, CONSCIOUSNESS, AND THE SELF

So what exactly *is* required for conscious awareness? Kihlstrom (1984, 1987) holds that conscious awareness requires that a mental representation of an event be connected with some mental representation of the self as agent or experiencer—an idea derived from William James. In his discussion of the stream of consciousness, James wrote that "the first fact for . . . psychologists is that thinking of some sort goes on." He also wrote, immediately thereafter, that "thought tends to personal form," i.e., that every thought (by which James meant every conscious mental state) is part of a personal consciousness: The universal conscious fact is not "feelings exist" or "thoughts exist" but "I think" and "I feel."

In other words, an episode of ongoing experience, thought, and action becomes conscious if, and only if, a link is made between the mental representation of the event itself and some mental representation of the self as the agent or experiencer of that event. This mental representation of self resides in working memory, as a memory structure, along with coexisting representations of the current external environment (Anderson, 1983; Kihlstrom and Cantor, 1984; Kihlstrom, Cantor, Albright, et al., 1988). Both self and context representations are necessary for construction of a full-fledged conscious perception, which according to James always takes the following form: "*I see* (or hear, smell, taste, etc.) *this, now.* Because memory is the residual trace of perceptual activity, these elements are necessary for reconstruction of a full-fledged conscious recollection as well.

Consider the following variations on Anderson's (1983) famous sentence, *The hippie touched the debutante.*

1. I saw the hippie touch the debutante in the park on Thursday.
2. I was the hippie who touched the debutante in the park on Thursday.
3. I was the debutante whom the hippie touched in the park on Thursday.

In each case we have a proposition representing the raw description of a particular event, a hippie touching a debutante; it is linked to a proposition representing the self as the agent or experiencer of this event and a further proposition (or two, depending on how you count) representing the context in which the event took place.

In a generic associative theory of knowledge representation, this entire episodic memory would be represented by one node connecting three others: the event node, the context node, and the self node. Conscious recollection of such an event occurs only when the representation of the self is retrieved along with some other information about the event. The inability to retrieve the links among all three types of propositions accounts for some of the peculiarities in conscious memory (Reed, 1988).

Two personal anecdotes from the life of one of us (J.F.K.) may help make the point.

> *1. A simple memory failure.* I remember that I once saw a new Woody Allen movie in the company of my former student Judith Harackiewicz and her husband Cliff Thurber. It was opening night, the midnight show, at the Beeckman Theatre in Manhattan; we sat in the balcony, and afterward we took the bus up Broadway back to their apartment. This event is a vivid personal recollection, confirmed by Judy and Cliff, but I do not remember the title of the movie, nor can I recollect any particular scene that I viewed that night. With Judy's aid (she keeps a diary of all the movies she has ever seen, at least since graduate school) I have been able to narrow it down to either *A Midsummer Night's Sex Comedy* (1982) or *Zelig* (1983). Maybe I fell asleep, which I have been known to do at movies, but I do not think so because I remember individual scenes from both films clearly, without benefit of subsequent videotape replays. I simply cannot say which film I saw that night.

> *2. A case of déjà vu.* In July 1976, while attending a hypnotists' convention, I visited the Philadelphia Museum of Art with Kenneth and Patricia Bowers to view an exhibit of American painting and sculpture on the occasion of the Bicentennial of the American Revolution. While standing in one of the basement galleries I had the strong impression that I had been there before. Of course, I *had* been in that room many times before, during the 5 years I had lived in Philadelphia as a graduate student. But my feeling was that this *particular* room, with this particular exhibit in place, was familiar. It was not until more than a year later, sitting in the Stanford medical library (in fact, preparing a lecture on déjà vu), that I remembered that in fact I *had* seen the Bicentennial exhibit the previous May, when I had attended a wedding out on the Main Line. I was aware of this fact even in July because I had encouraged Ken and Pat to see the exhibit on the basis of my previous visit. The recollection was not false at all but, rather, one whose source I failed to remember.

In both cases there is an explicit, conscious, episodic memory based on the retrieval of only partial information: in the first instance about self and context, and in the second about self and event. The point is that a conscious recollection is possible without the information represented by the context or event nodes, one or the other; but it is inconceivable without the information represented by the self node.

Thus in consciousness a connection is made between the mental representation of an event and the mental representation of the self as agent or experiencer of that event. In conscious experience, thought, and action the mental representation of self is explicitly connected to whatever is being experienced, thought, or done. This procedure makes the person a part of the event that he or she is perceiving, remembering, or thinking about. In consciousness, everything rises or falls on the link to the self.

What unites the various phenomena of the cognitive unconscious—automatic processing and the various forms of implicit perception, memory, and thought—is that the link to self either does not become forged in the first place or it is subsequently lost. With some disorders of consciousness the link between the fact node and the context node(s) also fails, but that is of secondary importance. Thus automatized procedural knowledge is executed without being represented in working memory at all, although its goals and the conditions of action presumably are (or may be). Hence, so far as the procedure itself is concerned, there is not even the possibility of a link to the self. Procedural knowledge is unconscious, in the proper sense of the word, because it is impossible to make the link to the self under any circumstances.

Preconscious processing concerns declarative rather than procedural knowledge, and thus the link to the self is possible at least in principle. In the usual case of implicit perception, however, in which stimuli are presented for brief periods of time, it may be that the event is never represented in working memory at all—perhaps because attention is focused elsewhere, not enough time is afforded to focus attention on the item, or not enough activation has been built up before the stimulus disappears. In the amnesic syndrome the stimuli are represented in working memory all right, but a permanent link to the self nevertheless fails to be encoded in a manner that supports its later retrieval, perhaps because of damage to certain brain structures. With subconscious processing, the stimulus information is not degraded in any way and is subject to substantial cognitive processing, but it nonetheless fails to make a proper link to the self. Preconscious and subconscious percepts, memories, and thoughts can have effects on ongoing experience, thought, and action, depending on the amount of processing they have received at the time of encoding, but these effects are not accompanied by the phenomenal experience of conscious thought, in James's (1890) sense, because that experience requires links to the mental representation of the self.

A Mechanism for Awareness of Deficits

How can we conceptualize unawareness of deficits in terms of the information-processing models described earlier? It is relatively easy to talk about perception or memory without awareness. The blindsight patient is unaware of visual forms, the prosopagnosic patient is unaware that certain faces are familiar, and the amnesic patient is unaware that certain events have occurred, even though at some level he or she processes the relevant percepts and memories. To account for this state of affairs, all one has to do is assume that complex mental processing can occur in the absence of a link in working memory between the mental representation of some object or event and a mental representation of the self. Thus Claparede (1911/1951) wrote of the amnesic syndrome:

> If one examines the behavior of such a patient, one finds that everything happens as though the various events of life, however well associated with each *other* in the mind, were incapable of integration with the *me* itself. [p. 71, emphasis in original]

It is somewhat more difficult to conceptualize *unawareness of deficits,* in contrast to deficits of awareness. Hemianopic patients with anosognosia are not unaware of seeing; rather, they are unaware of *not* seeing. Similarly, patients who are anosognosic for their amnesia are unaware of *not* remembering; those who are anosognosic for their aphasia are unaware of *not* communicating (see Chapter 3); and those who are anosognosic for their hemiplegia are unaware of *not* moving. What seems to escape the awareness of anosognosic patients is the discrepancy between their expectations and intentions on the one hand and their actual cognitive-behavioral performance on the other. The anosognosic patient does not consciously appreciate the discrepancy between what *should be,* in terms of cognition and behavior, and what *is.*

How do we then become aware of our deficits when we have them? It seems that there are two sources of information available to us. First, there is feedback from the environment: the dismayed expressions on the faces of observers when we make an error, the tone of voice in the examiner who repeats a request we have failed to carry out satisfactorily. Second, there is feedback from ourselves, a mismatch between what we intend and what actually happens; alternatively, there is a mismatch between what we can do or experience now and what we could do or experience in the past.

We assume that anosognosia is not merely a matter of poor interpersonal communication. Nevertheless, from a social-psychological point of view, aspects of the interpersonal context may contaminate some diagnoses. Consider, first, the frequent failure of physicians and other medical personnel to give patients adequate feedback about their examinations. When we conduct a mental status examination, an aphasia battery, or an IQ test, we are trained to behave in an impersonal, nonjudgmental, objective fashion, which effectively forbids us from telling the patient that he or she has made an error in performance. If we do not tell them, how are they ever going to find out? Maybe from other people, but that is not likely in fact. Common courtesy prevents us from pointing out others' errors to them: Consider the anguish we go through before we tell someone that his nose is running, or he has egg on his beard, or that her lipstick is smeared. Such a dilemma poses a test of true friendship. Rather than say a word, we usually try to behave as if nothing at all is wrong and passively allow the person to humiliate himself.

Therefore if even our best friends do not tell us, how are we to find out? The answer, of course, is by monitoring ourselves. In anosognosia the problem is really one of self-perception or, as Johnson (Johnson and Raye, 1981; see also Chapter 10) would put it, of reality monitoring and metacognition. How would you know you were blind? If you had never been able to see, it would be only after someone else pointed out your deficiency to you. However, if you had been able to see once, you would immediately notice the discrepancy between what happens now when you open your eyes and look around and what used to happen. You know you are amnesic when you recognize a gap between what you do remember and what you know you ought to be able to remember. You know you are aphasic when you recognize the difference between what you intend to say and what actually is articulated. Awareness of such discrepancies is the cognitive, in contrast to the environmental, basis of anosognosia.

The situation is somewhat reminiscent of the Test–Operate–Test–Exit (TOTE) mechanism of Miller, Galanter, and Pribram (1960) or, in more contemporary terms, the production system apparatus of Newell and Simon (1972;

see also Anderson, 1983). In the TOTE system, "action is initiated by an 'incongruity' between the state of the organism and the state that is being tested for" (Miller et al., 1960, pp. 25–26). In a production system architecture, a procedure is executed when there is a discrepancy between a representation of the present conditions and some goal state. It is the conscious recognition of such incongruities and discrepancies that is the basis of awareness of deficits. When we open our eyes, we expect to see something, unless we know it is pitch dark; when we do not see something, even though there is adequate light to support vision, we may begin to think that something has happened to our eyes. When we intend to move our limbs, we expect to see (or feel) them move; and when they do not, we know something is wrong. [In *Kings Row* (1942), the character played by Ronald Reagan discovers that his legs have been amputated and cries, "Where's the rest of me?"] When we try to remember, it is usually because metamemory processes have already indicated that the attempt might be successful—that we ought to be able to recollect the fact or event; and when we recognize failure, in the face of our knowledge (or belief) that we ought to succeed, we begin to suspect we are losing our minds.

Implicit Cognition of Deficits

If anosognosics fail to show conscious awareness of their deficits, do they show *implicit* appreciation of them? Anosognosia, as described, is a phenomenon of explicit cognition: The patient's cognitive-behavioral deficits are not represented in his or her phenomenal awareness. However, as we have seen in cases of implicit perception, memory, and thought, just because something is not registered in awareness does not mean that it is not registered at all or that it cannot influence ongoing experience, thought, and action outside awareness. Therefore the question is whether anosognosic patients might not show changes in task performance that are attributable to the registration of their deficits at some nonconscious level. As McGlynn and Schacter (1989; see also Weinstein, Cole, Mitchell, and Lyerly, 1964) have noted, certain aspects of the routine behavior of anosognosic patients indicate that they do appreciate their deficits at some level of awareness. Thus a patient who denies any psychological deficit may nonetheless remain in bed or otherwise enact the patient role.

For example, Bandura (1977, 1986) has argued that a person's behavior is, in part, determined by his or her belief that he or she can successfully meet the requirements of some situation. In a number of experiments, Bandura and his colleagues have shown that people's confidence that they can execute some behavior is a highly accurate predictor of their actual performance. Decisions involving the choice of situations and the activities to take place within them, the amount of effort and persistence to be devoted to a task, and one's emotional reaction to success and failure are determined, at least in part, by the person's beliefs about his or her operative capabilities. Self-efficacy is not the same as self-esteem, which depends largely on how the culture values the person's self-perceived attributes. However, it is closely linked to concepts of effectance motivation (White, 1959) or competence motivation (Harackiewicz, Abrahams, and Wageman, 1987). Individuals derive information about self-efficacy from various sources, including vicarious experience and persuasion by others. By far the most important source of self-efficacy information, however, is the person's history of mastery experiences—of repeated success in meeting task demands.

Viewed from this perspective, brain damage should have profound effects on perceived self-efficacy, at least in situations that are relevant to the lesion in question. It is what the catastrophic reaction is all about. We know of no empirical literature on brain damage, and there is little literature from other domains that might be relevant. There are reasons to believe that the elderly may show declines in perceived self-efficacy by virtue of persuasion by a culture that believes in age-related performance declines, vicarious learning from age peers, and comparison with their own levels of performance at an earlier point in life. Anosognosic patients, who are unaware of their deficits, are denied much of this information. No matter how much they may be told by others about their deficits, apparently they lack the personal experience of incapacity that Bandura (1986) suggested is the most important source of self-efficacy judgment. The prediction, then, is that anosognosic patients' self-efficacy judgments are more positive and less accurate than those of patients with comparable brain damage who are aware of their deficits. However, are their judgments as positive as those of intact controls? Perhaps not. Are their self-efficacy judgments totally orthogonal to actual performance? Again, probably not. Pessimism about performance coupled with any degree of accuracy in performance-related predictions might count as evidence of implicit cognition of deficits.

We might obtain additional evidence of implicit acknowledgment of deficits if we examined anosognosics' self-ratings of anxiety, depression, and other personality characteristics. For example, if anosognosics were in no sense cognizant of their deficits, we might expect them to score less on indices of the catastrophic reaction—anxiety, depression, and the like—than patients with comparable brain lesions who are aware of their deficits. Such evidence would be especially compelling if anosognosics proved to score normally, with respect to appropriate controls, in terms of dimensions that are unrelated to their deficits, e.g., agreeableness and friendliness.

TOWARD A NEUROPSYCHOLOGY OF CONSCIOUSNESS

These speculations aside, one achievement of contemporary cognitive psychology is a clear theoretical framework for studying the nonconscious mental structures and processes that so interested our nineteenth century forebears. With the development of a new class of psychological theories and a corresponding set of new experimental paradigms, we have revealed a topography of nonconscious mental life that is different from the seething unconscious of Freud and more extensive than the unconscious inference of Helmholtz. Work must now begin to clarify the nature of the processes by which cognitive and motoric procedures are automatized, the scope of preconscious processing of implicit percepts and memories, and the mechanisms underlying dissociation.

Historically, cognitive and clinical neuropsychology have played an important role in this work by revealing relations between conscious and unconscious mental processes that might well have gone unrecognized in more conventional laboratory work involving subjects who were not brain-damaged. This area is clearly one of the contributions to work on the amnesic syndrome, blindsight, and prosopagnosia, all of which classify in some sense as deficits of awareness rather than merely as deficits of perception or memory. Anosognosia counts even more clearly as a deficit of awareness, a pure deficit that can be attached, as it were, to a wide variety of other cognitive-behavioral deficits. With the beginning of serious experimental work on anosognosia, we can say that we are one step closer to uncovering the biological basis of consciousness and the experience of selfhood that is the essence of human nature.

ACKNOWLEDGMENTS

The point of view represented herein is based in part on research supported by grants MH-35856 and MH-44739 from the National Institute of Mental Health. We thank Jeffrey Bowers, Marcia K. Johnson, Susan M. McGlynn, Elizabeth Merikle, Mary A. Peterson, Daniel L. Schacter, and Douglas J. Tataryn for their comments.

REFERENCES

Anderson, J. R. (1982). Acquisition of cognitive skill. *Psychol. Rev.* 89:369–406.

Anderson, J. R. (1983). *The Architecture of Cognition.* Cambridge: Harvard University Press.

Andreason, N. C. (1982). Negative symptoms in schizophrenia: definition and reliability. *Arch. Gen. Psychiatry* 39:784–787.

Andreason, N. C., and Olson, S. A. (1982). Negative versus positive schizophrenia: definition and validation. *Arch. Gen. Psychiatry* 39:789–794.

Atkinson, R. C., and Shiffrin, R. M. (1968). Human memory: a proposed system and its control processes. In K. W. Spence and J. T. Spence (eds.), *The Psychology of Learning and Motivation.* Vol. 2. New York: Academic Press.

Babinski, M. J. (1914). [Contribution to the study of mental disturbance in organic cerebral hemiplegia (anosognosia)]. *Rev. Neurol. (Paris)* 1:845–848 [French].

Babinski, M. J. (1918). [Anosognosia.] *Rev. Neurol. (Paris)* 31:365–367 [French].

Bandura, A. (1977). Self-efficacy: toward a unifying theory of behavior. *Psychol. Rev.* 84:191–215.

Bandura, A. (1986). *Social Foundations of Thought and Action: A Social Cognitive Theory.* Englewood Cliffs, NJ: Prentice-Hall.

Bisiach, E., Vallar, G., Perani, D., Papagno, C., and Bertil, A. (1986). Unawareness of disease following lesions of the right hemisphere: anosognosia for hemiplegia and anosognosia for hemianopia. *Neuropsychologia* 24:471–482.

Bowers, K. S. (1981). Do the Stanford scales tap the "classic suggestion effect"? *Int. J. Clin. Exp. Hypn.* 29:42–53.

Bowers, K. S. (1984). On being unconsciously influenced and informed. In K. S. Bowers and D. Meichenbaum (eds.), *The Unconscious Reconsidered.* New York: Wiley-Interscience.

Bowers, K. S. (1987). Revisioning the unconscious. *Can. Psychol.* 28:93–104.

Bowers, K. S., and Meichenbaum, D. (eds.) (1984). *The Unconscious Reconsidered.* New York: Wiley-Interscience.

Bowers, P. G. (1982). The classic suggestion effect: relationships with scales of hypnotizability, effortless experiencing, and imagery vividness. *Int. J. Clin. Exp. Hypn.* 30:270–279.

Brady, J. P., and Lind, D. I. (1961). Experimental analysis of hysterical blindness. *Behav. Res. Ther.* 4:331–339.

Browne, M. W. (1988, August 16). The benzine ring: was it just a dream? *New York Times.*

Campion, J., Latto, R., and Smith, Y. M. (1983). Is blindsight an effect of scattered light, spared cortex, and near-threshold vision? *Behav. Brain Sci.* 6:423–486.

Claparede, E. (1911/1951). [Recognition and "me-ness."] In D. Rapaport (ed.), *Organization and Pathology of Thought.* New York: Columbia University Press.

DeHaan, E. H. F., Young, A., and Newcombe, F. (1987). Face recognition without awareness. *Cogn. Neuropsychol.* 4:385–415.

Ellenberger, H. F. (1970). *The Discovery of the Unconscious: The History and Evolution of Dynamic Psychiatry.* New York: Basic Books.

Evans, F. J. (1979). Hypnosis and sleep: techniques for exploring cognitive activity during sleep. In E. Fromm and R. E. Shor (eds.), *Hypnosis: Developments in Research and New Perpsectives.* New York: Aldine.

Freud, A. (1936/1966). *The Ego and the Mechanisms of Defense.* Rev. Ed. In *The Writings of Anna Freud.* Vol. 2. New York: International Universities Press.

Freud, S. (1899/1962). Screen memories. In J. Strachey (ed.), *The Standard Edition of the Complete Psychological Works of Sigmund Freud.* Vol. 3. London: Hogarth Press.

Freud, S. (1901/1960). The psychopathology of everyday life. In J. Strachey (ed.), *The Standard Edition of the Complete Psychological Works of Sigmund Freud.* Vol. 6. London: Hogarth Press.

Goldstein, K. (1948). *Language and Language Disturbances.* Orlando: Grune & Stratton.

Harackiewicz, J. M., Abrahams, S., and Wageman, R. (1987). Performance evaluation and intrinsic motivation: the effects of evaluative focus, rewards, and achievement orientation. *J. Pers. Soc. Psychol.* 53:1015–1023.

Heilman, K. M., and Valenstein, E. (eds.) (1985). *Clinical Neuropsychology.* 2nd Ed. New York: Oxford University Press.

Heilman, K. M., Bowers, D., and Valenstein, E. (1985). Emotional disorders associated with neurological diseases. In K. M. Heilman and E. Valenstein (eds.), *Clinical Neuropsychology.* 2nd Ed. New York: Oxford University Press.

Hilgard, E. R. (1969). Levels of awareness: second thoughts on some of William James' ideas. In R. B. MacLeod (ed.), *William James: Unfinished Business.* Washington, DC: American Psychological Association.

Hilgard, E. R. (1977). Controversies over consciousness and the rise of cognitive psychology. *Aust. Psychol.* 12:7–26.

Hilgard, E. R. (1980). Consciousness in contemporary psychology. *Annu. Rev. Psychol.* 31:1–26.

Hilgard, E. R. (1987). *Psychology in America: A Historical Survey.* San Diego: Harcourt Brace Jovanovich.

Hilgard, E. R., and Marquis, D. G. (1940). *Conditioning and Learning.* New York: Appleton-Century-Crofts.

Holender, D. (1986). Semantic activation without conscious identification in dichotic listening, parafoveal vision, and visual masking: a survey and appraisal. *Behav. Brain Sci.* 9:1–66.

Jacoby, L. L., and Dallas, M. (1981). On the relationship between autobiographical memory and perceptual learning. *J. Exp. Psychol.* [*Gen.*] 110:306–340.

James, W. (1890). *Principles of Psychology.* New York: Holt.

Janet, P. (1901). *The Mental State of Hystericals: A Study of Mental Stigmata and Mental Accidents.* New York: Putnam.

Janet, P. (1907). *The Major Symptoms of Hysteria.* New York: Macmillan.

Johnson, M. K., and Raye, C. L. (1981). Reality monitoring. *Psychol. Rev.* 88:67–85.

Kahneman, D., and Triesman, A. (1984). Changing views of attention and automaticity. In R. Parasuraman and D. R. Davies (eds.), *Varieties of Attention.* New York: Academic Press, pp. 29–61.

Kihlstrom, J. F. (1980). Posthypnotic amnesia for recently learned material: interactions with "episodic" and "semantic" memory. *Cogn. Psychol.* 12:227–251.

Kihlstrom, J. F. (1984). Conscious, subconscious, unconscious: a cognitive view. In K. S. Bowers and D. Meichenbaum (eds.), *The Unconscious Reconsidered.* New York: Wiley-Interscience.

Kihlstrom, J. F. (1985a). Hypnosis. *Annu. Rev. Psychol.* 36:385–418.

Kihlstrom, J. F. (1985b). Posthypnotic amnesia and the dissociation of memory. In G. H. Bower (ed.), *The Psychology of Learning and Motivation.* Vol. 19. Orlando: Academic Press, pp. 131–178.

Kihlstrom, J. F. (1987). The cognitive unconscious. *Science* 237:1445–1452.

Kihlstrom, J. F. (1989). Cognition, unconscious processes. *Neuroscience Year: The Yearbook of the Encyclopedia of Neuroscience.* Boston: Birkhauser Boston, pp. 34–36.

Kihlstrom, J. F. (1990a). Dissociative disorders. In P. B. Sutker and H. E. Adams (eds.), *Comprehensive Handbook of Psychopathology.* 2nd Ed. New York: Plenum, in press.

Kihlstrom, J. F. (1990b). Unconscious processes in personality. In L. Pervin (ed.), *Handbook of Personality Theory and Research.* New York: Guilford.

Kihlstrom, J. F., and Cantor, N. (1984). Mental representations of the self. *Adv. Exp. Soc. Psychol.* 17:1–47.

Kihlstrom, J. F., and Harackiewicz, J. M. (1982). The earliest recollection: a new survey. *J. Pers.* 50:134–148.

Kihlstrom, J. F., and Hoyt, I. P. (1988). Hypnosis and the psychology of delusions. In T. F. Oltmanns and B. A. Maher (eds.), *Delusional Beliefs: Interdisciplinary Perspectives.* New York: Wiley-Interscience, pp. 66–109.

Kihlstrom, J. F., and Schacter, D. L. (1989). Anesthesia, implicit memory, and the cognitive unconscious. Read at the First International Symposium on Memory and Awareness in Anesthesia, Glasgow.

Kihlstrom, J. F., Cantor, N., Albright, J. S., Chew, B. R., Klein, S. B., and Neidenthal, P. M. (1988). Information processing and the study of the self. *Adv. Exp. Soc. Psychol.* 21:145–178.

Ludwig, A. J., Brandsma, J. M., Wilbur, C. B., Bendfeldt, E., and Jameson, D. H. (1972). The objective study of a multiple personality; or, are four heads better than one? *Arch. Gen. Psychiatry* 26:298–310.

Marcel, A. (1983a). Conscious and unconscious perception: experiments on visual masking and word recognition. *Cogn. Psychol.* 15:197–237.

Marcel, A. (1983b). Conscious and unconscious perception: an approach to the relations between phenomenal experience and perceptual processes. *Cogn. Psychol.* 15:238–300.

McClelland, J. L., Rummelhart, D. E., and the PDP Research Group (1986). *Parallel Distributed Processing: Explorations in the Microstructure of Cognition. Vol. 2: Psychological and Biological Models.* Cambridge: MIT Press.

McGlynn, S. M., and Schacter, D. L. (1989). Unawareness of deficits in neuropsychological syndromes. *J. Clin. Exp. Neuropsychol.* 11:143–205.

Miller, G. A., Galanter, E., and Pribram, K. H. (1960). *Plans and the Structure of Behavior.* New York: Holt, Rinehart, & Winston.

Myers, G. E. (1986). *William James: His Life and Thought.* New Haven: Yale University Press.

Neal, P. (1988). *As I Am: An Autobiography.* New York: Simon & Schuster.

Nelson, T. (1978). Detecting small amounts of information in memory: savings for nonrecognized items. *J. Exp. Psychol.* [*Hum. Learn. Mem.*] 4:453–468.

Newell, A., and Simon, H. A. (1972). *Human Problem Solving.* Englewood Cliffs, NJ: Prentice-Hall.

Peirce, C. S., and Jastrow, J. (1884). On small differences of sensation. *Mem. Natl. Acad. Sci.* 3:73–83.

Reed, G. (1988). *The Psychology of Anomalous Experience.* Rev. Ed. Buffalo, NY: Prometheus Books.

Rummelhart, D. E., McClelland, J. L., and the PDP Research Group (1986). *Parallel Distributed Processing: Explorations in the Microstructure of Cognition. Vol. 1: Foundations.* Cambridge: MIT Press.

Sandler, J. and Freud, A. (1985). *The Analysis of Defense: The Ego and the Mechanisms of Defense Revisited.* New York: International Universities Press.

Schacter, D. L. (1987). Implicit memory: history and current status. *J. Exp. Psychol.* [*Learn. Mem. Cogn.*] 13:501–518.

Schacter, D. L., and Kihlstrom, J. F. (1989). Functional amnesia. In F. Boller and J. Graffman (eds.), *Handbook of Neuropsychology,* Vol. 3. Amsterdam: Elsevier, pp. 209–231.

Shiffrin, R. W., and Schneider, W. (1984). Automatic and controlled processing revisited. *Psychol. Rev.* 91:269–276.

Spelke, E. S., Hirst, W., and Neisser, U. (1976). Skills of divided attention. *Cognition* 4:215–230.

Tranel, D., and Damasio, A. R. (1985). Knowledge without awareness: an autonomic index of facial recognition by prosopagnosics. *Science* 228:1453–1454.

Tulving, E., Schacter, D. L., and Stark, H. A. (1982). Priming effects in word-fragment completion are independent of recognition memory. *J. Exp. Psychol.* [*Learn. Mem. Cogn.*] 8:336–342.

Weinstein, E. A., and Kahn, R. L. (1955). *Denial of Illness: Symbolic and Physiological Aspects.* Springfield, IL: Charles C Thomas.

Weinstein, E. A., Cole, M., Mitchell, M. S., and Lyerly, O. G. (1964). Anosognosia and aphasia. *Arch. Neurol.* 10:376–386.

Weiskrantz, L. (1980). Varieties of residual experience. *Q. J. Exp. Psychol.* 32:365–386.

Weiskrantz, L., Warrington, E. K., Sanders, M. D., and Marshall, J. (1974). Visual capacity in the hemianopic field following a restricted occipital ablation. *Brain* 97:709–728.

Weitzenhoffer, A. M. (1974). When is an "instruction" an instruction? *Int. J. Clin. Exp. Hypn.* 22:258–269.

White, R. W. (1959). Motivation reconsidered: the concept of competence. *Psychol. Rev.* 66:297–333.

Whyte, L. L. (1960). *The Unconscious Before Freud.* New York: Basic Books.

12
Role of Psychological Factors in Disordered Awareness

LISA LEWIS

A difficult question in the quest for knowledge is how we come to have any knowledge at all. As stated by John Locke, common sense provides a straightforward answer: "Perception is the first step towards knowledge, and the inlet of all of the materials of it." Yet this response raises more questions than it answers: If it is so, where does the knowledge come from, and how and where is it received (Young, 1988)? Does it arrive in ready-made packets of high-fidelity reproductions of the external world, or is the process a more active one in which the perceiver takes part in a construction of reality? If the latter is true, to what extent does each of us create our own private realities with idiosyncratic perceptions determined by our unique personality makeup? These are classic questions for philosophers, but they are also of intense interest to those in the broadly defined field of psychology.

The purpose of this chapter is to elucidate the psychological causes of distortions in awareness. Because the concept of motivated or psychological denial of reality emerged from psychoanalytical investigations, greatest emphasis is given to psychoanalytical formulations. Cognitive theories, as well as relevant empirical and clinical literature, are reviewed.

PSYCHOANALYTICAL PERSPECTIVE

Psychoanalysis, in each of its applications—as a theory of the mind, a form of treatment, and a method of obtaining knowledge applicable to a variety of fields including literature and anthropology—has as its aim the discovery of meanings intrinsic to human behavior and functioning. Its questions are straightforward and primarily consist in "how" questions, answered in terms of mechanisms and processes, and "why" questions, answered in terms of reasons and motives (Wallerstein, 1976). *Why* are people unaware of an aspect of themselves that is obvious to everyone else? *How* are they able to maintain this curious gap in self-awareness? These questions are important for the psychoanalytical approach. Our inquiry is based on the assumption that underlying issues/conflicts can motivate perceptions, thoughts, and actions. Although the link between the underlying and the obvious often remains mysterious, the psychotherapist, much like the novelist, attempts to bring it forth (Jacobsen, Beardslee, Hauser, et al., 1986). The concept of defense represents the gatekeeper between underlying and overt, between conscious and unconscious, and is thus pivotal in our efforts to understand distortions in awareness and other such symptoms. In the quest for insight and knowledge in a clinical setting, what one hopes the patient gains is not so much a cure as freedom, a liberation from those unconscious aspects of the mind that create distortions and blind spots in knowledge about oneself and the world (Freud, 1937/1961; Wheelis, 1971).

For the most part, then, we seek to understand the reasons for and mechanisms behind distortions in everyday awareness. The obstacles to obtaining undistorted awareness of ourselves and our environment probably do not spring from deficiencies in intelligence, technique, or education. As Rangell (1985) so eloquently theorized:

> Resistance is a defense against insight. This is not to be confused with obstacles to knowledge. Defenses are not inert barriers but psychic configurations with dynamic force. Insight is not blocked but actively opposed. And the knowledge that is kept from consciousness in the case of resistance is not out of reach because of its complexity, beyond man's cognitive capacity to encompass or comprehend, but by virtue of its unacceptability to the ego. . . . It is not the cognitive complexity but the affective accompaniments . . . with their anticipated retaliatory punishments . . . which constitute the building blocks of the psychic armor around the forbidden thoughts or feelings which need to be kept captive, out of sight or conscious awareness.

According to psychoanalytical theory, then, the obstacles to knowledge principally derive from a split within the self—between a part that wants to know and a part that fears the pain such knowledge would bring. Deficit, illness, and trauma may be denied because awareness would cause too much emotional pain and dissonance. In addition to the threat of pain awareness would bring, knowledge of unconscious wishes and motives may be resisted because bringing them into awareness would make us responsible for them (Freud, 1925/1961). As Blum (1979) pointed out,

> The quest for insight has always been paralleled by the "bliss of ignorance." The hero of the oedipal myth moves and wavers between insight and blindness. Oedipus seeks the truth while asserting innocence of his guilt and ignorance of his identity. Analogous to the analytic process, the oedipal myth depicts the struggle between insight and resistance to insight.

CLINICAL EXAMPLE

A case vignette illustrates the way that denial is typically manifest in the psycho-therapeutic situation with medically and neurologically healthy psychiatric patients.

> Libby, a 27-year-old woman, had come to therapy because of long-standing and intensifying depression that made it increasingly difficult for her to function in life as a factory worker and wife. She had only sketchy memories of her childhood, but I made mental note of the fact that her mother had been married and divorced three times, with each divorce preceded by her having an affair with a married man she subsequently married. Libby was a product of the first marriage. My efforts to help her talk about how she felt toward her mother were met with increasingly irritated protestations that she had no negative feelings toward her mother whatsoever. All negative feelings were steadfastly denied. According to the patient's version, her mother should be canonized as a saint, so pervasive and uniform were her idealized positive feelings for her. In contrast, she accused herself of being a miserable excuse for a woman, incapable of having true love or nurturant feelings for anyone. I sus-pected the patient was turning her anger and hateful feelings toward her mother back against herself, accusing herself of things she more truthfully felt toward her mother, but for months the patient was nowhere near ready to entertain such an interpretation.
>
> One day in therapy Libby seemed more than usually agitated and uneasy. With great trepidation and requiring much support from me, the reasons for her uneasiness gradually emerged over the next five sessions: She said she had seen me riding in a car with another doctor from the Clinic. She said she happened to know that the other doctor was married, and what was I doing in the car with him? She hated to say it but she had grown convinced that I was having an affair with this married man. How could she trust me to help her when I was nothing more than a faithless home-wrecker, cheating on my own husband, and destroying this other man's happy home life? How could I presume to be a role model for her efforts to develop the capacity for genuine love, loyalty, and nurturance? In one particularly heated moment of expressing her sense of bitter betrayal and despair she spat out, "You're no better than my mother!" Her exclamation stunned her and for a moment she stared at me in shocked silence, the blood draining from her face. She stammered, "I didn't meant that. It wasn't true, and I'm sorry I said it. I'm just a liar or a fool." It took a great deal of patience and support, but over the course of the next several weeks she was able to talk about her long-denied feelings of anger, shame, and despair toward her mother who had three times turned the family upside down by having affairs with married men. With her denial lifted and the negative feelings directed toward their rightful object, her depression gradually subsided and her feel-ings about herself as a wife and potential mother improved considerably.
>
> [Incidentally, the man she saw me with in the car and with whom she accused me of having an affair was indeed a married doctor at the Clinic. Unbeknownst to her, however, he is married to me.]

We have all likely had the experience of behaving as though some aspect of reality about ourselves or our environment did not exist and realized it only in retrospect when we "came to our senses." The numbing of awareness following the death of a loved one, which is increasingly shattered by sudden surges of realization of their death, the casual and light-hearted conversations that take place so often beside mangled cars after a car accident, the dawning realization of having behaved irritably and unfairly toward a spouse all the while insisting that nothing was the matter—these instances indicate that our perceptions are not always close approximates of reality. We can learn several lessons from studying these everyday examples of distorted awareness as well as dramatic counterparts that occur in psychiatric and medical populations.

First, we are reminded that our minds or brains, unlike computers or other mechanical information processors, do not simply register reality in pure form but distort perception to greater or lesser degrees. Second, we are led to suspect that the process of distortion goes on outside our awareness and is not the product of conscious intent (i.e., is different from lying or malingering). When we are made aware of the illusion we have created, the process of distortion is experienced as ego dystonic, as though we do not quite believe we are responsible for it. It is always humbling to learn that there are realms of our experience that are not entirely subject to conscious control. Third, we learn that such distortions are not random or meaningless events. They nearly always follow a comprehensible pattern that is typically obvious to everyone but the person engaging in the distortion. The pattern often entails protecting ourselves from some aspect of truth or reality that is offensive or too painful to be acknowledged. Fourth, we learn that though these distortions play a protective role and thereby have adaptive value, they are not without cost. The price that is paid always includes reduced cognitive and perceptual efficiency. These cognitive and perceptual limitations are descriptively not unlike those caused by actual lesions of the central nervous system and are sometimes mistaken for them. The etiology is quite different, however, in that these distortions are entirely psychogenic.

In short, studying such examples suggests a reasonable working definition of denial and other mechanisms of defense. They can be defined as protective mechanisms that are motivated unconsciously and serve the dynamic purpose of enhancing conscious pleasure and minimizing pain, thereby promoting the most adaptive equilibrium attainable at the time (Menninger, Mayman, and Pruyser, 1963). They may operate unconsciously; their presence is "typically" unknown to the person who uses them, and they are frequently beyond the person's capacity to control through volitional means. We are also led to hypothesize that reliance on denial and other mechanisms of defense is universal. It is not the presence of defense mechanisms that signals neurosis or psychopathology; indeed, the complete absence of ego mechanisms of defense would be closer to psychosis than to normality.

HISTORICAL OVERVIEW

Freud began his professional career as a basic scientist, and recent writers have gone so far as to depict him as a biologist of the mind (Sulloway, 1979). His early efforts at theory development culminated in the *Project for a Scientific Psychology* (1895/1961), a monograph that has since been reviewed and reexamined in the light of current knowledge by Pribram and Gill (1976). In it, Freud attempted to create a theory of mental functioning that was solidly based in neural events. Although a thorough-going biological explanation for mental events was subsequently abandoned, neural conceptualizations continued to appear throughout Freud's career. For example, in *Beyond the Pleasure Principle* (1920/1961), while discussing cell membranes in the "cortical layer" of the brain and sensory organs, Freud noted that protection against stimuli is an almost more important function for the living organism than reception of stimuli. He used such theorizing to promote the view that the human organism is created with a built-in defensive function to protect against being inundated by too many external stimuli or by stimuli that would create an experience of unpleasure. For him, psychological denial was the equivalent of this biological capacity.

The term "defense" is the earliest representative of the dynamic viewpoint in psychoanalytical thinking (Freud, 1946) and is perhaps Freud's most original contribution to human psychology (Vaillant, 1986). Ego mechanisms of defense, including denial, are the focal point in psychoanalytical theory. In his earliest theory, the topographical model, Freud repeatedly observed that patients evidenced blind spots or scotomas, as he termed them, for certain aspects of their inner and outer reality. At the time, he believed that these blind spots resulted from the conscious mind's attempt to defend itself against unconscious impulses pressing for expression and fulfillment.

Freud's attention shifted increasingly from the id (the seat of instincts and repressed mental contents) to the ego, particularly the ego's role in mediating conflict with the id, the superego, and the external world. In Freud's final conceptualization (1940/1961), the ego was depicted as mediating between the id below and the external world above. The processes used by the ego in the management of conflict were identified as ego mechanisms of defense. Initially, two generic forms of defense were identified: repression, the defense process employed to modulate internal stimuli from the id, and denial, the defense process used to manage stimuli emanating from the external world.

It remained for Anna Freud (1946), Sigmund Freud's daughter and intellectual heir, to do with defenses what her father had done so thoroughly with instincts (Rangell, 1985). She began to define defenses in the context of the ego's broader range of functions, introducing the school of ego psychology to which important contributions were made by Reich (1933), Hartmann (1939), Rapaport (1951), and Erikson (1950). Importantly, the ego psychologists explicated the emergence of defenses in the context of ego development and the subsequent impact of defenses on "conflict-free" ego functions such as memory, judgment, and perception. The perspective of ego psychologists is particularly relevant to neuropsychology because of their focus on adaptive cognitive functions. In their view, defenses as such are not inborn; rather, the infant's neuropsychological capacity to adapt and respond to environmental conditions is innate. This viewpoint is consistent with Freud's (1905) suggestion that defenses are the intermediate state between reflexes and conscious acts of judgment and were viewed as the psychical equivalent of those reflexes designed to avoid the experience of unpleasure.

Specifically, Spitz (1961), on the basis of direct observation of infant behavior, traced a continuous series beginning with physiological prototypes (e.g., eyelid closing in response to noxious visual stimulation of bright lights) and ending with what appear to be familiar defenses (e.g., denial in which aspects of painful reality are psychologically eclipsed). Benjamin (1965), in infant observation studies, documented that the passive stimulus barrier created by neuroimmaturity at birth and resulting in failure of stimuli to be transmitted to the cortex is replaced at 8 weeks of age by an active stimulus barrier. When this change occurs, sensory input, by virtue of being overly intense or inherently noxious, is actively screened from reaching consciousness (often through the act of the infant's falling asleep). The same process of actively screening out external stimulation was investigated in older, disturbed children by Shevrin and Taussieng (1965). They monitored psychophysiological measures and found that these children dealt with psychological conflict by raising their sensory thresholds for all external stimuli, resulting in periods of numbness and anesthesia. The authors related this psychophysiological reaction to the ego's mechanism of defense and went on to speculate that its persistent use could underlie the clinical phenomena of apathy, withdrawal, and depersonalization so often seen in children and adults exposed to chronically stressful environments.

Hartmann (1939) sought to extend the scope of psychoanalysis by documenting the fact that the ego's function is not solely defensive and not wholly confined to the management of conflict. He documented and described the many functions of the conflict-free sphere of the ego, including motility, perception, memory, and reasoning. Although these primary autonomous ego functions may be diverted into the management of conflict (repression of memories, denial of percepts), the primary purpose of all ego functions is to promote adaptation to reality, and the management of conflict always has its adaptive purpose. Indeed, some defenses against instinctual drives (such as intellectualization) actually result in heightened intellectual achievement, demonstrating that certain conflict situations may guarantee a greater degree of adaptation. In short, Hartmann delineated the ways in which maturation of functions in the conflict-free ego sphere affects the scope of resources available to the individual coping with conflict and how this situation in turn influences subsequent maturation of the conflict-free ego functions.

Shapiro (1965) described the ways in which this interaction of biologically based abilities and the psychological management of conflict produces characteristic cognitive styles: The obsessive-compulsive person, tempted to unusual enthusiasm or optimism, experiences this state of mind as recklessness that portends a loss of control; he feels compelled to look for the fly in the ointment and to anticipate all of the various ways in which the event could go wrong. The paranoid person, momentarily inclined to a less guarded action, discovers a suspicious clue just in the nick of time (resulting in the constriction of perception of the external environment). The hysterical man who begins to assert a sharply defined position suddenly becomes aware of the insufficiency of his qualifications and, in a rush of embarrassment, forgets what he had said altogether (resulting in a spotty memory for factual detail and a global and impressionistic style of thinking). Rapaport, Gill, and Schafer (1968) elaborated the ways in which these habitually employed defenses result in characteristic changes in cognition, motoric behavior, and perception as assessed by traditional psychological tests.

These ego psychologists promoted a shift in thinking about defense mechanisms from the earlier "marionette" view of defenses as passively and automatically protecting the individual to a view in which the individual actively participates in the process of defense, not by choice but simply by virtue of who he or she is (Shapiro, 1965; Valenstein, 1985). The paranoid individual does not decide to scrutinize his environment for signs of threat; but for someone who feels so vulnerable, what is there to do but to check once more? From the ego psychological point of view, the interplay between defensive functioning and neuropsychologically mediated cognitive functions is a matter of considerable interest.

CURRENT CONCEPTUALIZATIONS AND EMPIRICAL FINDINGS

During the decades that have elapsed since the publication of Anna Freud's seminal volume, *The Ego and The Mechanisms of Defense* (1946), numerous authors have offered definitions and schemes for grouping the mechanism of defense. Yet no consensus has been reached on a common list of defenses, on consensually shared definitions of the defense mechanisms, or on the pathological implications of certain defenses. In 1977 a prominent group of psychiatrists and psychologists who were committed to developing an axis for coding defenses as part of the *DSM-III* schema, met with its chief architect, Robert Spitzer, but were unable to come to any agreement (Vaillant, 1986).

One current way of conceptualizing defenses is to view them developmentally. Early efforts to create a developmental hierarchy of defenses grew out of psychosexual stage theory in which libidinal instincts were successively cathected to oral, anal, and genital body regions (Abraham, 1927; Fenichel, 1945), with each stage of development characterized by a particular set of defenses. Defenses employed by the ego early in life, such as denial, projection, and introjection, are referred to as primitive defenses, whereas others that come into use later when a greater degree of ego organization is present, such as intellectualization and sublimation, are referred to as mature defenses (Willick, 1985). Primitive and mature defenses are also differentiated on the basis of the danger that calls them into operation. Higher order defenses such as reaction formation are called into operation against the later developmental anxieties of separation and superego punishment, whereas the more profound dangers of threats to perseveration of the self and loss of identity are defended against by denial, projection, and so on (Frosch, 1970). Thus one way of conceptualizing defenses along developmental lines is to categorize them in terms of when they make their appearance during early childhood development and, relatedly, the severity of psychopathology with which they are associated in adult life (Gedo and Goldberg, 1973; Kernberg, 1975).

Clinical and empirical studies indicate that denial is a primitive defense in that it is one of the first defenses to make its appearance during childhood development. As stated earlier, Spitz, Benjamin, and other ego psychologist researchers have traced a developmental line for defenses. The neuroimmaturity of the central nervous system at birth and subsequent emergence of an active stimulus barrier at 8 weeks are the physiological and behavioral precursors of denial. Between the ages of 1 and 2, denial as we recognize it in adults begins to appear. A 2-year-old who is afraid of monsters in his bedroom at night pulls the covers over his head, believing that if the monster cannot be seen, it does not exist. A 3-year-old whom we have just observed hitting his sister looks at us wide-eyed and guileless and says, "No, I didn't hit Katherine." A 4-year-old becomes a bit more sophisticated, saying, "Yes, I hit Katherine, but I didn't mean to." The 4-year-old has developed enough cognitive capacity to have the savvy to appreciate that external reality is perceived by everyone and is therefore difficult to deny. In contrast, internal reality—the realm of intention and motive—is easier to deny. The 6-year-old is more sophisticated still and says, "Yes, I hit Katherine, but it was an accident. I was just swinging around and she stepped in front of me." Thus the 6-year-old bolsters denial with the defense of rationalization.

As suggested in these examples, each mechanism of defense can be viewed as having its own line of development. Breznitz (1983) posits such a developmental line for the defense of denial, relating seven forms of denial to progressive means of protecting against danger by resorting to different cognitive strategies. The ordering of these forms of denial is based on the extent of reality distortion involved, ranging from denial of information to denial of personal relevance. Denial of information can be most clearly seen in psychosis, as for example the depressed woman described by Freud who, following the death of her baby, carried around a piece of wood to which she related as though it were her living infant. Denial of information is also seen during the period immediately after neurological trauma when a patient may flatly deny having had a car accident and head injury or a stroke. Denial of personal relevance can be seen in normal and neurotic individuals, as for example when smokers deny the personal relevance of the Surgeon General's report on smoking, believing that the risks are not present for them or at least not for the moment and that they will quit before any danger materializes.

Another useful way of conceptualizing defenses that has its roots in Freud's early writings is provided by Dorpat (1985). Dorpat integrated psychoanalytical theory with Piagetian concepts of cognitive development and with information processing theory. He defined denial as the unconscious repudiation of some or all of the meanings of an event in order to allay anxiety or unpleasurable affects. Used in this way, denial refers to the reality-repudiating aspects of all defensive operations rather than to a discrete mechanism; defense always contains an aspect of denial but also represents something more than denial.

According to Dorpat (1985) defensive operations are carried out in two stages, with the first stage entailing a form of "cognitive arrest" based on denial. In this stage, denial prevents the formation of conscious representation of an aspect of threatening reality. This gap in the symbolic representation of reality results in the need to create a cover story or screen to hide the discontinuity caused by the cognitive arrest phase. The content of the screen is often the exact opposite of the reality that has just been negated, and it is in this second phase that other mechanisms of defense are called into being to bolster denial. For example, denial of hatred is bolstered by reaction formation when a husband who is bitterly resentful of his hypochondriacal wife's nonfunctional state adopts an attitude of exaggerated solicitousness and protectiveness towards her. Denial is bolstered by identification when a young woman, unable to accept emotionally the death of her mother who suffered from Parkinson's disease, develops a shuffling gait. In a clinically rich volume, Dorpat (1985) elaborated the consequences of denial in the failure to develop fully reality testing and a sense of one's own experience of personal agency and responsibility; he detailed the ways in which denial is manifest in the clinical situation and can be treated therapeutically.

These conceptualizations of ego mechanisms of denial have received empirical support. Bond (1986), in a factor analytical study of the defensive functions of 111 nonpatients and 98 psychiatric patients, found that defenses can be grouped into four factors that correlate with ego strength, ego development, and maturity, providing support for the notion of a developmental line of defenses. Perry and Cooper (1986) documented that defensive functioning can be assessed reliably from psychoanalytical interviews as well as from observations of actual life events. They concluded that defenses are powerful predictors of clinical symptomatology, level of psychosocial functioning, and future defensive functioning 2 to 3 years after the initial interview. Vaillant (1986) documented empirically the validity of ego mechanisms of defense in a prospective 40-year follow-up of 307 men and demonstrated that defensive style is an enduring facet of personality functioning rather than being solely situationally determined. Interestingly, they demonstrated that although the type of defense employed is related to emotional maturity or health the relation is complex. Specifically, those men who came from warm childhoods could attain good mental health without benefit of reliance on mature defenses, whereas men raised in bleak childhood environments achieved good mental health only by employing mature defenses. These authors also provided support for the idea that biological factors in part determine defensive functioning in that defenses become increasingly mature with development and increasingly less mature under the impact of organic brain disease and hereditary mental illness.

The clinical and empirical literature also supports the conceptualization of denial as an unconscious protective measure that is employed by a wide range of personality types in response to a broad range of intrapsychic and external dangers. Denial has been observed to be at least transiently employed by patients suffering from a wide range of psychiatric disorders. Habitual reliance on denial is commonly seen among patients with eating disorders who deny their hunger and need for food, deny their emaciated state, and instead insist they are grotesquely obese and indeed deny any illness at all (Halmi, 1983; Giles, 1985; Panepinto and Simmons, 1986; *Diagnostic and Statistical Manual III-R,* 1987). Habitual reliance on denial is also commonly seen among alcoholics who deny their true level of consumption, deny being out of control of their drinking, and deny their need for treatment (Smith, 1986).

Denial of deficit, symptoms, and illness is also manifest in patients suffering from a wide range of medical conditions including cancer (Lonnqvist, 1981; Silberfarb and Greer, 1982; Dougherty, Templer, and Brown, 1986), acquired immunodeficiency syndrome (AIDS) (Nichols, 1983; Buhrick and Cooper, 1987), and cardiac conditions (Dimsdale and Hackett, 1982; Havik and Mae- land, 1986; Levine, Warrenburg, Kerns, et al., 1987). The prevalence of denial in these nonneurological medical conditions led McGlynn and Schacter (1989) to conclude that psychological denial plays a potentially significant role in unawareness of illness and deficit in some cases of clear-cut neurological disease.

The implications of denial in medical illness have been found to be com- plex. In some instances, denial of disease symptoms has resulted in misdiagnosis and misapplied treatment (Reiser, 1987). In other instances, denial of physical symptoms has been associated with noncompliance with treatment and high relapse rates (Boehnert and Popkin, 1986; Levine, et al., 1987). In addition, denial of emotional stress has been posited to play a contributing role to the development of presumably psychosomatic or autoimmune diseases such as sys- temic lupus (Reiter and Penzel, 1983) and cancer (Dattore, Shontz, and Coyne, 1980). Finally, Willick (1985) drew attention to the fact that in cases of medical illness patients who rely on some degree of denial often fare better than those experiencing significant anxiety and depression.

With terminal or life-threatening illness, denial of symptoms and disease has been found to defend against depression and death anxiety as well as at times being a symptom of the central nervous system effects of the illness itself (Devins, Binik, Mandin, et al., 1986; Dougherty et al., 1986). In chronic medical conditions in which severe and debilitating symptoms are denied and tolerated for many years, the denial of treatment need may reflect the fact that being ill serves an organizing function for the patient by sheltering him or her from the demands of everyday life and establishing a tolerable identity (Douglas and Druss, 1987). Denial of medical illness can also serve the adaptive purpose of preserving hope in the face of adversity, thereby sustaining sufficient optimism to persevere with treatment and general life involvements.

Lest the reader believe that denial is confined to medical and psychiatric populations, it is important to reiterate that denial is manifest by healthy, nor- mal individuals as well. For example, denial has been found not only among alcoholics but among family members as well (Henderson, 1984), not only among neurologically impaired patients but in their symptom-free children (Power, 1984), and not only by patients but in their doctors and other profes- sionals who treat them (Dewald, 1982; Halpert, 1982; Corradi, 1983; Homer, 1984). Trauma can evoke denial in a wide range of individuals. After a review of clinical and empirical studies, Horowitz (1976) concluded that major stressful life events are followed by involuntary intrusive recollections alternating with periods of successful warding off through denial and emotional numbness. This pattern was observed across a wide variety of traumas including rape, bereave- ment, combat, and holocaust experience; and it occurred across a wide range of personalities.

In short, denial has been demonstrated to be a psychologically motivated defense against intrapsychic threat as well as objective external trauma. It has been observed across a wide range of psychological, medical, and neurological conditions. It is likely that the defense of denial is potentially at everyone's disposal and that character makeup and acutely threatening life events are determining factors in bringing about its use.

CONCLUSIONS AND IMPLICATIONS

Ego mechanisms of defense, including denial, are powerful unconscious processes that have both adaptive and negative consequences. Psychoanalytically oriented psychologists have shown increasing interest in incorporating the rich findings generated in the field of neuropsychology into their conceptualizations of the diagnosis and treatment of psychological dysfunction. For example, Palombo (1979), Buchholz (1987), Pickar (1986), Kafka (1984), and Allen, Colson, and Coyne (1988) have focused on the impact of developmental learning disabilities on the development of defenses, self and other representations, identity, and self-esteem as well as the implications for psychotherapeutic and hospital treatment. Lewis (1986; 1990), Stern (1985), Prigatano, Fordyce, Zeiner, et al. (1984), and Athey (1986) have made similar efforts to understand the impact of more severe, acquired neurological disorders on these same psychological processes and their treatment. Such integrative efforts are crucially needed, as there is nothing about a brain lesion that ablates an individual's psyche or renders him or her free from reliance on mechanisms of defense, instinctual impulses, and other such psychic functions. For our understanding of patients to be complete, there must be adequate comprehension of both the physical and mental determinants of their functioning (Galin, 1974; Reiser, 1984).

Descriptively, there appears to be little difference between the denial that follows neural damage and denial that evolves from unconscious psychological efforts to repudiate a painful reality. A psychologically troubled woman manifesting a conversion reaction may deny ability to move her left arm and maintain this denial in the face of medical evidence to the contrary. A patient suffering a right hemispheric infarct may similarly evidence denial, stating that her left arm is not her own despite her doctor's compelling demonstrations to the contrary. Thus the denial managing psychological conflict and the denial following neurological insult are grossly similar. However, three factors are useful for differentiating psychogenic and neurogenic denial (see Chapter 2). First, the time course is relevant. Anosognosia, or neurologically based denial of deficit, is not uncommon following damage to anterior brain regions, particularly in the right hemisphere. These patients typically deny that the affected limb is their own as, for example, a man who complained it was unfair to charge him for a hospital bed if he continued to be forced to share it (he attributed his affected limbs to a fictional bed partner). These instances of denial of deficit generally, though not invariably, remit within hours or days of the neurological event. Psychological denial, except as a reaction to acute trauma or disease, generally is more persistently manifest across time.

Second, in those instances where denial in large part reflects disrupted brain functioning, it is not an isolated symptom. Neurological examination, neuroradiological studies, and neuropsychological testing reveal a pattern of functional deficits and structural findings implicating central nervous system dysfunction as the primary etiological factor. In cases of psychological denial, the pattern of diagnostic findings indicates that the alteration in awareness and other symptoms and deficits conform to a pattern of chronic or acute psychological distress.

Third, clinical experience indicates that the patient relying on denial for psychological reasons is likely to become increasingly agitated when confronted with the denied reality. In contrast, the neurologically impaired patient evidencing denial typically remains bland or perplexed (Prigatano, 1988). These factors are illustrated by the following clinical vignette.

> A middle-aged man suffered three mild to moderate head injuries across a span of 19 months in work-related accidents. The third accident also caused extensive damage to the muscles and tendons of his right arm. After two surgical repairs of his arm and 5 months after discharge from the hospital, he was noted to have memory problems as well as angry outbursts. He was referred to a neurologist. Neurological examination, computed tomographic scanning, and neuropsychological testing revealed an infarcted area situated subcortically in the left parietal lobe and documented mild to moderate deficits in left-handed tactile sensitivity, language comprehension, recent verbal memory, and arithmetic computation. Neuropsychological testing also indicated that the patient's long-standing self-esteem problems had been compensated for by overreliance on work, productivity, physical prowess, and hypermasculine behaviors. His accident had severely curtailed his ability to rely on these coping mechanisms, and he was depressed. Moreover, he was denying his own limitations and maintaining an illusion of himself as robust and fully recovered. His denial, bolstered by projection, led him to blame others for all of the problems actually caused by the damage to his arm and brain. As a result, he was engaging in a number of angry altercations with others that at times escalated to fist fights. His angry displays thus reflected a complex interplay of psychological and neurological factors: His neurologically based impairment of recent memory left him vulnerable to forget what his doctors told him about his deficits and their causes; his psychological reliance on denial and projection led him to blame others for his difficulties; and he was relying on his long-standing coping mechanism of machismo behavior to bolster his self-esteem. Pharmacotherapy, brief focal psychotherapy, and repeated educational sessions about his neurological and physical limitations led to resolution of his depression, denial, and angry outbursts.

There are several diagnostic implications that follow from the existing literature on denial and ego mechanisms of defense. First, the way in which an individual responds to trauma, whether it is a head injury or the death of a loved one, is in large part predictable on the basis of how he has coped with past trauma. Thus it is worthwhile to obtain a historical account of how the patient has attempted to cope in the past and to thoroughly assess his or her character makeup through psychological testing as well as psychiatric interviews with the patient and family. In this process, one must appreciate that defenses have an impact on cognition, perception, and motoric behavior. Thus the pattern of performance on psychological and neuropsychological tests must be analyzed in a fashion that takes account of interplay between psychological and neurological factors in contributing to a pattern of deficits and strengths. One must sort out the relative contributions of neurological and psychological factors to impaired memory, denial of deficit, slowing of motoric functioning, and so on.

The above literature on ego mechanisms of defense carries additional clinical implications. Patients utilizing denial are doing so unconsciously, and one cannot expect exhortation for the patient to stop it to be successful. Engaging in therapeutic efforts to induce the patient to use will power, volitional means of self-control, and so on to acknowledge the denied aspects of reality are likely to result in frustration for both the patient and the clinician, a lesson learned by Freud nearly a century ago. In addition, denial must not be viewed as a simple obstacle to treatment to be overcome as quickly as possible but, rather, as a motivated process that has adaptive value and meaning. The patient is attempting to avoid awareness of some aspect of reality that would cause more pain than he or she can currently tolerate. The specific danger to the patient needs to be understood by the clinician before any efforts are made to lessen the denial. Perhaps acknowledgment of the denied aspect of reality would lead to overwhelming guilt (e.g., for having injured one's self in a car accident while drinking), fear of loss of love (e.g., abandonment by spouse who until then has been overly reliant on the patient to be competent and strong), precipitous loss of self-esteem (e.g., as when a particularly treasured ability is lost, such as motor functioning for an athlete), and so on.

The more the denial distorts reality, the more serious one can assume the subjective sense of the threat to be. In some instances, patients truly deny external reality and state flatly that they did not have a stroke or brain tumor. More typically, one sees milder forms of disavowal of the personal significance of reality. The patient acknowledges that he or she suffered a head injury or stroke but asserts that there have been no lasting consequences and that he or she is now back to normal. As with the therapeutic management of all defenses, the formation of a trusting and safe interpersonal relationship is requisite, and the therapist always begins by interpreting the defense before interpreting what is being defended against. It entails a process of gently and repeatedly bringing the patient's attention to the form in which denial is manifest across a variety of situations.

Finally, as pointed out by Dorpat (1985), denial is frequently bolstered by the presence of other defenses. In part based on preexisting character traits, the second stage of creating a cover story to bolster the denial can include obsessional defenses (intellectualization, isolation of affect, compulsive and rigid reliance on behavioral rituals and prescribed rules of social etiquette), narcissistic defenses (belief in personal omnipotence, devaluation of others in order to elevate one's self), and immature-infantile defenses (clinging, dependent behavior, refusal to do for one's self what is well within one's ability level, somatization-hypochondriasis, acting out as a means of avoiding toleration of painful feelings). Again, both the adaptive intent behind the defenses and the fact that they are being carried out unconsciously need to be appreciated when attempting to resolve distortions of awareness in the therapeutic situation.

REFERENCES

Abraham, K. (1927). *Selected Papers.* London: Hogarth Press.

Allen, J. G., Colson, D. B., and Coyne, L. (1988). Organic brain dysfunction and behavioral dyscontrol in difficult-to-treat psychiatric hospital patients. *Integr. Psychiatry* 6:1–6.

American Psychiatric Association (1987). *Diagnostic and Statistical Manual of Mental Disorders, Third Edition, Revised.* Washington, DC: American Psychiatric Association.

Athey, G. I. (1986). Implications of memory impairment for hospital treatment. *Bull. Menninger Clin.* 50:99–110.

Benjamin, J. D. (1965). Developmental biology and psychoanalysis. In N. S. Greenfield and W. C. Lewis (eds.), *Psychoanalysis and Current Biological Thought.* Madison: University of Wisconsin Press.

Blum, H. P. (1979). The curative and creative aspects of insight. *J. Am. Psychoanal. Assoc.* 27:41–69.

Boehnert, C. E., and Popkin, M. K. (1986). Psychological issues in treatment of severely noncompliant diabetics. *Psychosomatics* 27:11–20.

Bond, M. (1986). An empirical study of defensive styles. In G. E. Vaillant (ed.), *Empirical Studies of Ego Mechanisms of Defense.* Washington, DC: American Psychiatric Press.

Breznitz, S. (1983). The seven kinds of denial. In S. Breznitz (ed.), *The Denial of Stress.* New York: International Universities Press.

Buchholz, E. S. (1987). The legacy from childhood: considerations for treatment of the adult with learning disabilities. *Psychoanal. Inquiry* 7:431–452.

Buhrick, N., and Cooper, D. A. (1987). Requests for psychiatric consultation concerning 22 patients with AIDS and ARC. *Aust. N.Z. J. Psychiatry* 21:346–353.

Corradi, R. B. (1983). Psychological regression with illness. *Psychosomatics* 24:353–362.

Dattore, P. J., Shontz, F. C., and Coyne, L. (1980). Premorbid personality differentiation of cancer and noncancer groups: a test of the hypothesis of cancer proneness. *J. Consult. Clin. Psychol.* 48:388–394.

Devins, G. M., Binik, Y. M., Mandin, H., Burgess, E. D., Taub, K., Letourneau, P. K., and Buckle, S. (1986). Denial as a defense against depression in end stage renal disease: an empirical test. *Int. J. Psychiatry Med.* 16:151–162.

Dewald, P. A. (1982). Serious illness in the analyst: transference, countertransference and reality response. *J. Am. Psychoanal. Assoc.* 30:347–363.

Dimsdale, J. E., and Hackett, T. P. (1982). Effect of denial on cardiac health and psychological adjustment. *Am. J. Psychiatry* 139:1477–1480.

Dorpat, T. L. (1985). *Denial and Defense in the Therapeutic Situation.* New York: Jason Aronson.

Dougherty, K., Templer, D. I., and Brown, R. (1986). Psychological states in terminal cancer as measured over time. *J. Counsel. Psychol.* 33:357–359.

Douglas, C. J., and Druss, R. G. (1987). Denial of illness: a reappraisal. *Gen. Hosp. Psychiatry* 9:53–57.

Erikson, E. H. (1950). *Childhood and Society.* Rev. Ed. New York: Norton.

Fenichel, O. (1945). *The Psychoanalytic Theory of Neurosis.* New York: Norton.

Freud, A. (1946). *The Ego and the Mechanisms of Defense.* New York: International Universities Press.

Freud, S. (1895/1961). Project for a scientific psychology. *The Standard Edition of the Complete Psychological Works of Sigmund Freud.* Vol. 1. London: Hogarth Press, pp. 281–343.

Freud, S. (1905/1961). Three essays on the theory of sexuality. *The Standard Edition of the Complete Psychological Works of Sigmund Freud.* Vol. 7. London: Hogarth Press, pp. 125–245.

Freud, S. (1908/1961). Character and anal eroticism. *The Standard Edition of the Complete Psychological Works of Sigmund Freud.* Vol. 9. London: Hogarth Press, pp. 169–175.

Freud, S. (1920/1961). Beyond the pleasure principle. *The Standard Edition of the Complete Psychological Works of Sigmund Freud.* Vol. 18. London: Hogarth Press, pp. 3–64.

Freud, S. (1925/1961). Moral responsibility for the content of dreams. *The Standard Edition of the Complete Psychological Works of Sigmund Freud.* Vol. 19. London: Hogarth Press, pp. 131–134.

Freud, S. (1937/1961). Analysis terminable and interminable. *The Standard Edition of the Complete Psychological Works of Sigmund Freud.* Vol. 23. London: Hogarth Press, pp. 209–253.

Freud, S. (1940/1961). An outline of psychoanalysis. *The Standard Edition of the Complete Psychological Works of Sigmund Freud.* Vol. 23. London: Hogarth Press, pp. 141–207.

Frosch, J. (1970). Psychoanalytic considerations of the psychotic character. *J. Am. Psychoanal. Assoc.* 18:24–50.

Galin, D. (1974). Implications for psychiatry of left and right cerebral specialization. *Arch. Gen. Psychiatry* 31:572–583.

Gedo, J., and Goldberg, A. (1973). *Models of the Mind.* Chicago: University of Chicago Press.

Giles, G. M. (1985). Body image: anorexia nervosa patients and occupational therapy students. *Br. J. Occup. Ther.* 48:216–217.

Halmi, K. A. (1983). Advances in anorexia nervosa. *Adv. Dev. Behav. Pediatr.* 4:1–23.

Halpert, E. (1982). When the analyst is chronically ill or dying. *Psychoanal. Q.* 51:372–389.

Hartmann, H. (1939). *Ego Psychology and the Problem of Adaptation.* New York: International Universities Press.

Havik, O. E., and Maeland, J. G. (1986). Dimensions of verbal denial in myocardial infarction. *Scand. J. Psychol.* 27:326–339.

Henderson, C. D. (1984). Countering resistance to acceptance of denial and the disease concept in alcoholic families: two examples of experimental teaching. *Alcohol. Treat. Q.* 1:117–121.

Homer, L. (1984). Organizational defenses against the anxiety of terminal illness: a case study. *Death Educ.* 8:137–154.

Horowitz, M. (1976). *Stress Response Syndromes.* New York: Jason Aronson.

Jacobsen, A. M., Beardslee, W., Hauser, S. T., Noam, G. G., and Powers, S. I. (1986). An approach to evaluating adolescent ego defense mechanisms using clinical interviews. In G. E. Vaillant (ed.), *Empirical Studies of Ego Mechanisms of Defense.* Washington, DC: American Psychiatric Press.

Kafka, E. (1984). Cognitive difficulties in psychoanalysis. *Psychiatr. Q.* 56:533–550.

Kernberg, O. (1975). *Borderline Conditions and Pathological Narcissism.* New York: Jason Aronson.

Levine, J., Warrenburg, S., Kerns, R., Schwartz, G., et al. (1987). The role of denial in recovery from coronary artery disease. *Psychosom. Med.* 49:109–117.

Lewis, L. (1986). Individual psychotherapy with patients having combined psychological and neurological disorders. *Bull. Menninger Clin.* 50:75–87.

Lewis, L. and Rosenberg, S. J. (1990). Psychoanalytic psychotherapy with brain-injured adult psychiatric patients. *J Nerv Ment Disease* 178:69–77.

Lonnqvist, J., (1981). Adaptation to cancer. *Psychiatr. Fenn.* 00(suppl.):179–188.

McGlynn, S. M., and Schacter, D. I. (1989). Unawareness of deficits in neuropsychological syndromes. *J. Clin. Exp. Neuropsychol.* 11:143–205.

Menninger, K., Mayman, M., and Pruyser, P. W. (1963). *The Vital Balance.* New York: Viking Press.

Nichols, S. E. (1983). Psychiatric aspects of AIDS. *Psychosomatics* 24:1083–1089.

Palombo, J. (1979). Perceptual deficits and self-esteem in adolescence. *Clin. Soc. Work J.* 7:34–61.

Panepinto, W. C., and Simmons, L. (1986). Treating the illness, not the mandate: techniques for successful referral, engagement, and treatment of alcoholic persons. *Alcohol. Treat. Q.* 3:37–48.

Perry, J. C., and Cooper, S. H. (1986). What do cross-sectional measures of defense mechanisms predict? In G. E. Vaillant (ed.), *Empirical Studies of Ego Mechanisms of Defense.* Washington, DC: American Psychiatric Press.

Pickar, D. B. (1986). Psychosocial aspects of learning disabilities: a review of the research. *Bull. Menninger Clin.* 50:22–32.

Power, P. W. (1984). Adolescent reaction to parental neurological illness: coping and intervention strategies. *Pediatr. Soc. Work* 3:45–52.

Pribram, K. H., and Gill, M. M. (1976). *Freud's "Project" Re-assessed.* New York: Basic Books.

Prigatano, G. P. (1988). Anosognosia, delusions and altered self-awareness after brain injury: a historical perspective. *BNI Q.* 5:40–48.

Prigatano, G. P., Fordyce, D. J., Zeiner, H. K., Roueche, J. R., Pepping, M., and Wood, B. C. (1984). Neuropsychological rehabilitation after closed head injury in young adults. *J. Neurol. Neurosurg. Psychiatry* 47:505–513.

Rangell, L. (1985). Defense and resistance in psychoanalysis and life. In H. P. Blum (ed.), *Defense and Resistance: Historical Perspectives and Current Concepts.* New York: International Universities Press.

Rapaport, D. (1951). Toward a theory of thinking. In D. Rapaport (ed.), *Organization and Pathology of Thought.* New York: Columbia University Press.

Rapaport, D., Gill, M. M., and Schafer, R. (1968). *Diagnostic Psychological Testing.* New York: International Universities Press.

Reich, W. (1933). *Character Analysis.* New York: Pocket Books.

Reiser, L. W. (1987). Denial of physical illness in adolescence: collaboration of patient, family and physicians. *Psychoanal. Study Child* 42:385–402.

Reiser, M. F. (1984). *Mind, Brain, Body: Toward A Convergence of Psychoanalysis and Neurobiology.* New York: Basic Books.

Reiter, H. H., and Penzel, F. (1983). Psychological aspects of systemic lupus erythematosus. *Asian J. Psychol. Educ.* 11:5–18.

Shapiro, D. (1965). *Neurotic Styles.* New York: Basic Books.

Shevrin, H., and Taussieng, P. W. (1965). Vicissitudes of the need for tactile stimulation in instinctual development. *Psychoanal. Study Child* 209:310–339.

Silberfarb, P. M., and Greer, S. (1982). Psychological concomitants of cancer: clinical aspects. *Am. J. Psychother.* 36:470–478.

Smith, A. R. (1986). Alcoholism and gender: pattern of diagnosis and response. *J. Drug Issues* 16:407–420.

Spitz, R. (1961). Some early prototypes of ego defenses. *J. Am. Psychoanal. Assoc.* 9:626–651.

Stern, J. M. (1985). The psychotherapeutic process with brain-injured patients: a dynamic approach. *Isr. J. Psychiatry Relat. Sci.* 22:83–87.

Sulloway, F. (1979). *Freud: Biologist of the Mind.* New York: Basic Books.

Vaillant, G. E. (1986). Introduction. In G. E. Vaillant (ed.), *Empirical Studies of Ego Mechanisms of Defenses.* Washington, DC: American Psychiatric Press.

Valenstein, A. F. (1985). Working through and resistance to change: insight and the action system. In H. P. Blum (ed.), *Defense and Resistance: Historical Perspectives and Current Concepts.* New York: International Universities Press.

Wallerstein, R. S. (1976). Psychoanalysis as a science: its present status and its future tasks. In M. M. Gill and P. S. Holzman (eds.), *Psychology Versus Metapsychology: Psychoanalytic Essays in Memory of George S. Klein.* New York: International Universities Press.

Wheelis, A. (1971). *The Illusionless Man.* New York: Harper & Row.

Willick, M. S. (1985). On the concept of primitive defenses. In H. P. Blum (ed.), *Defense and Resistance: Historical Perspectives and Current Concepts.* New York: International Universities Press.

Young, J. Z. (1988). Hunting the homunculus. *New York Review* February 4, pp. 24–26.

13
Anosognosia and Denial of Illness

EDWIN A. WEINSTEIN

Neurological studies of anosognosia and denial go back a century to Von Monakow (1885), Anton (1896), and Babinski (1914). After these classic descriptions, anosognosia for hemiplegia was attributed to a lesion in the nondominant parietal lobe, thalamus, or corticothalamic connections and was explained as a disruption of the body image (Cobb, 1947; Critchley, 1953), as a hemispatial agnosia (Hécaen, Penfield, Bertrand, and Malmo, 1956), and as a failure to integrate sensory stimuli at the cortical level (Denny-Brown and Banker, 1954). Anton (1899) regarded his patients' inability to recognize their blindness as the result of pathology in association areas, disconnecting vision from "general perceptual synthesis."

Supporters of the focal lesion view pointed to the much more frequent occurrence of anosognosia for left hemiplegia than right hemiplegia and noted that many of the patients appeared to be mentally clear. As expressed by Gerstmann (1942), "it [anosognosia] does not necessarily entail lowering of general cortical or mental function. Indeed, the patients are not as a rule demented. Their sensorium, orientation, attention, and judgment are good except for the amnestic agnosic disturbance in the sphere of body awareness and recognition."

Other writers held that anosognosia was but one manifestation of a more widespread disturbance of function. It was noted that denial of hemiplegia could occur with pathology in areas other than the parietal lobe and thalamus, and that denial of blindness might be associated with lesions anywhere in the visual pathway. Redlich and Dorsey (1945) reported patients who denied both hemiplegia and blindness, and Sandifer (1946) commented that the condition was often preceded by a period of coma, confusion, or both. Redlich and Bonvicini (1908) regarded denial of blindness not as an agnosia but as a Korsakoff syndrome occurring in a blind person.

Some authors emphasized motivational and adaptive factors. Schilder (1932) spoke of "organic repression" whereby the patient excluded the unpalatable facts of hemiplegia or blindness from consciousness. Kurt Goldstein regarded anosognosia as a defense against the catastrophic reaction. Babinski remarked how the relatives of his patients considered their delusions providential.

In psychiatry before World War II, denial of external reality was seen in the context of a delusion: as a manifestation of psychosis and regression to an infantile state. In psychoanalysis, denial was considered mainly in terms of defenses against inner drives and repressing alien impulses and keeping them out of consciousness. World War II and the Holocaust did much to change this orientation in that these events directed attention toward adaptation to external stresses and the dynamics of survival. It became increasingly evident that denial was a mechanism by which normal persons coped with stressful life events. During the 1950s and 1960s, reports on denial and other forms of adaptation to traumatic life experiences such as those of the concentration camp and to physical illnesses and injuries, bereavement, and other forms of deprivation began to appear. Other developments in psychiatry were the growth of ego psychology, with its emphasis on relations with the outer world and problem solving, and interest in the phenomena of depersonalization and derealization, which indicated that the perception of reality was a more complex process than had hitherto been recognized.

CLINICAL DEFINITION

Operationally, denial is the product of a dyadic interaction in which the observer interprets the patient's behavior, particularly his responses to questions about disability and his behavior in situations in which his capacities are being tested. So regarded, denial takes many forms and is expressed in various spheres of function. A hemiplegic patient may say that he is not paralyzed and claim that he is perfectly well; or he may admit some weakness and assign it a trivial cause. He may not deny the paralysis explicitly but express delusions about the affected member, disowning it or referring to it as a foreign body. Some patients respond to questions about their disabilities with jokes and puns, such as the man with a left hemiparesis who said his main trouble was a "malicious wife." Others caricature their disabilities as did the man with a pituitary tumor who walked about with a lordotic gait and claimed he was pregnant. Others ignore questions about illness or reply in irrelevant fashion, or they respond in dysarthric, inaudible tones. When discussing Babinski's original paper, Souques described the behavior of a physician patient with a left hemiplegia who "forgot" his left side and when the word "hemiparesis" was mentioned to him seemed not to pay attention. Denial is thus a concept that provides unity to phenomena that might otherwise be regarded as discrete disturbances in cognition, perception, attention, or affect.

I have preferred the term denial rather than anosognosia for several reasons. One is that anosognosia has become synonymous with nonrecognition of hemiplegia to the exclusion of other disabilities. Second, anosognosia literally means lack of knowledge of disease, and patients often demonstrate such knowledge at some level of awareness. For example, a woman who admitted that she could not move her limbs on one side denied that she was paralyzed, and another patient denied that he had had a craniotomy but complained of the sawing and hammering on his head. Another aspect is that the type of interview can influence the degree of denial (Jaffe and Slote, 1958). Moreover, there is the matter of selectivity. When a patient with a left-sided weakness is asked to raise his left hand, he may lift the right hand but carry out other tests of left-right orientation correctly. Patients are delusional only about a member of the body the function of which is in some way impaired. They do not disown or otherwise misdesignate normally functioning limbs. Moreover, the delusions and metaphors are usually pejorative, such as "a piece of rusty machinery" or "dead wood," indicating knowledge that something is amiss. Finally, the word denial itself suggests that the patient's behavior has meaningful, motivational, and adaptive aspects.

There is denial of many types of disability other than blindness, left hemiplegia, and hemianopia. Those reported include denial of right hemiplegia, right hemianopia, aphasia, alexia, deafness, involuntary movements, paraplegia, loss of an amputated limb, the scars and contractures following severe burns with associated encephalopathy, incontinence, the fact of a craniotomy or head injury, and illness itself. Thus the deficit the patient denies is not necessarily the direct result of a lesion of the brain.

A patient may deny multiple disabilities, as illustrated strikingly in a case reported by Fink (1956). The patient was a 56-year-old man who had a cutdown right carotid angiogram after 6 months of headaches and episodes of ptosis of his right lid. During the procedure he suddenly developed a left hemiplegia and blindness and became drowsy and irrelevant in speech. The next day he denied not only his hemiplegia and loss of vision but also the cutdown despite a large bandage on his neck.

Patients with Huntington's disease commonly deny both their memory loss and the involuntary movements (Caine and Shoulson, 1983). Other patients with multiple deficits and traumatic experience do not deny them all. As noted by Cutting (1978), patients who deny or appear unaware of a hemiplegia may admit that they had a stroke. Our patient who joked about being pregnant agreed that his failing vision was due to his pituitary tumor. Alternatively, a patient may use one form of denial for one incapacity and another for some other deficit. A man who had suffered a skull fracture resulting in a bitemporal hemianopsia along with a fractured wrist denied his visual loss and, when questioned about his arm, was likely to tell a joke about playing pinochle and masturbating, in which the punch line was, "If you have a good hand, you don't need a partner."

As Babinski noted in his characterization of anisodiaphoria, some hemiplegic patients admit to their paralyses but show no interest or concern. Such patients do not seem to regard the affected limbs or other deficits as part of the self. They may admit that the limbs do not move but claim that they (the patients) themselves, are well and capable of working. They may refer to the paralyzed arm as an inanimate object or personify it as a living being, as "a little baby." Patients frequently refer to an affected extremity or even themselves in the third person, as "he," "she," or "it." The patient who admitted that he had a pituitary tumor said later that he had felt that he had been talking about someone else. A wide range of emotions may be expressed. Some patients give a paralyzed limb a nickname such as "Charley" or "Little Joe"; Critchley reported the case of a man who called his paralyzed left arm "the Communist" because it would not work. A patient may even express revulsion and shout abuse at the bad side (Critchley, 1974). When one of our patients dropped something from his left hand, he swore, "I'll make that son of a bitch behave." Cutting (1978) has grouped such delusions, personifications, and other misdesignations of the affected limb under the heading anosognosic phenomena.

Patients with explicit verbal denial are usually bland, affable, and unconcerned. They persist in their beliefs despite repeated demonstration of their disabilities; and despite the denial, they accept medication and submit to procedures without protest. Those with partial and implicit forms of denial or anosognosic phenomena are more apt to be overtly disturbed, displaying euphoric, depressive, and paranoid attitudes. It must be pointed out that the various forms of denial are not mutually exclusive, and a patient during the course of an illness may show more than one form.

ADAPTIVE ASPECTS

Denial is more than the "vision nulle" of a negative scotoma but has positive, adaptive value. A patient may complain bitterly of blindness but, as the pathological process progresses, may claim that he can see. As denial clears during the course of clinical recovery, patients may become agitated and depressed. This sequence of events is exemplified in the following case.

> A 22-year-old Korean War paratrooper veteran developed a subdural hematoma of the left cerebral hemisphere as the consequence of a car accident that left him comatose for 2 weeks. On examination 19 days after the accident, he was ambulatory and had a right homonymous hemianopia and a selective jargon aphasia. There was little visual neglect. He understood conversational speech and denied any difficulty speaking or with vision. When asked what had happened to him he replied, "I don't know, some form of malformation of the transmission." When asked where he was, he said he was in "a store for boys." Neutral questions were answered correctly. When naming objects he used pseudomilitary terminology for several objects, such as calling a magazine an "organizational file." In an interview 5 days later, he again denied trouble with his speech and boasted that he could speak four languages: English, Japanese, Russian, and "Kentuckian." When asked about his injury, he confabulated that he had been hurt in a parachute jump. Five days later he used no jargon, admitted that he had trouble understanding people, and said his right eye was weak. He was no longer euphoric but depressed and agitated to the point that he was transferred to a psychiatric floor. His disturbed state lasted for a week, after which his hospital behavior was unremarkable except for the lasting presence of a reduplicative delusion. He claimed that two girls had been in the car with him [actually one girl, who had sustained a fractured arm] and that the "other" girl was

uninjured because he had kept her head from striking the windshield (Weinstein, Cole, Mitchell, and Lyerly, 1964).

DENIAL AND CONFABULATION

Confabulations, defined as fictitious narratives without intent to deceive, may be classified in a number of ways. Some are fantastic and bizarre; others are mundane and plausible. Some are associated with memory loss; others are not. Some appear relevant to the patient's situation; others are not related. Although some confabulations, particularly fantastic ones, may be spontaneous, the great majority offered by brain-injured subjects are elicited in response to questions about illness and disability. These patients may negate, minimize, rationalize, or dramatize the traumatic aspects of the situation. Although such confabulations are ostensibly references to *past* events, they are also metaphorical or symbolic representations of *current* problems and disabilities.

For example, a soldier with a third nerve palsy caused by a ruptured aneurysm confabulated that he had been punched in the eye in a fight over a girl. The day after a painful carotid angiogram, an officer gave a fictitious account of having conducted the hanging of a deserter during World War II. An elderly officer hospitalized for cardiorespiratory difficulties did not explicitly deny them but told stories of having been gassed in World War I and of having ordered the bulldozing over of caves on Okinawa in World War II so thousands of civilians were suffocated. When he went on to say that he had been in a shell explosion and had his intestines blown out of his rectum "like a bunch of grapes you could have made a barrel of wine from," I asked him if he had hemorrhoids. He had. In general, the more elaborate and fantastic the confabulation, the less apt the patient is to explicitly deny injury and disability.

Patients may continue to confabulate even while indicating knowledge of the actual events, as in the case of the man who said, "I know it says in my [hospital] record that I was in an automobile accident but what happened was. . . ." A few patients, although confabulating in formal interviews, did not do so when questioned by members of their families. Veridical events may serve in lieu of confabulated ones in the sense that they may be symbolic representations of the patient's problems. A soldier who had sustained a crushing head injury in combat in Korea had been committed to a mental hospital by his wife over his protests. When asked about his injury he would go into a long story of his courtship of his wife, invariably including the fact that on their first date they had gone to see the film "Samson and Delilah."

The content of the confabulations that follow brain injury is determined by a number of factors. One, as has been indicated, is the nature of the patient's disability and traumatic experience. The second has to do with stimuli from the immediate environment. Thus a patient undergoing a lumbar puncture following a head injury caused by falling downstairs confabulated that he had come to the hospital to have shrapnel from a war wound removed from his back. A third factor is related to popular current events. The officer who confabulated after his carotid angiogram about a hanging did so when the book *The Trial of Private Slovik* (about the only American soldier executed for desertion during World War II) was a best seller and prominent in the news. The fourth determinant concerns past experience and values, particularly those themes that have been important sources of identity, and elements of patterns of social relatedness. Thus paratroopers who sustained head injuries in car accidents often confabulated that they had been hurt jumping.

A study of the confabulations of 58 patients recovering from brain injury (Weinstein and Lyerly, 1968) showed that the most common confabulatory theme was that of family, such as a story that a brother had been in the accident or that the patient had come to the hospital for his wife to be operated on. Confabulations of violence—someone killed or shot, or "I was in a fight"—were next in frequency. Confabulation about minor illnesses such as the patient claiming that he came to the hospital for a sprained ankle were common but were brief and not sustained. Confabulations about play and sports were also brief, whereas those about work and occupation were the longest and most elaborate. These categories were arbitrary, and most confabulations fell under more than one heading. An officer admitted to Bethesda Naval Hospital after a head injury sustained in a car accident in Spain said he had come to the hospital to enter his son in some athletic contests.

The following case illustrates the adaptive role of confabulation.

A 68-year-old retired officer was admitted to Walter Reed Army Hospital after a stroke that left him with a right hemiparesis, sensory loss, and a mild aphasia. He did not deny these impairments but told the story that he had been riding in the back of an open truck when his right side became frozen [it was winter]. He said he had ordered the sergeant in the driver's cab to stop but because of the roaring of the wind he could not be understood.

For this patient the fictional account may have imparted a *feeling* of belief because it gave order and predictability to a catastrophic event and preserved his sense of identity. In any case the "inner reality" expressed in the military metaphor took precedence over the external reality. This aspect of confabulation helps to explain why patients persist in their fictitious accounts despite the obvious disbelief of their auditors and all arguments to the contrary. An otherwise apathetic patient may become animated during a confabulatory narrative.

Confabulations clear in the course of time, but they may not vanish without trace. The themes may persist in the patient's emotional attitudes and social relationships. For example, a patient who confabulated that a silver plate had been put into his head became obsessed with repairing the roofs of his farm property. He insisted on going ahead against the advice of his colleagues, even though, prior to his head injury, he had decided that the expensive project was not worth the cost. His judgment in other areas was not impaired. In another case a patient confabulated that two of his children had been with him in the car. He made a good clinical improvement except for some residual diplopia. After his return home he became extremely protective of his children. He forbade them to watch television for fear of eye strain and did not permit his daughter to ride her horse because she might fall off (Weinstein and Lyerly, 1968).

DENIAL AND AMNESIA

There is also a relation between denial and retrograde amnesia, defined as the statement that the person does not remember a traumatic experience and contiguous preceding events (Weinstein, Marvin, and Keller, 1962). A soldier injured in a car crash may state that he does not remember the accident or anything over the prior 2 weeks or even being in the army. No one who has been knocked unconscious recalls the impact—there are exceptions, notably among persons who develop conversion reactions—but when the nonamnesic patient is asked what happened to him he says that he was in a car accident, even though he does not remember the actual impact. When questioned further, he goes on to give the gist of what occurred. The amnesic patient on the other hand is likely to persist with, "I don't know" or "I don't remember," despite having been told many times and even though he is in a hospital bed, perhaps with a bandage on his head and a cast on a limb.

These patients seem to have lost the sense of the reality of their experience, much as the anosognosic patient with anosognosia for hemiplegia does not believe he is really paralyzed or that the affected limb belongs to him. A man who had received a head wound in Korea refused to accept a Purple Heart decoration, stating that if he had really been wounded he would have known it. Patients sustaining head injuries in car accidents commonly insist on seeing a photograph of the wreck before they believe it really happened.

As with anosognosia and confabulation, patients often show implicit knowledge of events from the amnesic time period. Thus soldiers who did not remember having been in the army used army slang and showed familiarity with military procedures, such as knowing how to get paid. During clinical recovery patients recalled aspects of their military service—not usually in chronological order—but spoke of not remembering if they had been drafted or had enlisted or even the exact type of work they had done, indicating a feeling of unfamiliarity and a sense of noninvolvement. Confabulation of events that never occurred may fill such an anomic void.

Retrograde amnesia is also related to denial and confabulation in that the last thing the patient remembers before his accident and finding himself in the hospital may be a symbolic representation of current disabilities and problems. The "last memory" may be a veridical occurrence, an actual event displaced in space and time, or a confabulation. The "last memory" of a soldier who was left with a severe visual loss after a car accident was of looking at Hitler's castle in Berchtesgaden through a telescope. Particularly poignant "last memories" were given by patients who had head injuries in accidents in which someone had been killed. Here the last thing the patient remembered was "going to sleep the night before," "falling asleep in the back seat of the car," "passing out at drill." These symbolic representations of death were made by patients who apparently did not know of the fatality.

DENIAL AND REDUPLICATION

Delusional reduplication, like confabulation, may serve as a vehicle for denial and various forms of symbolic representation of deficits. With reduplication of place, the patient states that there are two or more places of the same name although only one exists. Reduplication of persons, objects, events, animals, and parts of the body also occurs, and one form commonly accompanies another provided the examiner specifically questions the subject. A patient who sustained bifrontal contusions in a car wreck claimed that there were three Bethesda Naval Hospitals, and that the nurse on the floor also worked for the doctor in his home town. A woman who reduplicated objects said another bed had been substituted for hers. Reduplication for event or time is an enduring déjà vu experience, as a patient awaiting surgery may say he has had the operation before. Hemiplegic patients may claim that they have two or more left (or right) arms.

The two or more places, persons, objects, events, or parts of the body are never identical but differ in some way that is germane to the patient's experiences, motives, feelings, or problems. The "extra" place or person can be thought of as a reification of emotionally significant experience, not simply as a disturbance of memory as the term "paramnesia" implies. Following Pick (1903), one of the first cases was described by Head (1926). The patient was a British soldier who had sustained a frontal missile wound during World War I. He thought that there were two towns of Boulogne in France, one you passed on the way to the front and the other you traversed on the way home. Head remarked that the man was rational in all other respects except that he wrote letters to his mother even though she had been dead for many years.

Reduplication for place in hospitalized patients usually involves the hospital, and the fictitious substitution is apt to be "convalescent place," "a branch" or "annex," or be located in the patient's home town or neighborhood. A man hospitalized with multiple fractures thought that there were three Walter Reed Hospitals: one for head injuries, one for fractures, and one for plastic surgery. A patient with reduced vision caused by a pituitary tumor compressing the optic chiasm claimed that his private nurse had a daughter who took care of him on alternate days. He said that mother and daughter looked exactly alike except that the "mother" wore eyeglasses. (His vision was good enough to identify famous faces.) A patient of Ullman (1960) with a left hemiplegia told him that her own left arm was all right, but that the "other left arm" felt so strange that it must belong to her dead husband. We (Weinstein and Kahn, 1955) have cited the case of the man who claimed that he had several heads. He had had a craniotomy for a posterior fossa tumor following which he developed purulent drainage from the operative site. He said that his own head had bad drainage, but that the other ones were fine and functioning well. When I commented that it was unusual to have more than one head, he replied that if a person could have a number of hats he could have lots of heads.

Feelings of unreality and depersonalization may precede the appearance of reduplication and be associated with them in a manner similar to the concurrence of jamais vu and déjà vu experience. A patient reported by Staton, Brumback, and Wilson (1982) had feelings of unreality during the months after his head injury, followed 4 years later by déjà vu phenomena; 8 years after his accident he reported the belief that his close relatives were doubles and not the people he had known. Even his cat was not real because of a new scar on the animal's ear.

Capgras syndrome, the illusion of doubles, is a form of delusional reduplication in which the patient claims that someone, usually a person or persons close to him, has been replaced by an impostor(s). As with other types of reduplication, the difference between the "original" and the "other" is a representation and reification of the patient's own experience. The Capgras phenomenon was once regarded as a rare, exotic phenomenon confined to paranoid schizophrenics, but in more recent years there have been reports of its occurrence after head injuries, in dementing conditions, and strokes. Alexander, Stuss, and Benson (1979) described the case of a 44-year-old man who developed grandiose paranoid delusions and auditory hallucinations over a period of several months and then sustained a head injury when he was struck by a car. A craniotomy revealed a large subdural hematoma and necrotic right frontal lobe. A later CT scan showed right frontal and temporal atrophy and decreased density in the left inferior medial frontal lobe. Ten months after his accident he had marked retrograde amnesia and expressed the reduplicative delusion that he now lived with a "different" family that was identical with his "original" family in all respects but one: The children of his first family were about 1 year younger than those in the second family. These differences appear to be the patient's symbolic representation of his own feelings of being different and the length of his disability, which he estimated as 18 months. The authors noted that the patient expressed positive feelings toward "both" wives, showing no anger or distress over the first wife's desertion. In a case reported by Christoudoulou (1977) a depressed woman developed Capgras syndrome after a bout of pneumonia with high fever and disorientation. She thought that her two daughters were dead and had been replaced by doubles. She also had nonaphasic misnaming, referring to her bedclothes as "shrouds." The idea that features of the putative double are a symbolic representation of the patient's own feelings helps to explain why, despite ideas of impersonation and deceptive masquerading by the double, patients are usually friendly or indifferent toward the putative imposters.

As with confabulation, the occurrence and character of the reduplicative delusion depends not only on the milieu of brain dysfunction but the patient's problems and disabilities as well as on past experience. Whereas with confabulation the referential and experiential symbolic aspects are ostensibly merged, with reduplication they are separate in that the real hospital or person is a referential designation, and the fictitious one represents the patient's idiosyncratic experience.

DISORIENTATION AND NONAPHASIC MISNAMING

Disorientation for place and misidentification of objects, like confabulation and reduplication, are often associated with denial and may be ways of expressing it. Hospitalized patients do not often deny that they are in a hospital but usually give the name of a hospital associated with home or work. Patients seen at Walter Reed Hospital were apt to say they were in Fort Jackson or Camp Lee Station Hospital, depending on their post of duty. Some used euphemisms such as "Walter Reed Rest and Rehabilitation Center." The name offered may also express the patient's feelings, as "Mount Sinai Butcher Shop," or represent the patient's disability in condensed metaphorical fashion. A hemiplegic patient seen at the Bronx Veterans Hospital near the Kingsbridge Armory referred to it as the "Veterans Armless Hospital."

Patients are apt to persist in their misidentifications despite corrections, cues, and clues, such as having the correct name in full view on a name tag, desk plate, or bed linen. Moreover, as in the case of the patient at Mount Sinai who called the hospital "Mount Cyanide," there may be evidence that he "knows" the proper name. A patient who is disoriented for place is not necessarily confused in the sense in which that term is often misused. I recall an officer at Walter Reed who maintained that he was at Fort Sill—he would cross out the Walter Reed inscription on the Red Cross stationery—but who otherwise showed no behavioral disorders. A patient may name and locate the hospital correctly but greatly condense the distance between the hospital and his home or place of business (Weinstein and Kahn, 1951). One of our subjects correctly named and located the hospital and accurately estimated the distance from his home as 400 miles "on the map." When then asked how long it would take him to get home, he replied he could get there in 5 minutes.

Patients selectively misname objects having to do with illness, hospitalization, and occupation while correctly identifying items of equal familiarity and complexity, such as calling a head bandage a "turban," a doctor's bag an "attaché case," or a wheelchair an "arm chair." Moreover, subjects do not accept correction, as in the case of the woman who said, "I know you call it a hospital bed, but I call it a chaise lounge." Dr. Stefan Shanzer observed a patient who identified a "chair with wheels" but refused to call it a wheelchair. Such behavior cannot be attributed to a defect in memory or perception or to a variety of aphasia. As with confabulation and reduplication, the patient appears to be operating on two cognitive levels. Also, as pointed out by Zaidel (1987), the functional deficit that results in the cognitive error may be dissociated from the one that prevents the patient from correcting it.

DENIAL AND HEMINEGLECT

Anosognosia for hemiplegia and hemianopia and hemineglect have been traditionally associated (Critchley, 1953; Weinstein and Kahn, 1955) and share a number of features. They occur under similar conditions of brain dysfunction, with a predominance of right brain over left brain lesions. Each is frequently associated with other alterations of behavior: mood change, disorientation for place or time, and reduplicative phenomena. As with anosognosia, patients with hemineglect may display implicit knowledge of things and events on the affected side of the body and circumambient hemispace. The patient with hemineglect usually walks about the floor without colliding with objects or people. When

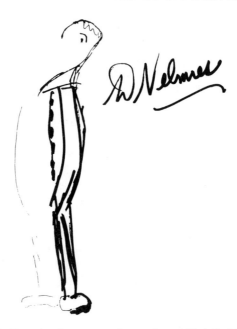

Figure 13–1. Drawing by a man who neglected his left side. See text.

reading words such as *brake* and *clever,* the patient with left-sided neglect is more apt to read *rake* and *lever* or *ever* than the nonwords *ake* or *ver.* On drawings he may selectively omit only one ear of a person. Figure 13–1, drawn by a man who neglected his left side, indicates an awareness of that side and suggests a recognition of its lifeless, ghostly quality.

Almost all patients with anosognosia for hemiplegia and hemianopia show some neglect, but most patients with marked hemineglect do not explicitly deny their disabilities. Weinstein and Friedland (1977) found explicit verbal denial in 12 of 30 patients with left hemineglect and 7 of 12 with right-sided neglect. Patients with conspicuous hemineglect are more apt to show forms of implicit denial with mood changes such as withdrawal and depression or comic tragic ludic behavior, often with sexual manifestations.

CONDITIONS OF BRAIN DYSFUNCTION

Brain damage is not a necessary prerequisite for denial. Rather, the state of brain function determines the *pattern* in which denial is expressed and maintained and, to some degree, the circumstances in which it is elicited. Denial is a major mode of adaptation to stress by people who do not have structural brain disease. Feelings of depersonalization, unreality, detachment from one's body, and lack of emotion are common among people exposed to life-threatening danger (Noyes and Kletti, 1976). Such experiences are analogous to the belief that a paralyzed limb does not belong to one's self, and that it is someone else who is sick. Moreover, these experiences may involve comparable changes in cortico-limbic relations on a biochemical level.

Although anosognosia following brain injury is commonly regarded as a manifestation of right cerebral hemisphere pathology, it is important to note that denial with left hemisphere lesions is not rare. In case series of anosognosia for hemiplegia, Nathanson, Bergman, and Gordon (1952) found a right hemisphere predominance of 2:1, whereas Cutting (1978) reported a ratio of 4:1 and Hécaen (1962) noted a right hemisphere predominance of 8:1. Cases of denial of aphasia are common (Weinstein et al., 1964; Sandson, Albert, and Alexander, 1986; Lebrun, 1987). In our initial study (Weinstein and Kahn, 1955), which included denial not only of hemiplegia and blindness but also of aphasia, involuntary movements, paraparesis, incontinence, loss of a limb, and craniotomy, there were three times as many right hemisphere as left hemisphere lesions. However, the number of patients with pathology involving both hemispheres exceeded those with lesions confined to a single hemisphere.

The lesions involving the hemispheres were extensive and most frequently involved the frontal and parietal lobes. Temporal lobe pathology, which was mainly neoplastic, extended into other areas and was associated with hemiparesis. Denial occurred with lesions of the cingulate area and other mesial paralimbic structures, basal ganglia, diencephalon, and upper brain stem. Almost all the pathology was of neoplastic, vascular, or traumatic origin. We concluded at the time that the necessary conditions for the existence of anosognosia were provided by lesions that, by reason of acute onset, progressive course, bilateral location, or association with edema or hemorrhage, involved corticolimbic connections and produced dysfunction of both hemispheres. We noted that enduring denial did not appear with focal lesions confined to the cortex, nor was anosognosia reported after right parietal cortical ablation (Hécaen et al., 1956; Weinstein and Cole, 1963) or even after hemispherectomy (Smith, 1969, 1972). These features indicate that the disordered neural mechanisms involved widely spaced networks and altered activity of both hemispheres.

A significant feature of anosognosia after strokes is its relatively transient nature. It is common for a patient with an acute hemiplegia to deny his paralysis on admission to the hospital but admit it a day or two later. A study of 41 patients with right hemisphere strokes by Hier, Mondlock, and Caplan (1983) showed denial in 14 patients with a median duration of 11 weeks compared to 19 weeks for hemineglect, 43 weeks for sensory extinction, and 64 weeks for arm and leg weakness. After delusional denial has cleared over the course of clinical recovery, it may again be elicited during the intravenous administration of Amytal Sodium (Weinstein, Kahn, Sugarman, and Linn, 1953; Weinstein, Kahn, Sugarman, and Malitz, 1953). All of these observations suggest that a bilateral neural substrate affecting cortical limbic relations is involved.

The delineation of the paralimbic cortex by Pandya and Seltzer (1982) and Mesulam (1985) is relevant to the subject of cortical limbic relations. The paralimbic cortex, which girdles the mesial and undersurfaces of the hemispheres connects with the other multimodal sensory association cortices and with primary limbic structures. The cingulate gyrus has extensive connections with the posterior parietal and prefrontal areas. The network is responsive to the affective relevance of stimuli—to the pleasures of food and the suffering of pain, as Broca suggested a century ago—with particular reference to those concerned with coping in the environment and survival. When this network is damaged in man, the brain registers the stimulus but not its conventional emotional significance. Thus the hemiplegic patient may recognize that his limbs on one side do not move but he does not believe that he is paralyzed or even that the limbs belong to him; yet another example is the patient who is shown the scar of a craniotomy but still does not regard the operation of having been part of her experience. [Pain asymbolia, in which the patient feels the sharpness of a pinprick but not its noxious quality, is often present in nonverbal denial syndromes (Weinstein, Kahn, and Slote, 1955).] The stimulus, however, is meaningful in the context of values and past experience, as in the case of the army officer for whom the novel events of a stroke made "sense" in a military setting.

Why are right hemisphere lesions more common than those of the left hemisphere? An aspect related to hemineglect is that the right hemisphere has more control of attentional-motivational processes, but it does not explain the cognitive features. The fact that many patients with left hemisphere damage are aphasic is not the entire reason because relatively few aphasic patients cannot comprehend and give a yes or no answer to a question of whether they have a paralysis or trouble speaking. Language, however, may play a role in that left hemisphere function is necessary for the production of the metaphors, similes, personifications, imagery, delusions, and confabulations that impart a feeling of validity to the denial. Thus the patient who develops denial after a left brain lesion is either not aphasic or only mildly so, or he has a jargon type of aphasia associated with disorientation, reduplication, confabulation, or nonaphasic misnaming, phenomena that may become clearer during the course of clinical recovery from aphasia (Weinstein et al., 1964). Rather than regarding anosognosia for hemiplegia as a defect in some specialized right hemisphere function localized in the posterior parietal lobe, it is more useful to think of it in terms of frontoparietal and interhemispheric relations.

The work on the modular organization of cerebral function (Mountcastle, 1979), ideas of parallel distributed processing (Rumelhart and McClelland, 1986), and Edelman's (1987) theories of neuronal group selection offer an approach to the adaptive aspects of denial and the role of past experience and premorbid personality factors. The way in which one responds to novel situations depends on the nature of the stimulus, the environmental conditions under which it is encountered, one's expectations based on past experience, and the pattern of brain activity that is set up. The brain is made up of a number of neural networks that can receive input from the same sensory receptor; and because each group of neurons has its own pattern of internal connections each may respond differently to identical stimuli. Synaptic networks are shaped by developmental maturation and experience. Neural structures carry information from the environment, but the environment also acts dynamically on the potential orderings already represented by neural networks. According to Edelman, there is Darwinian competition among neuronal groups in the interests of survival, and the perception of reality is both veridical and adaptive. In situations of stress in which the integrity of the organism is threatened, groups whose activities are correlated with signals arising from adaptive behavior are selected. Although Edelman eschewed homunculi and strict localization of higher mental functions, it is likely that the prefrontal area plays a predominant role in determining which networks are activated and which are inhibited.

PERSONALITY FACTORS

Past experience and values and habitual modes of structuring the social environment influence the positive aspects of denial, its forms, and the content of confabulations and reduplicative delusions. The meaning of illness varies among people and may be closely tied to other aspects of personality.

For patients who developed explicit verbal denial, illness had been seen as a kind of personal failure or weakness involving a loss of prestige and integrity. When asked about their previous health, relatives and colleagues were apt to say that they were "never sick," or if they were the ailments had not interfered with work. Informants described the subjects as orderly, conscientious, independent, self-disciplined, controlling, work-oriented persons with a need to achieve and improve themselves. They were not seen as emotional or particularly empathic. They were concerned with principles and being right and had the ability to rationalize events so that they fit the principles. They emphasized will power and the idea that the flesh is the servant of the spirit.

Woodrow Wilson, who sought a third term as president of the United States after sustaining a massive stroke that resulted in a left hemiplegia had a prototypical "anosognosic personality." He believed that good health depended on following the rules for right living and carrying out God's teachings, so that illness represented a moral dereliction. Wilson was fond of saying that when he was unable to think of a word he did not, like other professors, wait for the word to come to him, but he *made* the word come (Weinstein, 1981).

The emphasis on work, responsibility, and success suggests features of Max Weber's Protestant ethic. Gainotti (1975) compared the incidence of explicit denial in a group of Calvinistic Protestant demented patients seen in a clinic in Geneva with a group of Catholic patients in Perugia, Italy. He found more denial among the Protestants.

Some differences were found between patients who expressed complete verbal denial in serene, unruffled fashion and those with paranoid forms of partial denial, such as attributing weakness of limb to being beaten, starved, or sexually abused. These patients also might have had a good deal of compulsive drive and a need to deny imperfections but were less concerned with principles and values and had expressed their feelings in more concrete fashion. They had been openly fearful and resentful about illness, as in not being able to stand the sight of blood, the smell of hospitals, or the pain of an injection. Emphasis on the physical was also shown in concerns with looks, dress, odors, food and diets, and the overt attributes of masculinity and femininity. It is impossible to assign a set of character traits to each of the manifold forms of denial that appear after specified brain damage, but there is ample evidence that premorbid experience is one determinant (Weinstein and Kahn, 1953).

SEQUELAE OF DENIAL

We were interested in learning if the presence or absence of denial during the acute stage after head injuries affected subsequent behavior. We followed a group of 118 patients with a mean age of 25 years seen initially at Walter Reed Army Hospital: 96 were classified as severe and 22 as moderately severe depending on the duration of unconsciousness. They were followed for periods of 3 to 13 years and were rated on three categories: (1) work record; (2) social, marital, and sexual adjustment; and (3) the presence of so-called postconcussion symptoms: inability to concentrate, nervousness, episodes of temper and violence. Markedly aphasic patients were excluded. The major findings were as follows.

1. Forty-five percent of the severely injured and thirty-six percent of the moderately severely injured subjects expressed verbal denial of the accident or injury (or both) during the initial hospitalization. The denial was not related to age, education, or marital status.
2. On follow-up the severely injured were worse off in all three categories.
3. Comparing the deniers and the nondeniers, there were no significant differences in problem scores of social adjustment and symptomatology, but the verbal denial group had a worse record of employment. My guess is that the latter was because these men were more perfectionistic, more apt to be dissatisfied with their performance, and less able to adjust to diminished capacity. Denial may be adaptive or maladaptive.

CLOSING COMMENTS

1. Denial/anosognosia in brain-injured persons has negative and positive features. It not only involves deficits in cognition, perception, and affect but has motivational and adaptive aspects.

2. Denial takes many forms operating at different levels of awareness: negation, minimization, avoidance, selective forgetting, ludic caricaturization, and delusional misrepresentation.

3. The existence and form of denial/anosognosia are determined by the location and rate of development of the brain lesion, the situation in which the denial is elicited, the type of disability, and the way the patient perceives its meaning on the basis of his past experience.

4. The necessary conditions of brain dysfunction for the maintenance of delusional denial are provided by disruption of networks interconnecting cortical and paralimbic association areas and limbic structures. The patient does not appreciate the emotional significance of stimuli from the affected part of the body or from the traumatic situation and the relevance of the stimuli to the self. At the same time other synaptic connections transform stimuli into symbolic

representations of an "inner" reality expressed in metaphor, personification, reduplication, confabulation, and other types of delusional misidentification.

5. Anosognosia/denial, the amnestic confabulatory state, and the delusional misidentification syndromes (e.g., Capgras syndrome) share a number of features.

REFERENCES

Alexander, M. P., Stuss, D. T., and Benson, D. F. (1979). Capgras syndrome: a reduplicative pehnomenon. *Neurology* 29:334–339.

Anton, G. (1896). Blindheit nach beiderseitiger Gehirnerkrankung mit Verlust der Orienterung in Raume. *Mitteil. Vereines Arzte Steirmark* 33:41–46.

Anton, G. (1899). Ueber die Selbstwahrnehmung der Herderkrankungen des Gehirns durch den Kranken bei Rindenblindheit und Rindentaubheit. *Arch. Psychiatr.* 32:86–127.

Babinski, J. (1914). Contribution a l'etude des troubles mentaux dans hémiplégie organique cérébrale (anosognosie). *Rev. Neurol. (Paris)* 27:845–847.

Caine, M. D., and Shoulson, I. (1983). Psychiatric syndromes in Huntington's disease. *Am. J. Psychiatry* 140:727–733.

Christoudoulou, G. N. (1977). The syndrome of Capgras. *Br. J. Psychiatry* 130:356–364.

Cobb, S. (1947). Amnesia for the left limbs developing into anosognosia. *Bull. Los Angeles Neurol. Soc.* 12:48–52.

Critchley, M. (1953). *The Parietal Lobes.* London: Edward Arnold.

Critchley, M. (1974). Misoplegia or hatred of hemiplegia. *The Mt. Sinai J. Med.* 41:82–87.

Cutting, J. (1978). Study of anosognosia. *J. Neurol. Neurosur. Psychiatry* 41:548–555.

Denny-Brown, D., and Banker, B. Q. (1954). Amorphosynthesis from left parietal lesions. *Arch. Neurol.* 71:302–313.

Edelman, G. (1987). *Neural Darwinism: Theory of Neuronal Group Selection.* New York: Basic Books.

Fink, M. (1956). Denial of blindness following cerebral angiography. *J. Hillside Hospital* 5:238–245.

Gainotti, G. (1975). Confabulation of denial in senile dementia. *Psychiatr. Clin.* 8:99–108.

Gerstmann, J. (1942). Problem of imperception of disease and of impaired body territories with organic lesions. *Arch. Neurol. Psychiatry* 48:890–913.

Goldstein, K. (1939). *The Organism.* New York: American Book Co.

Head, H. (1926). *Aphasia and Kindred Disorders of Speech.* Cambridge: University Press.

Hécaen, H. (1962). Clinical symptomatology of right and left hemisphere lesions. In V. B. Mountcastle (ed.), *Interhemisphere Relations and Cerebral Dominance.* Baltimore: Johns Hopkins Press.

Hécaen, H., Penfield, W., Bertrand, C., and Malmo, R. (1956). The syndrome of apractognosia due to lesions of the minor cerebral hemisphere. *A.M.A. Arch. Neurol. Psychiatry* 75:400–423.

Hier, D. B. and Mondlock, J. (1983). Behavioral abnormalities after right hemisphere stroke. *Neurology* 33:337–344.

Jaffe, J., and Slote W. H. (1958). Interpersonal factors in denial of illness. *AMA Arch. Neurol. Psychiatry* 80:653–656.

Lebrun, Y. (1987). Anosognosia in aphasics. *Cortex* 23:251–263.

Mesulam, M-M. (1985). *Principles of Behavioral Neurology*. Philadelphia: F. A. Davis.

Mountcastle, V. B. (1979). An organizing principle for cerebral function: the unit module and the distribution system. In F. O. Schmitt and F. G. Worden (eds.), *The Neurosciences. Fourth Study Program*. Cambridge, MA: MIT Press.

Nathanson, M., Bergman, P. S., and Gordon, G. G. (1952). Denial of illness, its occurrence in one hundred consecutive cases of hemiplegia. *A.M.A. Arch. Neurol. Psychiatry* 68:380–387.

Noyes, R., and Kletti, R. (1976). Depersonalization in the face of life threatening danger: a description. *Psychiatry* 39:19–27.

Pandya, D. P., and Seltzer, B. (1982). Association areas of the cerebral cortex. *Trends Neurosciences* 53:386–390.

Pick, A. (1903). On reduplicative paramnesia. *Brain* 26:260–267.

Redlich, E., and Bonvicini, G. (1908). Ueber das Fehlen der Wahrnehmung eigenen Blindheit hei Hirnkrankheiten. *Jahr. Psychiatr.* 29:1–134.

Redlich, F. C., and Dorsey, J. F. (1945). Denial of blindness by patients with cerebral disease. *Arch. Neurol. Psychiatry* 53:407–417.

Rumelhart, D. E., and McClelland, J. L. (1986). *Parallel Distributed Processing. Explorations in the Microstructure of Cognition. Vol. 1: Foundations*. Cambridge, MA: MIT Press.

Sandifer, P. H. (1946). Anosognosia and disorders of body scheme. *Brain* 69:122–137.

Sandson, J., Albert, M. L., and Alexander, M. P. (1986). Confabulation in aphasia. *Cortex* 22:621–626.

Schilder, P. (1932). Localization of the body image (postural model of the body). *Assoc. Res. Nerv. Ment. Dis.* 13:466–484.

Smith, A. (1969). Nondominant hemispherectomy. *Neurology* 19:442–445.

Smith, A. (1972). Dominant and nondominant hemispherectomy. In W. L. Smith (ed.), *Drugs, Development and Cerebral Function*. Springfield, Ill.: Charles Thomas.

Staton, R. D., Brumback, R. A., and Wilson, H. (1982). Reduplicative paramnesia, a disconnexion syndrome of memory. *Cortex* 18:23–85.

Ullman, M. (1960). Motivational and structural factors in denial of hemiplegia. *Arch. Neurol.* 3:306–318.

Von Monakow, A. (1885). Experimentelle and pathologischanatomisch Untersuchungen über die Beziehungen der sogennanten Sehspare zu den infracorticalen Opticuscentren und zum Nervus opticus. *Arch. Psychiatr.* 16:151–199.

Weinstein, E. A. (1981). *Woodrow Wilson: A Medical and Psychological Biography*. Princeton: Princeton Univ. Press.

Weinstein, E. A., and Cole, M. (1963). Concepts of anosognosia. In L. Halpern (ed.), *Problems of Dynamic Neurology*. Jerusalem: Dept of Nervous Diseases, Rothschild Hadassah Hospital Hebrew University.

Weinstein, E. A., and Friedland, R. P. (1977). Behavioral disorders associated with hemi-inattention. In E. A. Weinstein and R. P. Friedland (eds.), *Hemi-inattention and Hemisphere Specialization*. New York: Raven Press.

Weinstein, E. A., and Kahn, R. L. (1951). Patterns of disorientation in organic brain disease. *J. Neuropathol. Clin. Neurol.* 1:214–225.

Weinstein, E. A., and Kahn, R. L. (1955). *Denial of Illness: Symbolic and Physiological Aspects*. Springfield, IL: Charles C Thomas.

Weinstein, E. A., and Lyerly, O. G. (1968). Confabulation following brain injury. *Arch. Gen. Psychiatry* 18:348–354.

Weinstein, E. A., Cole, M., Mitchell, M. S., and Lyerly, O. G. (1964). Anosognosia and aphasia. *Arch. Neurology* 10:376–386.

Weinstein, E. A., Kahn, R. L., and Slote, W. (1955). Withdrawal, inattention and pain asymbolia. *A.M.A. Arch. Neurol. Psychiatry* 74:235–246.

Weinstein, E. A., Kahn, R. L., Sugarman, L. A., and Linn, L. (1953). Diagnostic use of amobarbital sodium ("Amytal Sodium") in brain disease. *Am. J. Psychiatry* 109:889–894.

Weinstein, E. A., Kahn, R. L., Sugarman, L. A., and Malitz, S. (1943). Serial administration of the "Amytal test" for brain disease: its diagnostic and prognostic value. *A.M.A. Arch. Neurol. Psychiatry* 71:217–226.

Weinstein, E. A., Lyerly, O. G., Cole, M., and Ozer, M. (1966). Meaning in jargon aphasia. *Cortex* 2:165–187.

Weinstein, E. A., Marvin, S. L., and Keller, N. J. A. (1962). Amnesia as a language pattern. *Arch. Gen. Psychiatry* 6:259–270.

Zaidel, E. (1987). Hemispheric monitoring. In D. Ottoson (ed.), *Duality and Unity of the Brain*. London: Macmillan.

14
Forms of Unawareness

DANIEL L. SCHACTER
AND GEORGE P. PRIGATANO

The chapters in this volume testify to the rich variety of phenomena that can be observed and the questions that arise when considering unawareness of deficit after brain injury. The fact that such unawareness has been documented in at least some patients from virtually all the major neuropsychological syndromes underscores the clinical pervasiveness of awareness disturbances and their potentially widespread theoretical implications. Despite the seemingly boundless diversity of this subject, however, the preceding chapters suggest four main theoretical and clinical reasons why unawareness of deficits is a potentially revealing and rewarding topic for further investigation.

First, systematic study of the clinical phenomena should provide an empirical foundation for developing a neuropsychological approach to understanding the brain systems and neural mechanisms involved in awareness. Various aspects of this theme are developed in the chapters by Bisiach and Geminiani, Heilman, Stuss, McGlynn and Kaszniak, Prigatano, Schacter, and Goldberg and Barr. Second, research concerning unawareness of deficits can also contribute to the development of cognitive theories of awareness. Just as the study of patients with selective impairments of language, memory, perception, reading, or other neuropsychological deficits has influenced cognitive theories about normal function in each of these domains, investigation of anosognosia represents a potentially rich source of insight for cognitive approaches to awareness and consciousness. Although cognitive psychologists have thus far paid scant attention to the sort of unawareness phenomena discussed in this volume, the chapters by Bisiach and Geminiani, Rubens and Garrett, Schacter, Johnson, and Kihlstrom and Tobias indicate various ways in which cognitive theories about awareness could benefit from serious consideration of anosognosic phenomena. Third, unawareness of deficits has major implications for rehabilitation of brain-damaged patients: Patients who are unaware of their deficits are unlikely to seek or accept treatment. A number of these implications are delineated in Prigatano's chapter. Fourth, as discussed by Lewis and by Weinstein, defensive or motivated denial plays a role in manifestations of unawareness in some brain-damaged patients. Because defensive denial has been approached traditionally within a purely psychiatric framework, study of the subset of brain-damaged patients who exhibit defensive denial represents an opportunity to develop a neuropsychological approach to this important phenomenon.

The foregoing chapters illuminate various issues in each of these four key areas. They also remind us that programmatic research on unawareness of deficits has barely begun and that relevant phenomena remain poorly understood. It is clear that numerous key questions need to be addressed: How can unawareness of deficits be measured more adequately? What are the neural mechanisms that normally allow patients to become aware of their deficits, and what is the nature of the impairment that produces unawareness? What role does confabulation play in awareness disturbances? Does unawareness of deficit occur in patients with otherwise normal cognitive functions, or is it observed only in the context of broader intellectual impairment or confusion? What is the natural history of unawareness in different patient groups? What are the possibilities for developing effective remedial interventions for those patients in whom unawareness of deficit interferes with everyday functioning? The development of answers to these and other questions raised by the authors in this volume is essential to improving our currently meager understanding of awareness and unawareness of deficit after brain injury.

After considering this volume, however, we have become convinced that progress in understanding these questions likely depends on coming to grips with a fundamental, yet little discussed, issue that we refer to as the problem of *forms of unawareness*. One of the unfortunate consequences of the widespread tendency to describe patients as either "aware" or "unaware" of their deficits is that such terms imply that unawareness of deficit is a monolithic or unitary entity. Yet a number of chapters in this volume suggest that it is important to distinguish among various types or forms of unawareness of deficit. If different forms of unawareness can be distinguished, answers to any of the questions posed above will depend on the particular form of unawareness that is assessed. Thus the task of distinguishing among forms of unawareness must be undertaken to some extent logically prior to, and is perhaps a necessary condition of, answering various other questions concerning the nature and basis of unawareness phenomena.

FORMS OF UNAWARENESS: FIVE EXAMPLES

When reviewing the chapters for this book we found five distinct though partly related issues concerning the forms of unawareness.

1. *Levels of Unawareness.* A distinction can be made between unawareness of the existence of a neuropsychological deficit itself and unawareness of some of the conse-

quences of the deficit. For example, Rubens and Garrett (see Chapter 3) discussed research indicating that various aphasic patients have difficulties with on-line monitoring of linguistic errors; that is, patients are often unaware that they have made a linguistic error. Yet these patients may acknowledge the existence of their deficit. Thus they appear to be aware of their deficit at one level and unaware at another. Goldberg and Barr (Chapter 9) discussed a related distinction between global and local error detection. Although little attention has been paid to the distinction between unawareness of the deficit itself and unawareness of the consequences of the deficit, it is likely to be crucial for developing an adequate theoretical understanding of awareness disturbances because different mechanisms may be involved in these two types or levels of unawareness.

2. *Neural Bases of Unawareness.* Data concerning the neural bases of awareness disturbances also suggest that some sort of distinction between forms of unawareness must be made. As is well known, much of the early literature on anosognosia for hemiplegia and related disorders (e.g., Critchley, 1953) indicated that lesions to right inferior parietal regions are closely associated with unawareness of deficit, as noted by Bisiach and Geminiani (Chapter 2) and Heilman (Chapter 4). In contrast, awareness disturbances observed in cases of amnesia, dementia, head injury, and schizophrenia appear to be associated with damage to the frontal lobes, as discussed by Johnson (Chapter 10), McGlynn and Kaszniak (Chapter 6), Prigatano (Chapter 7), Schacter (Chapter 8), and Stuss (Chapter 5). The observation that these two brain regions are often associated with unawareness of deficit has led to the suggestion that psychologically distinct forms of unawareness may be observed in conjunction with parietal and frontal damage, respectively (Prigatano, 1988; McGlynn and Schacter, 1989). Careful comparative studies of the kinds of unawareness observed after damage to these two brain regions remain to be done. Nevertheless, the literature on neural bases of anosognosia is consistent with, and provides some support for, the general proposition that forms of unawareness need to be distinguished.

3. *Specificity of Unawareness.* Relatively little attention has been paid to the measurement of awareness disturbances, but two observations reported in this volume suggested that different measures may tap different aspects of unawareness. First, McGlynn and Kaszniak (Chapter 6) reported that Huntington's disease patients who exhibited diminished awareness of memory and motor deficits on a questionnaire measure showed relatively intact awareness when required to predict their performance on some, but not all, memory and motor tasks. If only the questionnaire data were considered, one would have concluded that Huntington's disease patients have impaired awareness of their deficits; if only the data from certain experimental tasks were considered, one would have concluded that Huntington's patients have intact awareness of their deficits. As McGlynn and Kaszniak pointed out, however, such observations are also consistent with the idea that different measures tap different aspects of awareness. Similarly, Schacter (Chapter 8) described a study in which an amnesic patient who was largely unaware of his memory deficit was given repetitive feedback concerning his poor performance on various memory tasks. After this intervention, the patient's general rating of the severity of his memory problem increased, but his responses to questions regarding the likelihood that he would be able to remember in particular situations did not change. Thus conclusions about whether the intervention increased the patient's "awareness" of his memory deficit depended on the specific measure that was used to assess it.

The foregoing results are suggestive rather than conclusive. They do, however, lend empirical support to the contention that different measures of awareness may tap distinct underlying processes, which in turn can support either "aware" or "unaware" performance, depending on the status of the specific processes that are tapped in particular patients (see Chapter 9 for further discussion). These results are thus consistent with the general idea that different forms of unawareness need to be distinguished.

4. *Partial/implicit knowledge of deficits.* A number of clinical observers have noted an intriguing and possibly important feature of anosognosic patients: Even when patients explicitly deny the existence of a deficit, certain aspects of their behavior (see Chapter 2) and linguistic expressions (Weinstein, Cole, Mitchell, and Lyerly, 1964) betray some knowledge of it. McGlynn and Schacter (1989) suggested that such phenomena could be thought of as *implicit* expressions of knowledge about the deficit (see Chapter 8 and Schacter, McAndrews, and Moscovitch, 1988, for general discussion of implicit knowledge in neuropsychological syndromes). This basic idea was discussed and elaborated by Kihlstrom and Tobias (Chapter 11), who considered the phenomenon in the broader context of research on implicit memory, perception, and cognition.

The evidence for implicit knowledge of deficits that are denied explicitly derives largely from uncontrolled clinical observations and hence must be treated with interpretive caution. These observations, however, are consistent with the idea that simply describing patients as "aware" or "unaware" of their deficits does not do full justice to the subtleties of awareness disturbances. Perhaps the degree to which patients exhibit implicit "awareness" of deficits that are not acknowledged explicitly can provide a basis for distinguishing among forms of unawareness.

5. *Defensive denial.* Students of anosognosia have long debated the role of defensive or motivated denial in awareness disturbances, and various aspects of the issue are discussed in the present volume by Lewis (Chapter 12), McGlynn and Kaszniak (Chapter 6), Prigatano (Chapter 7), and Weinstein (Chapter 13). Although most observers agree that defensive denial of a kind that can be observed in non-brain-damaged patients plays *some* role in the unawareness phenomena exhibited by *some* brain-damaged patients, the nature and extent of the contribution is still the subject of debate. For the present purposes, however, the notion that defensive denial must be distinguished from other awareness disturbances is consistent with our main thesis. The critical problem, of course, is to develop adequate criteria for distinguishing between defensive and nondefensive forms of unawareness and to delineate the underlying bases for them.

Each of the five foregoing examples illustrates a somewhat different aspect of the issues that need to be confronted in order to begin examining what we have referred to as the problem of forms of unawareness. Progress in clarifying these issues will not, of course, provide a complete understanding of all the numerous and complex problems associated with unawareness phenomena, but it may well represent a necessary step toward attaining such an understanding. One of the most fundamental tasks that confronts any scientific enterprise is to develop a useful *taxonomy* of relevant empirical phenomena. By delineating and discussing the problem of forms of unawareness, we are hopeful that students of anosognosia can develop an adequate taxonomy of awareness disturbances that can serve as the basis for real advances in understanding this important and perplexing phenomenon.

REFERENCES

Critchley, M. (1953). *The Parietal Lobes.* New York: Hafner.
McGlynn, S. M., and Schacter, D. L. (1989). Unawareness of deficits in neuropsycholog-ical syndromes. *J. Clin. Exp. Neuropsychol.* 11:143–205.
Prigatano, G. P. (1988). Anosognosia, delusions, and altered self awareness after brain injury. *BNI Q.* 4(3):40–48.
Schacter, D. L., McAndrews, M. P., and Moscovitch, M. (1988). Access to consciousness: dissociations between implicit and explicit knowledge in neuropsychological syn-dromes. In L. Weiskrantz (ed.), *Thought Without Language.* Oxford: Oxford Univer-sity Press, pp. 242–278.
Weinstein, E. A., Cole, M., Mitchell, M. S., and Lyerly, O. G. (1964). Anosognosia and aphasia. *Arch. Neurol.* 10:376–386.

Glossary

EDOARDO BISIACH
AND GIULIANO GEMINIANI

The following glossary was kindly provided by Drs. Edoardo Bisiach and Giu-liano Geminiani. For an extensive definition of these and related terms centering around phenomena of anosognosia, see the Glossary in Weinstein, E. A., and Friedland, R. P. (1977). *Advances in Neurology, Volume 18: Hemi-Inattention and Hemisphere Specialization.* New York: Raven Press.

Alloesthesia (allochiria): Perception of a stimulus addressed to one side of the body as being located in a mirror-symmetrical position with respect of the point that has actually been stimulated.

Anosodiaphoria: Lack of emotional reaction to a deficit caused by a brain lesion.

Anosognosia: Apparent unawareness, misinterpretation, or explicit denial of an illness. The term usually refers to the patient's behavior in relation to the consequence of a brain lesion.

Cortical blindness: Blindness due to a lesion of the visual cerebral cortex.

Cortical deafness: Deafness due to a lesion of the auditory cerbral cortex.

Dysphasia: Disorder of language due to a brain lesion.

Hemianesthesia: Anesthesia confined to one side of the body.

Hemianopia: Blindness confined to one side of the visual field.

Hemineglect (syn. **unilateral neglect**): Neglect of the side of the patient's body and environment contralateral to the side of a brain lesion.

Hemiplegia: Paralysis of the limbs of one side, with or without participation of the lower half of the same side of the face.

Jargon aphasia: Variety of fluent aphasia in which most of the patient's speech is totally incomprehensible.

Misoplegia: Contempt or hatred, sometimes associated with physical violence, exhibited by the patient with regard to limbs that are paralyzed as a consequence of a brain lesion.

Neglect dyslexia: Failure to correctly read the side of a word or the side of a string of words contralateral to the side of a brain lesion.

Somatoparaphrenia: Denial of ownership and other delusional beliefs related to the limbs contralateral to the side of a brain lesion.

Subject Index